CONGENITAL MALFORMATIONS OF THE FEMALE GENITAL TRACT

Diagnosis and Management

CONGENITAL MALFORMATIONS OF THE FEMALE GENITAL TRACT

Diagnosis and Management

Editors

Gita Gidwani, MD
*Departments of Gynecology and Obstetrics
  and Pediatrics
The Cleveland Clinic Foundation
Cleveland, Ohio*

Tommaso Falcone, MD
*Associate Professor
Department of Obstetrics and Gynecology
Ohio State University
Columbus, Ohio
Head, Section of Reproductive Endocrinology
  and Infertility
Department of Gynecology and Obstetrics
The Cleveland Clinic Foundation
Cleveland, Ohio*

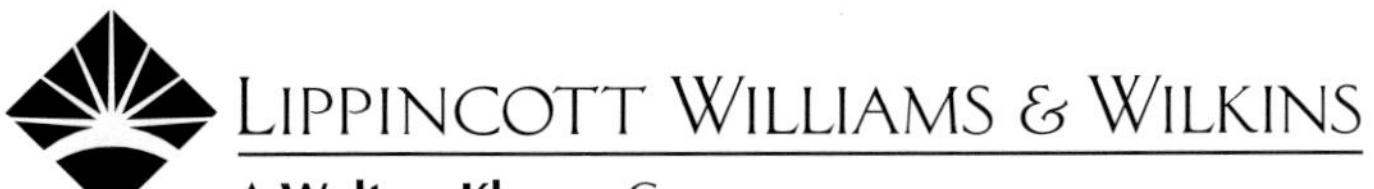

A **Wolters Kluwer** Company
Philadelphia • Baltimore • New York • London
Buenos Aires • Hong Kong • Sydney • Tokyo

Acquisitions Editor: Lisa McAllister
Developmental Editor: Jennifer Kowalak
Manufacturing Manager: Tim Reynolds
Production Manager: Liane Carita
Production Editor: Mary Ann McLaughlin
Cover Designer: Mark Lerner
Indexer: Kathleen Patterson
Compositor: Maryland Composition
Printer: Maple Press

Printed in the United States of America

9 8 7 6 5 4 3 2 1

Library of Congress Cataloging-in-Publication Data

Congenital malformations of the female genital tract : diagnosis
and management / [edited by] Gita Gidwani, Tommaso Falcone.
    p. cm.
  Includes bibliographical references and index.
  ISBN 0-7817-1725-6 (alk. paper)
    1. Generative organs, Female—Abnormalities. I. Gidwani, Gita
II. Falcone, Tommaso.
  RG211 .C656 1999
  618.1'043—dc21
                                 98-52913
                                     CIP

We wish to dedicate this book to
Sir John Dewhurst
excellent teacher, surgeon, and mentor.

Table of Contents

Contributors

Frederick Alexander, MD   *Associate Clinical Professor, Department of Pediatric Surgery, Ohio State University, Columbus; Ohio; Chief, Department of Pediatric Surgery, The Cleveland Clinic Foundation, 9500 Euclid Avenue, Cleveland, Ohio 44195*

Kimberly Applegate, MD   *Associate Staff Radiologist, Section of Pediatric Radiology, Children's Hospital of The Cleveland Clinic Foundation, 9500 Euclid Avenue, Cleveland, Ohio 44195*

Marjan Attaran, MD   *Department of Gynecology and Obstetrics/A81, The Cleveland Clinic Foundation, 9500 Euclid Avenue, Cleveland, Ohio 44195*

Mark E. Boyd, MD   *Associate Professor, Department of Obstetrics and Gynecology, McGill University; Director, Division of Gynecology, Women's Pavilion, Royal Victoria Hospital, 687 Pine Avenue West/Suite F4.29, Montréal, Canada, QC H3A 1A1*

E. Daniels, PhD   *Associate Professor, Department of Anatomy and Cell Biology, McGill University, Strathcona Anatomy and Dentistry, 3640 University Street, Montréal, Quebec, Canada, H3A 2B2*

D. Keith Edmonds, MD, FRCOG, FRACOG   *Honorary Senior Lecturer, Institute of Obstetrics and Gynaecology, Imperial College School of Medicine; Consultant Gynaecologist, Queen Charlotte's and Chelsea Hospital, Goldhawk Road, London, England W6 0XG*

Tommaso Falcone, MD   *Associate Professor, Department of Obstetrics and Gynecology, Ohio State University, Columbus, Ohio; Head, Section of Reproductive Endocrinology and Infertility, Department of Gynecology and Obstetrics/A81, The Cleveland Clinic Foundation, 9500 Euclid Avenue, Cleveland, Ohio 44195*

Gita Gidwani, MD   *Departments of Gynecology and Obstetrics and Pediatrics/A81, The Cleveland Clinic Foundation, 9500 Euclid Avenue, Cleveland, Ohio 44195*

Jeffrey M. Goldberg, MD   *Assistant Professor, Department of Obstetrics and Gynecology, Ohio State University, 1654 Upham Drive, Columbus, Ohio 43210; Staff Physician, Department of Gynecology and Obstetrics, The Cleveland Clinic Foundation, 9500 Euclid Avenue, Cleveland, Ohio 44195*

Marilyn J. Goske, MD   *Pediatric and Adolescent Radiology/HB-6, The Cleveland Clinic Foundation, 9500 Euclid Avenue, Cleveland, Ohio 44195*

Mark R. Gray, PhD *Assistant Professor, Obstetrics, Gynecology, and Reproductive Biology, Department of Obstetrics and Gynecology, Harvard Medical School; Director of Research, Division of Reproductive Endocrinology, Department of Obstetrics and Gynecology, Beth Israel Deaconess Medical Center, 330 Brookline Avenue, Boston, Massachusetts 02215*

Vanessa K. Jensen, PsyD *Head, Section of Pediatric Psychology, The Cleveland Clinic Children's Hospital, 9500 Euclid Avenue/Desk A-120, Cleveland, Ohio 44195*

Robert Kay, MD *Professor, Department of Surgery, Ohio State University, Columbus, Ohio 43210; Section of Pediatric Urology, The Cleveland Clinic Foundation, 9500 Euclid Avenue, Cleveland, Ohio 44195*

Craig S. Mitchell, DO *Associate Staff Radiologist, Department of Radiology, Children's Hospital of The Cleveland Clinic Foundation, 9500 Euclid Avenue, Cleveland, Ohio 44195*

Richard H. Reindollar, MD *Associate Professor, Department of Obstetrics, Gynecology, and Reproductive Biology, Harvard Medical School; Director, Division of Reproductive Endocrinology, Department of Obstetrics and Gynecology, Beth Israel Deaconess Medical Center, 330 Brookline Avenue, Boston, Massachusetts 02215*

Stephanie L. Reiter, PhD *Pediatric Clinical Psychology, The Cleveland Clinic Foundation, 9500 Euclid Avenue, Cleveland, Ohio 44195*

Ellen S. Rome, MD, MPH *Assistant Professor, Department of Pediatrics, Ohio State University; Clinical Assistant Professor, Pennsylvania State University School of Medicine; Head, Section of Adolescent Medicine, Department of Pediatrics and Adolescent Medicine, The Cleveland Clinic Foundation/Department A120, 9500 Euclid Avenue, Cleveland, Ohio 44195*

Jonathan H. Ross, MD *Head, Section of Pediatric Urology, The Cleveland Clinic Foundation, 9500 Euclid Avenue, Cleveland, Ohio 44195*

Joseph Salvatore Sanfilippo, MD *Professor, Department of Obstetrics and Gynecology, Allegheny University of the Health Sciences; Chairman, Department of Obstetrics and Gynecology, Allegheny General Hospital, 320 East North Avenue, Pittsburgh, Pennsylvania 15212*

Betsy Schroeder, MD *Fellow, Pediatric-Adolescent Gynecology, Department of Obstetrics and Gynecology, University of Louisville, Louisville, Kentucky 40292*

James R. Stelling, MD *Clinical Fellow, Department of Obstetrics, Gynecology, and Reproductive Biology, Harvard Medical School; Clinical Fellow, Department of Obstetrics and Gynecology, Beth Israel Deaconess Medical Center, 330 Brookline Avenue, Boston, Massachusetts 02215*

Foreword

To be born with a major malformation of any kind is a heavy burden to carry, but, when this malformation affects the genital organs, the implications are more serious. Without expert management, a patient so afflicted may be unable to lead a normal sex life and may be doomed to suffer sexual inadequacy and frustration as well as infertility. If properly treated, such disastrous consequences can be overcome, and a normal sex life and fertility can be made possible.

The investigation and management of congenital abnormalities of the genital organs in the female are thoroughly dealt with in this new book. The authors themselves are experts in the field; in addition, they have collaborated with an impressive group of co-authors of acknowledged excellence, so that every related aspect of the subject may be presented to the reader in as comprehensive a manner as possible. In this way, in addition to a thorough coverage of the diagnosis and surgical management of these complex problems, associated aspects are examined in detail, including recent embryological knowledge, endocrinology and molecular biology of normal and abnormal genital tract development, associated renal tract abnormalities, and the very important psychological management of these affected patients.

Here is a text that answers all the questions concerning these serious malformations. The editors and their collaborators are to be congratulated on the very high quality of their accomplishments.

Professor Sir John Dewhurst, FRCOG, FRCS (Ed)
Middlesex, England

Preface

For many years, we have used a multidisciplinary approach here at the Cleveland Clinic Foundation to diagnose and manage the medical and surgical problems of patients with Müllerian anomalies. Since 1980, Dr. James Kreiger, Dr. Lester Ballard, and Dr. Gita Gidwani have used pediatric urologists, plastic surgeons, pediatric surgeons, endocrinologists, radiologists, and psychologists in our clinical practices to continue this tradition. Dr. Tommaso Falcone added a further dimension by introducing minimally invasive surgery to the treatment of these disorders.

In the various chapters, the readers will find debatable views by recognized authorities from different disciplines, and we have purposely left these opinions unedited. We feel that it is important that the reader of the book gets a flavor of the controversies and questions, which continue to be faced by surgeons from different disciplines regarding these unusual anomalies.

Gita Gidwani, MD
Tommaso Falcone, MD

Acknowledgments

We wish to acknowledge the medical artist for this book
Nancy Heim, AMI.

Congenital Malformations of the Female Genital Tract: Diagnosis and Management, edited by
G. Gidwani and T. Falcone.
Lippincott Williams & Wilkins, Philadelphia © 1999.

1

Development of the Female Genital Tract and External Genitalia

Mark E. Boyd and *E. Daniels

*Department of Obstetrics and Gynecology, McGill University, Division of Gynecology,
Women's Pavilion, Royal Victoria Hospital, Montréal, Quebec, Canada, H3A 1A1, and
*Department of Anatomy and Cell Biology, McGill University, Strathcona Anatomy and
Dentistry, Montréal, Quebec, Canada H3A 2B2*

Embryology is a perennially fascinating subject and is especially interesting when it concerns the development of the female genitourinary system. The subject is full of surprises and mysteries. Consider, for example, the early embryo. Externally uncertain as to sex, it possesses a double set of all necessary internal sexual apparatus and a gonad, which is prepared to take one of two directions and will occasionally make half-hearted attempts at both. What happens next has never been fully explained. At a certain point, for reasons that remain imperfectly understood, it is as though the embryo finally makes its decision and embarks on an irreversible developmental path. That path, its imperfections, and its early abandoned efforts constitute the subject of this chapter. As for what the embryo leaves behind, there is nothing that needs to be added to an authoritative description of these remnants that compares them to the materials studied in archaeology: "Most of it is in ruins, some of it has been converted to new use; and much has vanished" (1).

The embryology of the female urogenital system has been studied from at least the time of Aristotle, and therefore an immense amount of information about the subject is readily available. Yet it is a mistake to ignore the importance of familiar information, particularly when the information can be used in a number of practical ways. Although it is obvious that the rational management of congenital abnormalities will depend on such knowledge, it is equally important that surgeons be familiar with the other uses for this knowledge. For that reason, this chapter will discuss the relationship between embryology and the surgical anatomy of the pelvis and will attempt to demonstrate how embryologic knowledge can make operative dissections both understandable and safe.

Therefore the purpose of this chapter is to foster an understanding of the genital tract development. No attempt will be made to present an exhaustive account of this complex process, which involves a series of simultaneous changes in a number of organ systems. What will be emphasized instead are the critical embryologic events that occur at each stage of its development. The aim will be to develop principles that can be used not only to rationalize the diagnosis and treatment of congenital anomalies of the female genital tract but to provide a better understanding of the wider applications of these principles.

Because the discussion will be limited to the embryology that is directly related to the formation of the female urogenital tract and of the external genitalia, nothing will be said concerning the preimplantation or early postimplantation events. For the most part we will describe the genitourinary development that occurs in the first trimester. At the end of the first trimester the development of the female genitourinary tract is nearly complete, even though some changes, such as the final canalization of the vagina and the repositioning of the gonads, will remain incomplete until a somewhat later date (2).

A word or two must be said concerning nomenclature. In embryologic literature, diction often serves to confuse rather than to clarify. The use of anatomic names and eponyms is a case in point. Mesonephric ducts may be referred to as Wolffian ducts, just as the paramesonephric ducts are called the Müllerian ducts in honor of Caspar Wolff and Johannes Müller, their eighteenth and nineteenth century discoverers. Confusion reigns, however, when these terms are used interchangeably in the same paper or even in the same paragraph. In order to avoid any ambiguity, the anatomic terms will be used in this chapter. For the sake of additional clarity, all anomalies will be described, and the use of unnecessary and confusing Greek or Latin words will be avoided. The term *uterine didelphys* is a case in point. Inasmuch as "di" means two and "delphys" means uterus, one of the two words in the phrase must be superfluous; in any case, the use of a Latin phrase does nothing to improve our understanding of the nature of the medical problem that it describes. Further confusion results from referral to the peritoneal cavity as the celomic cavity. In fact, the two cavities are identical; *celomic cavity* is an embryonic term for body cavity, and *peritoneal cavity* is the anatomic description of part of that cavity. Finally, the terms *mesoderm* and *mesenchyme* will be used interchangeably for the description of cells that are either arranged loosely (mesenchyme) or tightly (mesoderm).

THE UROGENITAL RIDGE

The formation of the three primary germ layers is rapidly followed by the lateral folding into a cylindric embryo, which contains a primitive gut and body cavity. As the endodermal gut forms it is suspended within the celomic cavity by mesenchyme to the dorsal body wall. As a result of lateral folding, two elongated ridges of mesenchyme (intermediate mesenchyme) are formed on either side of the mesentery (midline mesenchyme). The ridges are known as the urogenital ridges because they contain the mesenchymal precursors of the entire genital and urinary system except for the external genitalia, the lower vagina, the urethra, and the bladder. The position and longitudinal extent of the urogenital ridges are shown in Fig. 1. Note that they terminate in the lower abdominal wall in the labioscrotal folds.

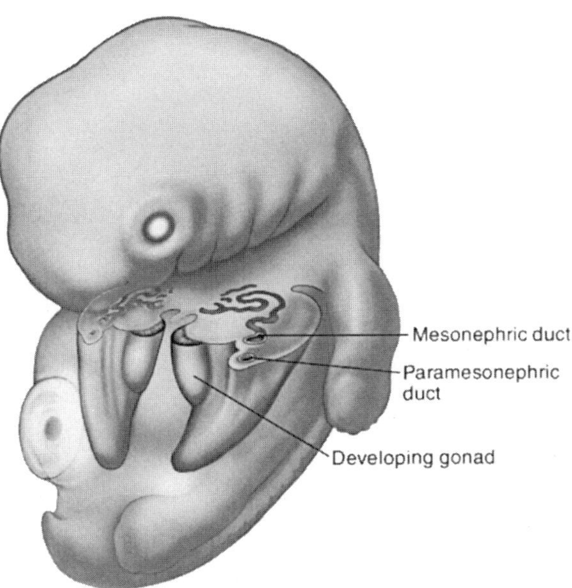

FIG. 1. Urogenital ridge that contains a medial fold (site of future gonad) and a lateral fold that contains the mesonephric and paramesonephric ducts.

Critical Embryonic Events

It is to be expected that tissue that is derived from the same germ layer will react to various stimuli in a similar fashion. For example, the uterus, ovaries, and most of the vagina are mesodermal in origin. They all have estrogen receptors and should respond to estrogen.

CLOACA

Formation of Cloaca

As described, the primitive gut runs from one end of the embryo to the other. At its distal end a diverticulum, the allantois, extends into the umbilicus. The distal gut expands at this point to form a reservoir, the cloaca (Fig. 2). As a result the endoderm of the gut is put in direct contact with the ectoderm. The point of contact is called the cloacal membrane. The cloacal membrane is initially located on the embryo's ventral body wall. The invading mesoderm, which forms the abdominal wall, displaces the membrane in a caudal direction.

Critical Embryonic Events

If the mesoderm does not invade the cloacal membrane it will break down, and the anterior wall of the abdomen and bladder will not form. Invasion by mesoderm is hin-

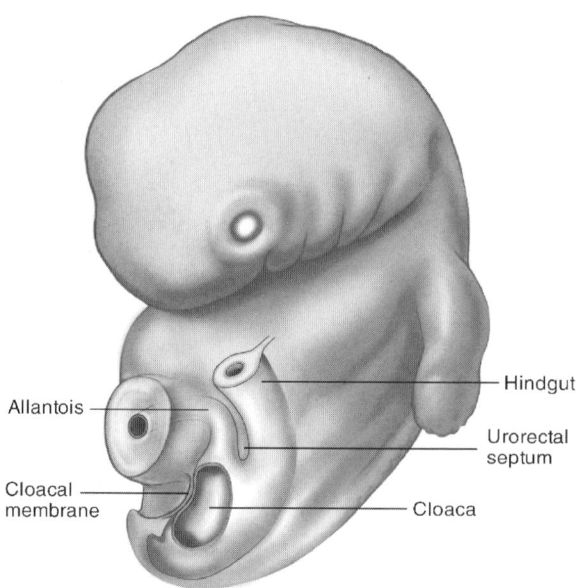

FIG. 2. Formation of the cloaca.

dered if the cloacal membrane is larger than usual or if the genital tubercle is displaced caudally at too early a stage (3,4). Exstrophy of the bladder results; the posterior wall of the newborn's bladder may be visible, and the pubic bones may be separated.

Subdivision of the Cloaca

The urorectal septum, which is mesodermal in origin, pushes against the roof of the cloaca and divides it into the urogenital sinus anteriorly and the anorectal canal posteriorly (Fig. 3). The upper part of the urogenital sinus, which is connected to the umbilicus by the allantois (future urachus), is the precursor of the bladder, urethra, and paraurethral glands. The lower part of the urogenital sinus will form the vestibule of the vagina. The perineal body develops at the point where the urorectal septum reaches the cloacal membrane. The perineal body divides the cloacal membrane into the anterior urogenital membrane and the posterior anal membrane. The anorectal canal will eventually connect with the anal pit.

Critical Embryonic Events

If the urorectal septum is defective the cloaca is not divided or is incompletely divided. As pointed out by Allen and Husmann, this results in a "spectrum of possible abnormalities" (5). For example, if the urorectal septum fails to reach the cloacal membrane, the anus will be absent, and its place will be taken by a fistulous opening of the

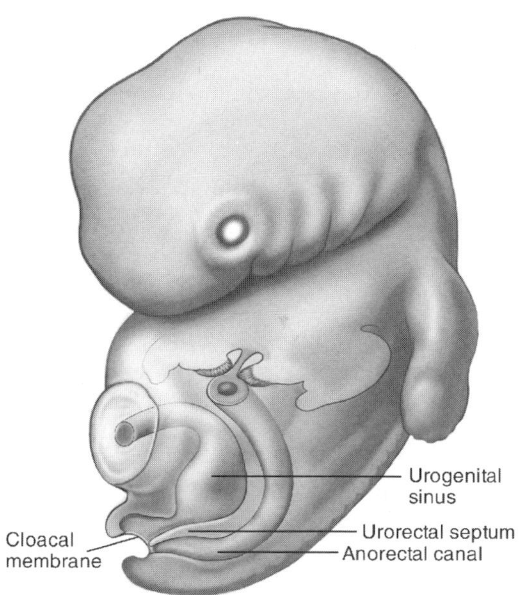

FIG. 3. Subdivision of the cloaca into the urogenital sinus and anorectal canal by the urorectal septum.

rectum into the vagina, or vestibule, or onto the anterior part of the perineum. Failure of the anorectal canal to connect with the anal pit will result in an imperforate anus.

THE MESONEPHRIC DUCT (WOLFFIAN DUCT)

The mesonephric tubules, glomeruli, and duct form along the lateral side of the urogenital ridge. The duct runs downward toward the urogenital sinus. Just before it enters the urogenital sinus, it gives off a bud, i.e., the ureteric bud (Fig. 4A). All of the mesonephric glomeruli and tubules disappear except for the remnants, the parovarian cysts, also known as the epoophoron and paroophoron, though portions of the duct persist. In the male embryo the mesonephric tubules will form the efferent ductules. The mesonephric duct will form the duct of the epididymis, ductus deferens, seminal vesicle, and ejaculatory duct.

The ureteric buds, the future calyces and ureter of the adult kidney first grow dorsally and then turn upward into the lower end of the urogenital ridge (Fig. 4B). At that point, they induce formation of the metanephros, which will form the cortex, and medulla of the adult kidney. As the embryo lengthens, the kidneys ascend from the pelvis (Fig. 4C). The ureters keep pace with the kidneys by elongating. As the kidneys develop, they acquire their new blood supply from higher segmental arteries of the aorta.

With further growth, the portions of the mesonephric ducts that are distal to the ureteric buds and the orifices of the ureteric buds are incorporated into the wall of the

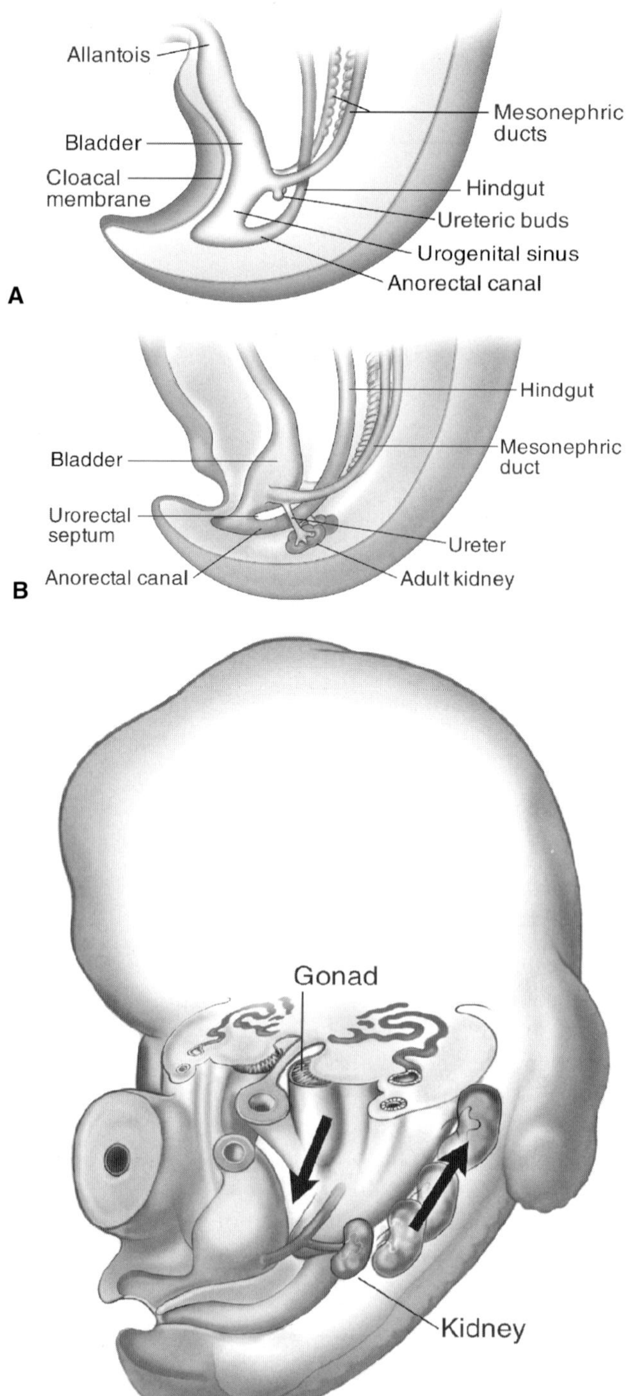

FIG. 4. **A:** Anatomic relationship of the mesonephric ducts with the urogenital sinus. **B:** Formation of the ureteric buds and adult kidney. **C:** Differential growth of the embryo results in ascent of the kidney and descent of the gonad.

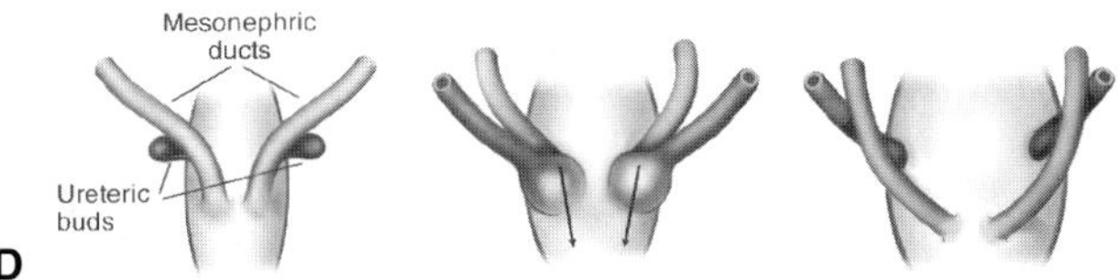

FIG. 4. *Continued.* **D:** Anatomic relationship of the mesonephric duct and ureters with the urogenital sinus.

urogenital sinus (Fig. 4D). Differential growth of the posterior wall of the bladder then carries the mesonephric duct orifices downward. In this way, the positions of the orifices belonging to the ureters and the mesonephric ducts are reversed. This results in the formation of the trigone of the bladder with the ureteral orifices in the upper lateral corners and the mesonephric duct orifices at the inferior point, where the urethra enters the vestibule of the urogenital sinus. The absorptive process has transposed a patch of mesoderm onto the mucosa of the bladder, which is endodermal in origin (6).

Critical Embryonic Events

The most common reason for renal agenesis is failure of the mesonephric duct to form a ureteric bud.

There is duplication of the ureter if the ureteric bud splits before reaching the metanephros.

A pelvic kidney results from failure of the kidneys to ascend. The pelvic kidney's blood supply is from segmental vessels at that level. Although they are called accessory renal arteries, they are in fact segmental vessels that have persisted.

Because the trigone and the posterior wall of the urethra are mesodermal in origin, they respond to estrogen. For that reason clinicians use estrogen in order to treat postmenopausal women with atrophy of the trigone or a posterior urethral caruncle. In the same way, the prolapsed urethral mucosa of preadolescent girls can be treated with estrogen cream.

Mesonephric duct remnants can be found in the mesosalpinx, alongside the uterus, deep within the cervix, along the anterolateral wall of the vagina, or near the urethra. Their names change with their location. Consequently, they are known as parovarian cysts, paratubal cysts, or Gartner duct cysts.

On occasion the mesonephric system keeps its urinary function. In such instances, the ureter may retain its connection with the mesonephric duct and have an ectopic opening into the vagina.

THE BIPOTENTIAL UROGENITAL SYSTEM

The early genital tract is described as bipotential because the gonads, mesonephric and paramesonephric duct systems, and external genitalia have the potential of adapting to either the male or the female phenotype. The basic sequence of change from the bipotential state is that chromosome sex determines gonad formation, which in turn favors the development of either the male or female duct system and external genitalia (7). It will be appreciated that in the final analysis all depends on the endocrine effects, not on chromosome sex.

This cascade of events is initiated by the arrival of the primordial germ cells in the genital ridge. The germ cells originate in the yolk sac and allantoic regions and then migrate through the hindgut mesenchyme to the genital ridge. At that site they cause proliferation of the adjacent celomic epithelium and underlying mesoderm (8,9). In the process of proliferating, the epithelial cells arrange themselves into cords and invade the mesoderm. The resulting bipotential gonad has an outer cortex and an inner medulla. In the male embryo, the medulla will predominate and the cortex will regress; the opposite occurs in the female embryo, with the cortex progressing and the medulla regressing.

In 1990 it was found that a 35-kilobase region on the short arm of the human Y chromosome was necessary for male sex determination (10). The DNA sequence that is responsible for this determination is called the sex-determining region on Y (*SRY* gene). The gene causes the bipotential gonad to secrete testis-determining factor (TDF) and a surface antigen, histocompatibility antigen Y (H-Y antigen), which are responsible for the formation of Sertoli cells (11,12). The Sertoli cells then secrete anti-Müllerian hormone (AMH), which acts locally; its first action is to cause degeneration of the paramesonephric system.

The second function of the anti-Müllerian hormone is to cause the formation of Leydig cells, which then produce testosterone. The development and maintenance of the mesonephric duct system require testosterone. If there is no testosterone the mesonephric duct system will regress.

The development of the ovary and of the paramesonephric duct system is the opposite of the development of the mesonephric duct system. As described earlier, the mesonephric duct system depends on the secretion of both anti-Müllerian hormone and testosterone. The paramesonephric duct system is the default system and is not dependent on the secretion of any active substance. In the absence of the testis-determining factor, the indifferent gonad forms an ovary. Because there is no testis, there is no anti-Müllerian hormone secretion, and the paramesonephric system is allowed to develop. In addition, there is no testis to secrete testosterone, and the mesonephric system atrophies.

Critical Embryonic Events

Chromosome sex is responsible for the development of either the testes or the ovaries. The gonads are then responsible for female or male sexual development.

Most XY females have mutations in the *SRY* gene, and some XX males have *SRY* gene content. The absence of anti-Müllerian hormone in XX embryos or XY embryos with a mutant *SRY* gene allows the paramesonephric ducts to develop.

True hermaphrodites may have ovarian tissue on one side and testicular tissue on the other. In such instances, there is no secretion of the anti-Müllerian hormone on the ovarian side, and a fallopian tube and uterine horn will develop on that side.

THE PARAMESONEPHRIC (MÜLLERIAN) DUCT SYSTEM

On the lateral surface of the urogenital ridges, a longitudinal series of ingrowths form a groove and then a tube. Because the tubes are in contact with the mesonephric ducts, they are called the paramesonephric ducts. In fact, the ducts are interdependent; the paramesonephric duct will not develop if the mesonephric duct is absent (13).

The paramesonephric ducts accompany the mesonephric ducts into the pelvis (Fig. 5). At a low level in the pelvis the paramesonephric ducts cross from the lateral to the front and then to the medial side of the mesonephric ducts. They then fuse with their opposite number as they abut against the posterior wall of the urogenital sinus between the orifices of the mesonephric ducts. The classical understanding of Müllerian development holds that the Müllerian duct crosses ventrally over the mesonephric ducts and their medial walls fuse in the midline at the caudal most aspect. Fusion would then continue cranially. Goldberg and Falcone reported a case of a double cervix and vagina with a normal uterus that challenges this classical view and supports the alternative view of Musset that fusion occurs at the level of the uterine isthmus and proceeds simultaneously in both directions (14). Midline resorption also begins at the isthmus and is first directed caudally, unifying the cervix and vagina, and later cephalad to eliminate the uterine septum.

The lower end of the fused paramesonephric ducts proliferates, giving rise to a downgrowth of tissue that invaginates the posterior wall of the urogenital sinus. The resulting prominence is called the Müllerian tubercle (Fig. 6). The tissue downgrowth separates the fused tip of the paramesonephric ducts from the posterior wall of the urogenital sinus. The vertical portions of the paramesonephric ducts that have fused will form the endometrium of the future uterus and the endocervix; the separated cranial ends of the ducts become the fallopian tubes; the most inferior part of the downgrowth is destined to form the upper two thirds of the vagina. The myometrium and the supporting tissue of the vagina originate from the surrounding mesoderm.

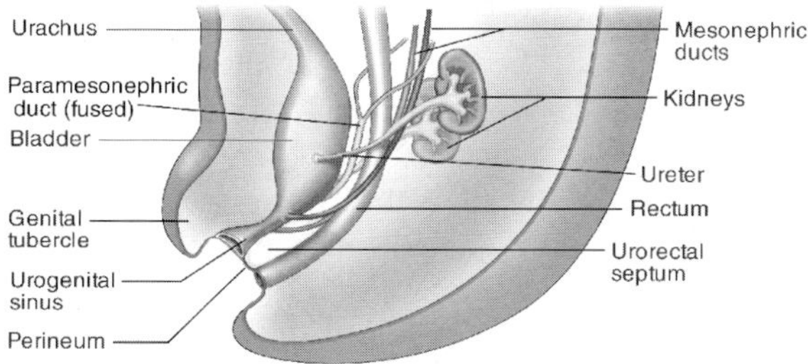

FIG. 5. Anatomic relationship of the mesonephric and paramesonephric ducts.

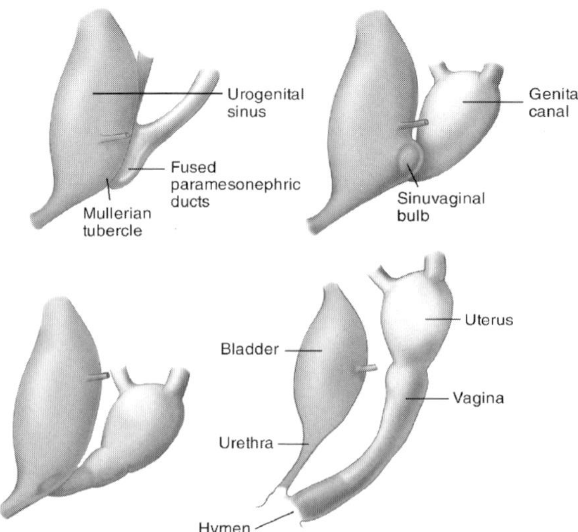

FIG. 6. Formation of the uterus and vagina from the paramesonephric ducts and urogenital sinus.

As this is happening, the epithelial cells of the urogenital sinus, which are in contact with the Müllerian tubercle, proliferate and organize themselves into columns of squamous tissue, the sinovaginal bulbs (15). The bulbs elongate by growing upward and in so doing further separate the fused ends of the paramesonephric ducts from the urogenital sinus (16). The upgrowths will form the lower third of the vagina.

The lower third of the vagina becomes hollow by the formation and then the amalgamation of vaginal lacunae. The downgrowth of tissue from the paramesonephric ducts and the fused ducts themselves break down in a similar manner. In this way, the lumina of the lower third and the upper two thirds of the vagina and uterus become contiguous.

A caudal growth of mesenchyme, the sinovaginal plate, will separate the bladder from the vagina (Fig. 6). The part of the urogenital sinus above the Müllerian tubercle forms the bladder and urethra; when the part of the urogenital sinus below the tubercle widens, it becomes the vaginal vestibule. As a result of the widening, the urethra and the vagina develop separate openings into the vaginal vestibule. The hymen represents the junction of the developing vagina with the urogenital sinus.

There are a number of possible origins for the stratified squamous epithelium of the vagina. The traditional explanation is that it originates from upgrowths of stratified squamous epithelium of the urogenital sinus. A more recent and more easily understandable explanation suggests that it forms as a result of squamous metaplasia of the columnar epithelium. The initiating cause is thought to be contact with the amniotic fluid (2).

Uterine and Vaginal Anomalies

Uterine and vaginal anomalies are of clinical interest. The anomalies range from a minor defect that has no clinical impact to the complete absence of the vagina and uterus or to any degree of impaired development of one or both sides of the uterus and vagina. There are a number of different ways of classifying these anomalies (17). In fact, all such classifications should be considered as different ways of describing a breakdown in the normal development of the uterus and vagina. When this principle is used, the nature of the anomalies can be understood.

Critical Embryonic Events

1. *The paramesonephric duct fails to form.* Developmental problems with mesonephric duct formation cause renal anomalies; these in turn cause uterine anomalies (18). The mesonephric duct serves as a guide for the paramesonephric duct. If the mesonephric duct is absent, the paramesonephric duct cannot descend into the pelvis, fuse, and proliferate. The urogenital sinus will be present, but the sinovaginal bulbs will not elongate as much as usual. The final result is that the uterus and upper vagina do not form, but a stump of vagina might be present. The failure to form the paramesonephric ducts is the commonest cause of vaginal atresia. In most such instances, there is no functional uterus or any trace of the vagina (19,20).
2. *The paramesonephric ducts on one or both sides form and then split.* This condition results in a duplication of the uterus and vagina. "True duplications" are extremely rare events and are not to be confused with the so-called fusion defects that are described in the following paragraphs.
3. *The early paramesonephric ducts fail to "fuse."* In the normal course of events, the paired paramesonephric ducts fuse at a very early stage. Thereafter, they develop into the uterus and upper vagina. It is important to realize that fusion defects represent a failure of part or of all the fused ducts to develop into the uterus or vagina. Congenital anomalies that are called fusion defects arise because of problems relating to the developmental part of this process. Müllerian anomalies do not recapitulate normal ontogeny. That is, none of the defects found clinically would be observed as critical events in the normal development of the female genital tract.

    Failure of the sinovaginal plate to divide the bladder from the vagina results in the distal vagina fused with the urinary tract.
4. *There is no development of the urogenital sinus.* This condition causes vaginal atresia that involves most of the vagina (21).
5. *The paramesonephric or sinovaginal bulb proliferations are not canalized.* The vaginal septum that results can be of any thickness, at any level, or at any position—transverse, vertical, or spiral (17). In the final analysis, it is difficult to say whether or not the so-called septa are the result of a failure of the vagina to canalize or to develop (22). In the extreme case, the patient suffers from vaginal agenesis.

THE VULVA

The development of the vulva is straightforward. As previously described, the urorectal septum in the process of forming the perineal body divides the cloacal membrane into the urogenital membrane anteriorly and the anal membrane posteriorly. The urogenital membrane will break down to expose the lower part of the urogenital sinus, the future vestibule of the vagina.

A double set of folds develops alongside the urogenital membrane (Fig. 7). Just lateral to the membrane and destined to become the labia minora are the urogenital folds. Further lateral are the labioscrotal folds, the future labia majora. It is unclear as to whether the genital tubercle, destined to become the clitoris, forms as a result of fusion of the urogenital or labioscrotal folds (23,24).

It is easy to surmise that the genital tubercle in the male embryo enlarges and forms the glans penis, that fusion of the urogenital folds leads to the formation of the penile urethra, and that closure of the labioscrotal folds will result in the formation of the scrotum.

The development of the external genitalia along male lines depends both on the availability of an androgen and on tissue sensitivity. In the usual circumstance, testosterone is changed to 5-dihydrotestosterone by 5α-reductase in the soft tissue of the genitalia. The 5-dihydrotestosterone then binds to an appropriate receptor in the cloaca and causes male differentiation. In addition, the timing of androgen stimulation is important. If the stimulation only occurs after the female genitalia are developed, the only result will be clitoral hypertrophy; the labia minora and majora will not fuse.

Critical Embryonic Events

Congenital abnormalities in sexual development normally present with ambiguous external genitalia.

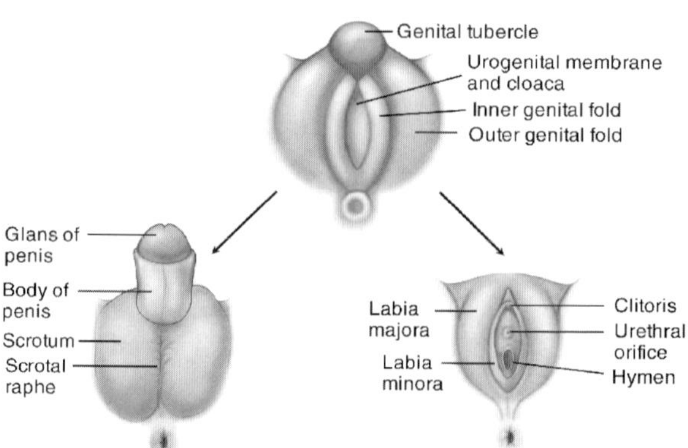

FIG. 7. Formation of the external genitalia.

The XY male embryo will have female external genitalia if there is gonadal failure and impaired androgen formation or lack of androgen receptors.

Congenital adrenal hyperplasia is a common cause of ambiguous genitalia.

THE MESENTERIES AND LIGAMENTS

The urogenital ridges continue downward on the posterior body wall and then turn forward to the anterior abdominal wall, the site of the future inguinal canals, where they end in the labioscrotal folds (25). The superior portion of the urogenital ridges divides longitudinally into a medial fold that contains the gonad and a lateral fold for the mesonephric and paramesonephric ducts (see Fig. 1). The projection of the urogenital ridge into the peritoneal cavity leads to the formation of a mesentery, the urogenital mesentery. The genital portion of the ridge acquires its own mesentery, which is continuous with the mesentery of the lower part of the ridge. The inferior continuation of the genital mesentery is called the *gubernaculum.* The gubernaculum plays an important role in the descent of the gonads (see Fig. 4C).

The paramesonephric ducts cross in front of the gubernaculum. The gubernaculum then fuses with the posterior wall of the future uterus at its junction with the fallopian tubes. In this way the gubernaculum is divided into two parts: the proximal part, between the ovary and the uterus, becomes the ovarian ligament; the distal portion, between the uterus and the inguinal canal, becomes the round ligament.

The gubernaculum attaches to the labioscrotal folds before the development of the abdominal musculature (26). The inguinal canal forms as a result of muscular development around the gubernaculum. The peritoneum partially surrounds the gubernaculum, covering it on the anterior and lateral sides. The female counterpart to the male *processus vaginalis* is the canal of Nuck, which extends into the labia majora and is usually obliterated after birth. If the *processus vaginalis,* which is an evagination of the peritoneal cavity, persists the patient will present with an indirect inguinal hernia.

Gubernaculum is a Latin word that translates as "helm" or "rudder." The embryologic implication is that it directs the ovary into the pelvis. It does so by differential growth of the embryo. Because the gubernaculum fixes the ovary, the rest of the embryo in effect grows away from it.

Critical Embryonic Events

If the canal of Nuck is not obliterated it presents as a mass in the labia majora.

THE RETROPERITONEUM OF THE PELVIS

Management of certain uterine anomalies, such as a rudimentary horn, might require extirpative surgery. Knowledge of the embryology of the retroperitoneum will aid in this surgery. The key to understanding regional anatomy is to build the anatomy around the development of a single structure. If its development is understood, the relationship between neighboring structures will also be understood. Moreover, the knowledge allows easy recall of these associations because there is no need to rely on memory. The anatomy of the pelvic retroperitoneum is determined in the embryonic stage when the predominant regional structures are the umbilical arteries. It is logical to use these vessels as the anatomic keys to the pelvic retroperitoneum.

The umbilical arteries play a crucial role in the establishment of anatomic relationships in the pelvis. In the first instance, they give rise to the vascular grid that supplies the primitive cloaca and the adjacent mesonephric and paramesonephric ducts. Second, they provide a structure for the development of the fascial supports of the pelvic viscera. The development of the umbilical arteries will be used both to give a rationale to the pelvic vascularization and in order to provide the orientation of the pelvic fascia.

Embryology of the Umbilical Arteries

The umbilical arteries are major vessels in the embryo and are well established by day 20 because of the early need for placental exchange (Fig. 8). The lower limb buds appear shortly thereafter; their blood supply is taken from the external iliac arteries which rise from the umbilical arteries. The portion of the umbilical arteries

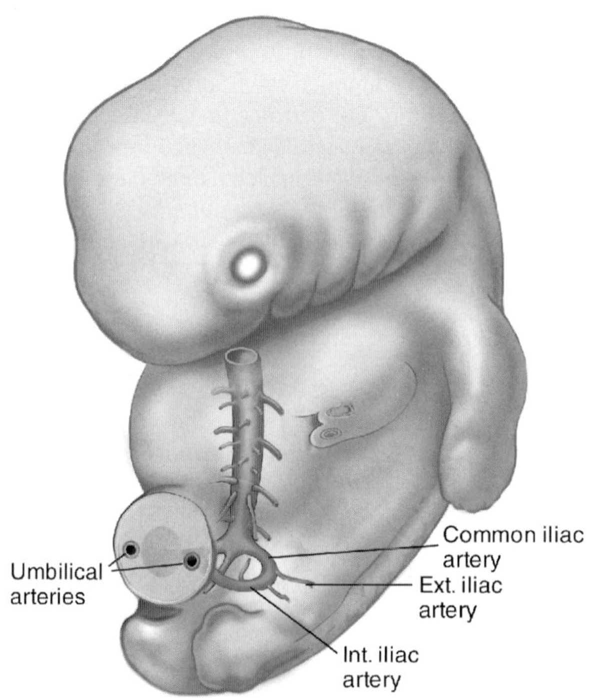

FIG. 8. Branches of the umbilical arteries.

dorsal to the external iliac arteries will become the common iliac arteries; the immediately proximal part will become the internal iliac arteries. The internal iliac arteries descend in a vertical direction along the pelvic side wall before giving branches to developing pelvic viscera. The remaining parts of the umbilical arteries maintain their original name, continue downward, and then turn in a horizontal direction to run along the lateral pelvic wall to the anterolateral corner of the bladder. Near the iliopectineal line, they pass upward, beneath the peritoneum of the anterior abdominal wall, to the umbilicus. Though there are many variations of the visceral branches, the constant features of the vascular arrangement are the umbilical arteries themselves.

Figure 8 illustrates the relatively large size of the embryo's umbilical arteries compared to the external iliac arteries. The portion of the umbilical artery that lies dorsal to it becomes the common iliac artery. The ventral portion of the umbilical artery becomes the internal iliac artery. The portion of the umbilical artery, which runs from the pelvis to the abdominal wall, is still called the (obliterated) umbilical artery. In the abdominal wall it is referred to as the lateral umbilical ligament.

The umbilical arteries lie immediately lateral to the distal portions of the urogenital ridges and the cloaca. That lateral position determines that the arteries and their branches will be lateral to the median umbilical ligament, the bladder, and the ureter. The blood supply of these structures is derived from small branches that run medially from the umbilical arteries. The final blood supply of the pelvic viscera, with the exception of the hindgut, originates from those branches.

The kidneys first appear in the embryo's pelvis and are then displaced upward by the differential growth of the caudal part of the embryo. Their original blood supply is derived from distal branches of the umbilical arteries. As the kidneys ascend, their blood supply is acquired from more superior branches of the umbilical arteries until they receive their definitive blood supply from the aorta (27). The branches of the umbilical arteries that supply the kidneys when they are in the pelvis remain in place and supply parts of the pelvic ureter. In the adult, they are recognized as the ureteric branches of the internal iliac and superior vesical arteries.

Fascia of the Umbilical Arteries

The fascia of the pelvis develops from one of two lines, namely, in relation to the umbilical arteries themselves or in relation to the venous drainage of the pelvic viscera which were supplied by the umbilical artery. The umbilical arteries are bound to the urogenital ridge by thin fascial mesenteries. The mesenteries form as a result of hyperplasia of areolar tissue around the small blood vessels that run between the umbilical arteries and the urogenital ridge (28). The ligaments that hold the pelvic organs in place are the result of areolar hyperplasia around venous pathways (29–31). Thus the cardinal ligament, the main lateral support of the uterus, develops about the veins that run obliquely from the uterus to the pelvic side wall (32,33). The ligaments that develop around veins are more substantial than those that accompany the umbilical arteries. The umbilical arteries' lack of accompanying vein(s) and their obliteration after birth may account for the difference in development.

The umbilical artery's fascial mesentery extends along the vessel's entire length, from the internal iliac artery to the umbilicus (Figs. 9,10). Three contiguous portions of this structure can be recognized. The first part of the fascial mesentery is the least well developed. It attaches the internal iliac and umbilical artery to the adjacent part of the ureter. It runs downward from the internal iliac artery to the cardinal ligament (34,35). This section of the fascia forms as a result of the mesenchymal hyperplasia around the blood supply of the embryo's pelvic kidney and ureter.

The second part of the fascial sheet is called the vesicohypogastric fascia, and it runs forward from the lateral cervical ligament in a nearly horizontal direction to the lateral corner of the bladder. The name is somewhat of a misnomer because it is difficult to recognize the portion of the fascia between the umbilical artery and the external iliac vessels. The part of the fascia that is readily identified runs between the umbilical artery and the lateral wall of the bladder (36).

The name of the last section of the fascial mesentery changes: it is now called the umbilical-vesical fascia. It is vertically placed on the anterior abdominal wall with its apex at the umbilicus; laterally, it is limited by the two umbilical arteries; it lies posterior to the transversalis fascia (37). In the midline, it encloses the remnant of the urachus, the median umbilical ligament, and is recognized at laparotomy as a flat sheet of fascia which lies immediately in front of the peritoneum and connects the remains of the urachus to the obliterated umbilical arteries (Fig. 9).

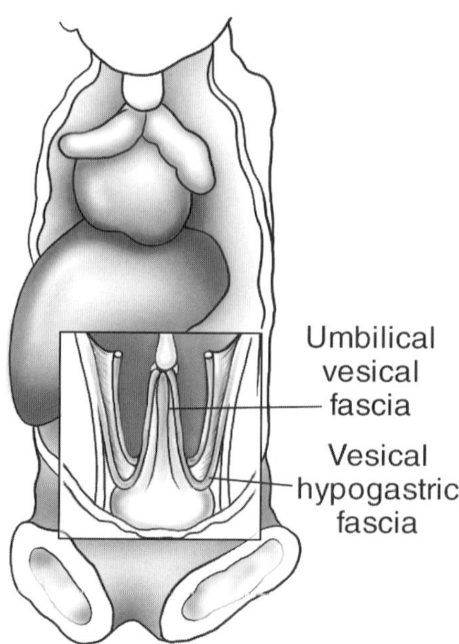

FIG. 9. Fascia of the umbilical arteries.

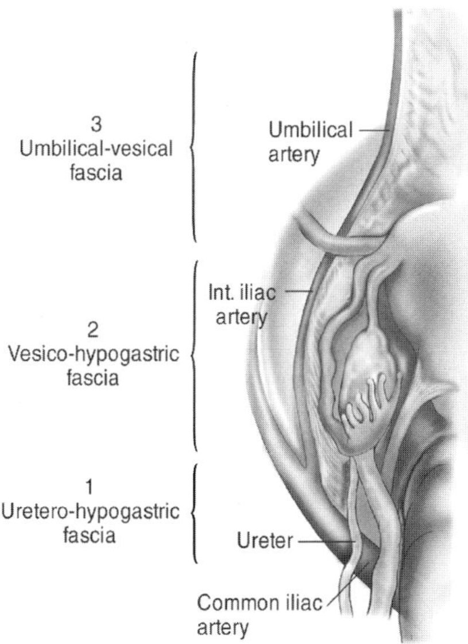

FIG. 10. Anatomic relationship of the different fascial layers with the umbilical artery and ureter.

Dry Spaces of the Retroperitoneum

The retroperitoneum is an important surgical plane because it is avascular. Thus there is a potential "dry space" in which the surgeon can dissect (Fig. 11). The whole of the retroperitoneum is a single entity, but those parts of the retroperitoneum that are adjacent to the umbilical artery's fascial mesentery are separately described.

The pararectal spaces lie beneath the descending portions of the umbilical vessels and their mesenteries on the posterolateral walls of the pelvis. The lateral limits of these spaces are formed by the internal iliac arteries, the medial by the ureters, and the distal by the cardinal ligaments. The roof of the pararectal space is formed by a connective tissue sheet (the fascial mesentery) that extends between the ureter and the internal iliac artery. The paravesical spaces are beneath the horizontal portions of the umbilical arteries and their mesenteries. The bladder forms the medial wall of the paravesical space; the lateral wall is formed by the external iliac vessels and the internal obturator muscle. The vesicohypogastric fascia (the fascial mesentery), with the accompanying umbilical arteries, form the roof of this space. They are limited posteriorly by and separated from the pararectal spaces by the cardinal ligaments. The prevesical space, the space of Retzius, is beneath the anterior ascending part of the umbilical arteries and its fascial mesenteries, now called the umbilical-vesical fascia. This space is the anterior and superior extension of the paravesical spaces. It extends upward to the umbilicus between the symphysis pubis, to which the transversalis fascia is attached, and to the anterior wall of the bladder. Because it is then lo-

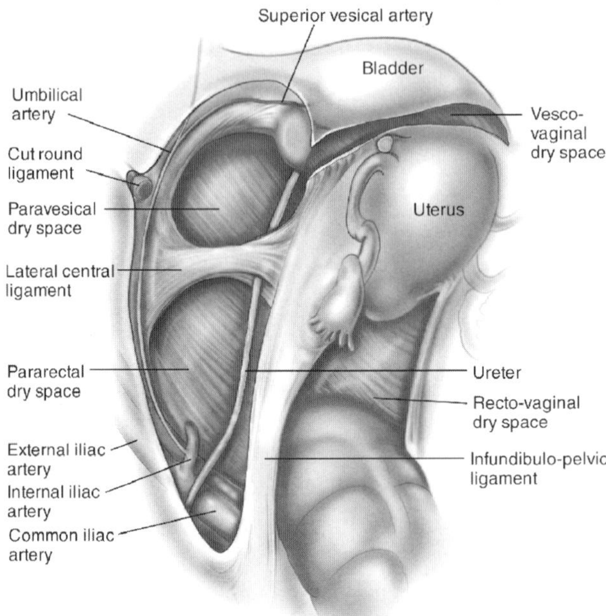

FIG. 11. Dry spaces of the retroperitoneum.

cated between the anteriorly placed transversalis fascia and the posterior umbilical-vesical fascia, it is the most anterior part of the retroperitoneal space (Fig. 11).

Critical Embryonic Events

The surgeon who understands the development of the umbilical artery and its fascia will be able to deduce the location and dimensions of the avascular spaces of the retroperitoneum, foresee the relationship between the pelvic blood supply and the genitourinary tract, and have an easy means of locating the origin of the uterine artery.

The umbilical arteries have a practical importance because they can also serve as surgical landmarks. In a word, if various operative procedures are undertaken with aims that clearly relate to the umbilical arteries, pelvic surgery can be effectively simplified.

REFERENCES

1. Gray S, Skandalakis J, Broecker B. The female reproductive tract. In: Skandalakis J, Gray S, eds. *Embryology for surgeons: the embryological basis for the treatment of congenital anomalies*, 2nd ed. Baltimore: Williams & Wilkins, 1994:816–847.

2. Terruhn V. A study of impression moulds of the genital tract of female fetuses. *Arch Gynecol* 1980;229:207–217.
3. Patten B, Barry A. The genesis of exstrophy of the bladder and epispadias. *Am J Anat* 1952;90:35–57.
4. Marshall V, Muecke E. Variations in exstrophy of the bladder. *J Urol* 1962;88:766–796.
5. Allen T, Husmann D. Cloacal anomalies and other urorectal septal defects in female patients: a spectrum of anatomical abnormalities. *J Urol* 1991;145:1034–1039.
6. Parmley T. Embryology of the female genital tract. In: Kurman R, ed. *Blaustein's pathology of the female genital tract*, 3rd ed. New York: Springer-Verlag, 1987.
7. Duncan S. Embryology of the female genital tract: its genetic defects and congenital anomalies. In: Shaw R, Soutter W, Stanton S, eds. *Gynaecology*, 2nd ed. New York: Churchill Livingstone, 1997:1–22.
8. Haqq C, King C-Y, Ukiyama E, *et al.* Molecular basis of mammalian sexual determination: activation of mullerian inhibitory substance gene expression by SRY. *Science* 1994;266:1494–1500.
9. Gillman J. The development of gonads in man, with a consideration of the role of fetal endocrines and the histogenesis of ovarian tumors. *Contrib Embryol* 1948;32:81–131.
10. Sinclair A, Berta P, Palmer M, et al. A gene from the human sex-determining region encodes a protein with homology to a conserved DNA-binding motif. *Nature* 1990;346:240–244.
11. Page D, Mosher R, Simpson E, et al. The sex determining region of the human Y chromosome encodes a finger protein. *Cell* 1987;51:1091–1104.
12. Wolf U. Genetic aspects of H-Y antigen. *Hum Genet* 1981;58:25–28.
13. Gruenwald P. The relation of the growing mullerian duct to the wolffian duct and its importance for the genesis of malformations. *Anat Rec* 1941;81:1–19.
14. Goldberg JM, Falcone T. Double cervix and vagina with a normal uterus: an unusual Mullerian anomaly. *Hum Reprod* 1996;11:101–2.
15. Koff A. Development of the vagina in the human foetus. *Contrib Embryol Carnegie Inst Wash* 1933;24:61–90.
16. Cunha G. The dual origin of vaginal epithelium. *Am J Anat* 1975;143:387–392.
17. Rock J, Schlaff W. The obstetric consequences of uterovaginal anomalies. *Fertil Steril* 1985;43:681–692.
18. Marshall F, Beisel D. The association of uterine and renal anomalies. *Obstet Gynecol* 1978;51:559–562.
19. McIndoe A. Treatment of congenital absence and obliterative conditions of the vagina. *Br J Plast Surg* 1950;2:254–267.
20. Bryan A, Nigro J, Counseller V. One hundred cases of congenital absence of the vagina. *Surg Gynecol Obstet* 1949;88:79–86.
21. Tarry W, Duckett J, Stephens F. The Mayer-Rokitansky-Küster-Hauser syndrome: pathogenesis, classification and management. *J Urol* 1986;136:648–652.
22. Jones H, Rock J. *Reparative and constructive surgery of the female genital tract.* Baltimore: Williams & Wilkins, 1983.
23. Spaulding M. The development of the external genitalia in the human embryo. *Contrib Embryol Carnegie Inst Wash* 1921;13:69–88.
24. Anderson J, Genadry R. Anatomy and embryology. In: Berek J, ed. *Novak's gynecology*, 12th ed. Baltimore: Williams & Wilkins, 1996:71–122.
25. Lytle W. The deep inguinal ring: development, function and repair. *Br J Surg* 1970;57:531.
26. Backhouse K. The gubernaculum testis Hunteri: testicular descent and maldescent. *Ann R Coll Surg Engl* 1964;35:15.
27. Tanagho E. Development of the ureter. In: Bergman H, ed. *The ureter.* New York: Springer-Verlag, 1981:1–12.
28. Cuneo B, Veau V. De l'origine péritonéale des aponévroses périvésicales. *Séances Memoires Soc Biol* 1898;10:202–203.
29. Curtis A, Anson B, Beaton L. The anatomy of the subperitoneal tissues and ligamentous structures in relation to surgery of the female pelvic viscera. *Surg Gynecol Obstet* 1940;70:643–656.
30. Curtis A, Anson B, Ashley F, Jones T. The blood vessels of the female pelvis in relation to gynecological surgery. *Surg Gynecol Obstet* 1942;75:421–423.
31. Uhlenhuth E, Day E, Smith R, Middleton E. The visceral endopelvic fascia and the hypogastric sheath. *Surg Gynecol Obstet* 1948;86:9–28.
32. Quinby W. The anatomy and blood vessels of the pelvis. In: Meigs J, ed. *Surgical treatment of cancer of the cervix.* New York: Grune & Stratton, 1954:26–62.

33. Richter K, Frick H. Die Anatomie der Fascia pelvis visceralis aus didaktischer Sicht. *Geburtshilfe Frauenheilkd* 1985;45:282–287.
34. Friedland G, De Vries P. Renal ectopia and fusion. *Urology* 1975;5:698–706.
35. Hawtrey C. Surgical anatomy. In: Buchsbaum H, Schmidt J, eds. *Gynecologic and surgical urology.* Philadelphia: WB Saunders, 1982:26–38.
36. Peham H, Amreich J. *Gynäkologische Operationslehre.* Berlin: Verlag Von S. Karger, 1930.
37. Hammond G, Yglesias L, Davis J. The urachus, its anatomy and associated fasciae. *Anat Rec* 1941;80:271–286.

Congenital Malformations of the Female Genital Tract: Diagnosis and Management, edited by G. Gidwani and T. Falcone.
Lippincott Williams & Wilkins, Philadelphia © 1999.

2

Endocrinology and Molecular Biology of the Female Genital Tract in Utero to Puberty

James R. Stelling, Mark R. Gray, and Richard H. Reindollar

Division of Reproductive Endocrinology, Department of Obstetrics and Gynecology, Beth Israel Deaconess Medical Center, Harvard Medical School, Boston, Massachusetts 02215

Human sexual differentiation is an intricate and extremely coordinated sequence of events that begins at conception. The embryo has the potential to develop along either male or female lines, possessing the primordia to develop either gender-appropriate gonad and reproductive tract ducts (Wolffian and Müllerian). The complete expression of gender is under both genetic and hormonal control. Male sexual development is a highly dependent developmental process, with distinct steps directed by products of single genes acting in a specific chronological order. In contrast, female development seems to be an independent process that occurs in the absence of male gonadal morphogenesis.

The developmental steps in male sexual differentiation have been well studied and characterized (1). A cascade of molecular events precedes the development of the testes, the Wolffian (mesonephric) ductal system, and the external male genitalia. The initial stimulus for these events is expression of the *SRY* gene on the short arm of the Y chromosome, discovered by the molecular genetic analysis of rare sex-reversed male and female patients (2). The *SRY* gene is present in 80% of sex-reversed 46,XX males and absent or mutant in some 46,XY females (3,4). The requirement for the activity of genes downstream from that of *SRY* is suggested by the absence of *SRY* gene mutations in most 46,XY sex-reversed females and the lack of the *SRY* gene in some 46,XX true hermaphrodites (2). Several genes and endocrine abnormalities that disrupt different steps of male sexual differentiation have been well characterized. Besides *SRY,* mutant genes causing abnormal sexual development in 46,XY individuals include those encoding Müllerian inhibiting substance *(MIS),* type 2 3 β-hydroxysteroid dehydrogenase, 17α-hydroxylase, type 2 5α-reductase, and the androgen receptor *(AR)* (5–10). Many of these findings demonstrate the importance of hormonal control in male sexual development. In the absence of *SRY* gene–initiated hormonal influences in 46,XY individuals, sexual development is directed to the female pathway, resulting in the female phenotype or undermasculinization of the male phenotype.

Virtually nothing is known about the genes that control normal mammalian female sexual differentiation. Observations from several animal models suggest that once female sexual development is initiated in the embryo, final differentiation proceeds with less dependence on intermediary gene and hormonal regulation than for male sexual development (11). Female differentiation ensues because of the lack of signals directing male differentiation. Observations that support this model include (a) ovarian development occurs in the absence of *SRY* gene expression, (b) the Müllerian system completely develops in the absence of *MIS* gene expression, and (c) the external genitalia feminize in the absence of androgens. Although there seems to be no regulation of Müllerian system development in females, reproductive system abnormalities are common, occurring in up to 3.2% of fertile females (12). The diversity of Müllerian system developmental anomalies suggests that numerous different genes are required for its complete development. Only rare patients have been identified with abnormal external genitalia in the absence of other abnormalities of female sexual differentiation, suggesting that few intermediary genes control external female genital development. This chapter will review the endocrinology and molecular genetics of female sexual development, from fetal life through puberty. Although the main focus of this review is the roles of factors that regulate normal genital development, it concludes with a brief summary of congenital malformations of the female reproductive tract.

ROLE OF HORMONES IN FEMALE REPRODUCTIVE DEVELOPMENT

The endocrine contribution to fetal sexual development has been well described (Fig. 1). Although the importance of hormones for normal male differentiation is well understood, there is no evidence for a requirement of normal endocrine function to

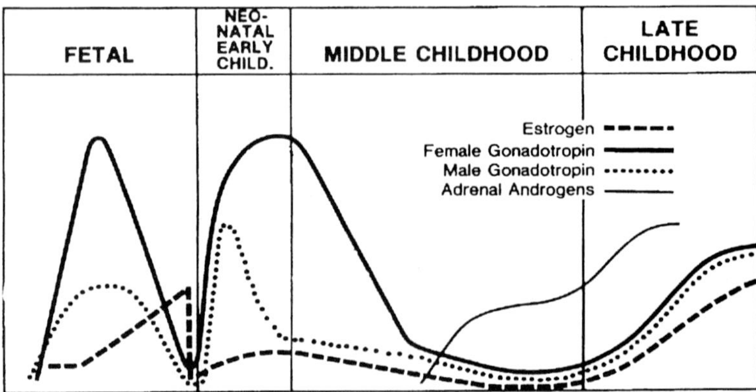

FIG. 1. Schematic representation of quantitative changes in secretion of gonadotropins, gonadal steroids, and adrenal androgens during phases of development and maturation. (Modified from ref. 2, with permission.)

achieve normal female fetal development (1). Fetal development of the hypothalamic-pituitary-ovarian (HPO) circuit occurs concomitant with, but independently of, the formation of the female genital tract (13). As early as the tenth week of gestation, luteinizing hormone (LH)–containing cells have been detected in the pituitary gland (14). Gonadotropin secretion increases through midgestational development (Fig. 1). The pulsatile release of gonadotropin-releasing hormone (GnRH) and LH has been demonstrated from the hypothalamus and pituitary at 20 weeks of gestation (15,16). Maturation of the negative feedback mechanisms of the HPO axis is demonstrated at midgestation by the decrease in gonadotropins secondary to increasing sex steroid levels (Fig. 1). In humans, an inverse relationship exists between levels of circulating testosterone and LH as early as 17 weeks in gestation in males, as demonstrated by analysis of serum samples obtained by percutaneous umbilical blood sampling (PUBS) from 114 normal fetuses, indicating maturation of negative feedback at this gestational age (17).

The female gonad is markedly different from the male gonad, both developmentally and functionally. The fetal testis is an endocrine organ during male sexual development; the ovary seems to have no significant endocrine function during intrauterine life. In late gestation, as demonstrated by *in vitro* experiments with cultured pituitary cells, females produce higher gonadotropin levels than males do, possibly because of the lack of feedback suppression by ovarian steroids and peptides (e.g., inhibin) (18). Fetal male castration in sheep leads to higher gonadotropin levels than those found in eugonadal or ovariectomized female fetuses (19). Sexual differences have also been observed in spontaneous human "genetic knockouts." Males with LH receptor mutations present with pseudohermaphroditism because of inadequate testosterone stimulation (20,21). Males lacking LH-β activity have normal genital tract development because of adequate androgen stimulation by human chorionic gonadotropin (hCG); LH and hCG bind to the same receptor (22). In addition, patients with follicle stimulating hormone–β (FSH-β) mutations also have developmentally normal reproductive tracts (23). Females with LH-β and inactivating LH receptor mutations have normal genital development, but experience anovulatory amenorrhea at the time expected for menarche (21,24,25).

The presence of central nervous system peptide hormone deficiencies further demonstrates the dispensability for GnRH and gonadotropin secretion in normal female genital development. Anencephalic female fetuses have normal Müllerian duct development (26). Females with inactivating GnRH receptor mutations also have developmentally normal reproductive tracts (27).

Despite the fact that female sexual differentiation occurs independently of HPO regulation, gonadotropin secretion may be important to maintain the normal complement of germ cells in the ovary (28). For example, patients with FSH deficiency have streak or hypoplastic ovaries (28). FSH receptor mutations have been found in patients with abnormal puberty and elevated gonadotropins (29). In Rhesus monkeys, germ cell numbers are decreased after fetal hypophysectomy because of atresia (30). If gonadotropins are necessary to prevent loss of germ cells, it is most likely an indirect effect because oocytes lack FSH receptors (31,32). In summary, fetal gonadotropins are not necessary for normal development of the female genital tract or germ cells but are necessary for the prevention of premature loss of germ cells.

If fetal gonadotropins are not needed for female genital development, it remains possible that maternal steroids supplied to the fetus in utero contribute to normal sexual differentiation independently of gonadotropin stimulation. The highest levels of estrogen in humans are produced during pregnancy by the placenta (8,300 pg/mL) (33). This placentally derived estrogen-rich state may be important for female genital system development independent of the estrogen potentially produced by the fetal ovary. Estrogen has well-recognized uterotropic effects. The estrogen receptor is present in the human fetal uterus by the fifteenth week of development and is also present in the external female genitalia (34,35). Estrogen responsivity has been documented in chick Müllerian ducts (36). The synthetic estrogen-like drug diethylstilbestrol causes the formation of a T-shape uterus in one half of females exposed in utero (37–39). Although estrogen may be needed for maturation and maximal growth of the Müllerian duct derivatives, both animal and human data suggest that estrogen is not required for their normal development. The gray-spotted hyena, deficient in aromatase activity and therefore estrogen-deficient, demonstrates the absence of the requirement for estrogen in mammalian female reproductive tract development. Female hyenas have normal internal genital development and are externally partially virilized secondary to excess androgens (40). Normal female genital development occurs in human pregnancies in spite of defects in maternal, placental, or fetal estrogen biosynthesis, including deficiencies in 17-hydroxylase and aromatase (41,42). Transgenic mice lacking the estrogen receptor gene have structurally normal but hypoplastic genital tracts (43). Human females with inactivating estrogen receptor mutations have normally developed reproductive tracts (44). In summary, it seems unlikely that the primary female sex steroid, estrogen, contributes significantly to female sexual development.

Deficiency of other steroids does not disrupt normal female sexual development. Congenital adrenal hyperplasia (CAH) patients who have 21-hydroxylase deficiency demonstrate that adrenal steroids are not needed for normal Müllerian development, although development of their external genitalia may be affected by excess androgens (45). Defects in androgen biosynthesis do not disrupt female sexual development. Female patients who are deficient for 17α-hydroxylase and unable to synthesize either androgens or estrogens have normal Müllerian derivatives (41). Patients with androgen insensitivity syndrome, who are unable to respond to androgens at the target organs, have normal female external genital development (10,46).

REPRODUCTIVE HORMONAL EVENTS DURING CHILDHOOD THROUGH PUBERTY

After birth, an intact and functional negative endocrine feedback system is already present. With the abrupt decrease in placentally derived steroids, synthesis and secretion of the pituitary gonadotropins increases in the newborn infant. Within 2 weeks of birth, the serum concentration of each of the gonadotropins, FSH and LH, is approximately 10 to 20 mIU/mL (47,48). In boys, the neonatal rise in gonadotropins is associated with an increase in testosterone to the lower limits of the adult range (47). In contrast, in girls, there is relatively little estrogen response from the ovaries because the pattern of gonadotropin release is different from that of the adult state (49). During female childhood, FSH levels are higher than LH levels and the bioactivity of the gonadotropins is low. Occasional periods of ovarian response to these elevated gonadotropins during childhood results in isolated precocious thelarche. In boys, the elevated gonadotropins become suppressed by approximately 4 to 6 months of age. In girls, the gonadotropins may remain elevated for up to 2 to 4 years, after which time the arcuate nucleus activity for GnRH release becomes suppressed (47). Once GnRH is suppressed, the negative feedback set point seems to be altered, so that feedback suppression by estradiol becomes very sensitive. At this time, a relative excess of FSH compared to LH develops (FSH = 1.0 mIU/mL, LH = 0.04 mIU/mL). The high FSH/LH ratio is maintained until puberty (50).

The maturation of negative feedback in the HPO axis is primarily of central origin (49). Gonadal dysgenesis patients have qualitatively similar patterns of prepubertal decreases in gonadotropin production, although the levels of FSH and LH are significantly higher (51). This suggests that much of the prepubertal gonadotropin suppression is under CNS control. Sensitive immunofluorometric assays for measurement of gonadotropins have revealed more information about gonadotropin levels during childhood (52,53). Several studies have reported GnRH-dependent sleep-entrained LH and FSH pulsatile secretion in prepubertal females even earlier than previously demonstrated. In addition, concomitant estradiol production has been demonstrated at low levels during prepubertal childhood (0.6 pg/mL) (54).

Puberty begins with the augmentation of the sleep-entrained LH pulses, the result of desuppression of GnRH production. This most likely is associated with removal of CNS inhibitors such as τ-aminobutyric acid (GABA), melatonin, dopamine, and endorphins. The nighttime increase in gonadotropins is then followed by an increase in the daytime levels of these hormones. The typical adult pattern of 90- to 120-minute pulse intervals becomes apparent late in puberty (53). Patients with gonadal dysgenesis undergo the same reemergence of the pulse generator, supporting the notion of central mediation (51). Evidence suggests that each component of the HPO axis functions appropriately when presented with the correct "higher level" stimulations. The prepubertal ovary responds to exogenous gonadotropins. The pituitaries of infantile Rhesus monkeys respond to exogenous GnRH, as do patients with Kallmann's syndrome (55,56). Even the hypothalamus is competent for stimulation to secrete pulsatile GnRH in response to the excitatory neurotransmitter *N*-methyl-D-aspartate (57). The adult FSH/LH ratio of approximately 1 is finally obtained at the time in puberty when all components of the HPO circuit are functional and driven by the adult pattern of GnRH release (52). The final step in pubertal maturation in females is the acquisition of the positive feedback response. The gonadotropin surge is elicited when estrogen levels peak at approximately 200 to 250 pg/mL for approximately 50 hours (58).

Menarche occurs after adequate stimulation of the endometrium by estrogen, and then subsequent estrogen withdrawal, producing menstrual shedding. This sequence is the result of the negative feedback mechanism of the HPO circuit. Relatively few of the initial menstrual cycles are the result of progesterone withdrawal. Approximately 15% of cycles in the first menstrual year are ovulatory; after nearly 5 years of menstrual activity, approximately 75% of cycles are ovulatory (49).

The timing of the onset of puberty is controlled by a wide array of factors; the exact mechanism remains elusive. Relevant factors include the amount and composition of body fat, nutritional state, level of exercise, and emotional status. Frisch suggested that a minimum body weight and/or amount of body fat (24%) is necessary to achieve puberty; in order to achieve regular ovulatory cycles, 28% body fat is required (59). This idea was later refined to include body proportions in an attempt to establish a link between the onset of puberty and the amount of subcutaneous abdominal fat accumulation (60). Most adolescents who have completed puberty do fit these criteria; however, cause and effect cannot be determined. With the discovery of the leptin gene, a potential endocrine signal has been hypothesized to link adipose tissue with the onset of puberty. Leptin is a protein hormone produced by peripheral adipose cells that feeds back to the CNS to regulate appetite and body weight (61). Leptin suppresses neuropeptide Y, a factor that modulates GnRH secretion (62). Mice deficient in leptin have pubertal delay that can be corrected with leptin replacement (63). Furthermore, normal mice administered leptin demonstrated accelerated pubertal onset (64). Homozygous missense mutations in the human leptin gene result in amenorrhea in girls and delayed puberty and hypogonadism in boys (65). In a small longitudinal study of peripubertal boys, an increase in circulating leptin was found during the few months prior to the increase in testosterone (66). This finding has not been confirmed in further human studies or in a Rhesus monkey model, and the role of leptin in pubertal onset remains speculative but promising (67).

Although many changes in the activity of the HPO circuit occur between birth and puberty, disruption of its maturation process in girls does not affect the development of Müllerian duct derivatives. Almost all patients with Müllerian developmental defects, including those with the most extreme anomalies, i.e., congenital absence of the uterus and vagina, have a normal and functional HPO axis, with normal ovulatory cycles (68).

ETIOLOGY OF CONGENITAL MALFORMATIONS OF THE FEMALE REPRODUCTIVE TRACT

The etiologies for the majority of congenital anomalies of the female reproductive tract are largely unknown (69). Although most patients with such anomalies are isolated cases, some familial clusters have also been found, including siblings with the same reproductive tract abnormality. Identical twins discordant for Müllerian anomalies have also been described (70,71). Taken together, these observations suggest that both genetic and environmental factors underlie Müllerian duct developmental defects. Some cases might be caused by *de novo* germline or somatic mutations in genes that normally direct reproductive system development. Also, the occurrence of Müllerian anomalies in well-recognized multiorgan birth defect syndromes also implicates genetic factors. A recently described example is a family affected by the hand-foot-genital (HFG) syndrome, a skeletal disorder that includes a bicornuate or didelphic uterus. Family members with both classes of defects had a germline mutation in the *HOXA13* gene (72). So far this case is the only example of a single gene mutation that has produced a Müllerian duct anomaly.

Environmental Influences

The sporadic occurrence of developmental anomalies of the female reproductive tract would suggest that teratogenic exposure might underlie many cases, as in many types of cancer. Two well-known teratogens can cause abnormal Müllerian duct development; both are synthetic pharmaceutical agents. One of them, diethylstilbestrol (DES), is specifically teratogenic to the female reproductive system. Others, such as thalidomide, produce severe developmental anomalies that include defects of the female reproductive tract. DES is a synthetic estrogen-like compound that was initially believed to prevent recurrent abortion and preeclampsia (73,39). Unfortunately, further studies did not support these benefits (74). Daughters of patients who had taken DES experienced an abnormally high incidence of clear cell adenocarcinoma of the vagina and cervix, an otherwise extremely rare tumor. Also, a T-shaped uterus was reported in up to 68% of women exposed to DES in utero (37,38). Abnormalities of the cervix and fallopian tubes have also been described in association with the other abnormalities after in utero DES exposure (39). Given the absence of a role for estrogen in genital development, the adverse effects of DES were unexpected based on the assumption that the teratogenic affect depends on its ability to bind to the estrogen receptor. Estrogen receptors may not be present in the Müllerian ducts until after differentiation is complete, after the period when DES exerts its teratogenic affect (34,75). The exact mechanism for DES teratogenicity remains unknown. DES has been demonstrated recently to change the normal pattern of *HOX* gene expression in the developing Müllerian system in mice (76). Expression of several *HOX* genes has been demonstrated in human fetal and adult Müllerian derivatives (77). DES may exert its teratogenic affect by altering the pattern of expression of one or more *HOX* genes. These genes encode a family of DNA-binding proteins that act as transcription regulators. Different combinations of *HOX* transcription factors define patterns of gene expression and development throughout the early embryo (78,79). The point mutation causing HFG syndrome in a large family is in the *HOXA13* gene, as noted above (72).

Thalidomide is a teratogen that causes developmental defects in mesodermal derivatives, including primordia of the limbs, the renal system, and the heart and circulatory system. Phocomelia is present in 100% of affected thalidomide-exposed patients. Approximately one third of female patients have genital tract abnormalities, including varying degrees of uterine fusion defects, ranging from aplasia to bicornuate uterus and longitudinal vaginal septa (80–82). The expression of a gene(s) required for normal genital and limb development may have been misregulated in some way by thalidomide or its metabolites. In spite of its notoriety, thalidomide has been approved by the United States Food and Drug Administration as a therapeutic agent to treat leprosy. Thalidomide is also being tested for its ability to fight certain types of tumors and acquired immunodeficiency syndrome (AIDS) because of its angiogenesis inhibition properties.

Genetic Factors

The presence of severe reproductive system developmental defects often results in infertility, preventing the genetic transmission of causative mutant genes. The reproductive tract anomalies of patients with mild uterine defects often go unnoticed because their pregnancies are often uncomplicated. Both of these factors complicate the study of the genetic transmission of mutant genes that cause reproductive defects. Before the advent of modern assisted reproductive technologies (ARTs), patients with congenital absence of the uterus and vagina (CAUV) were unable to produce children. A recent preliminary survey of children born to CAUV patients by uterine surrogacy has provided some clues for the mode of inheritance of this disorder (83). Because each of 17 female infants had no detectable Müllerian anomalies, it is likely that CAUV is not commonly transmitted as a dominant trait. On the other hand, mild uterine defects would not be detected easily. The genetic transmission pattern for CAUV is further complicated by the possibility that the Müllerian system defect is only one of many different abnormalities in a syndrome of developmental anomalies, such as in the case of the HFG syndrome discussed above. Retrospective analysis of phenotypic data for reproductive system defects is further complicated by incomplete analysis, poor follow-up, and scanty documentation.

Many studies of developmental defects in humans have been enhanced by the availability of an animal model for the disorder under investigation. The human is one of few species that normally develops a fused Müllerian tract. Failure to fuse the Müllerian ducts during early development is normal in most mammals, thus limiting their usefulness as models for the investigation of malformations of the human female reproductive tract. A disorder found in Holstein-Friesian cows, white heifer disease, is characterized by varying degrees of Müllerian duct aplasia and hypoplasia, along with a coat color change (84). This disorder is most likely transmitted in an autosomal recessive pattern. Although linkage analysis has been used to map the disorder close to the bovine *steel* locus, the causative mutant gene(s) has not been identified (85). The human homolog of the *steel* locus is *SCF,* a gene that encodes a mast cell growth factor. No patients with mutations in the *SCF* gene have been identified; patients with mutations in the gene encoding the *SCF* ligand's receptor, *C-KIT,* have not been reported to have reproductive system abnormalities (86).

Systematic genetic studies of abnormal human sexual differentiation are uncommon because of the difficulties in the clinical evaluation of relatives of the affected patients. In a study based on interviews of 24 patients with Müllerian fusion anomalies, only 1 patient was aware of a relative with a Müllerian derivative anomaly (87). Another survey of 23 patients with Müllerian aplasia failed to reveal any relatives with uterine anomalies (88). In one recent clinical study of 261 patients with malformations of the uterus and vagina, 39.8% were reported to have relatives with undefined reproductive system disorders (89). Examples of familial clusters of genital tract malformations have been reported; in one study, 10 of 13 women with complete Müllerian aplasia had similarly affected relatives (90). In these families, inheritance of the disorder was consistent with a sex-limited autosomal dominant pattern. Other families with affected siblings suggest an autosomal recessive pattern of inheritance for CAUV (91). Taken together, these observations support the hypothesis that most Müllerian fusion defects are caused by polygenic defects, with each patient having a new mutation in one of numerous unlinked genes required for normal Müllerian development.

Development of the portion of the female reproductive tract that arises embryologically from primordia outside of the Müllerian ducts may also be disrupted by mutations. A familial cluster of imperforate hymen has been identified with an apparent dominant mode of inheritance (92). Other studies have also found familial clusters of imperforate hymen, with an apparently recessive inheritance pattern (93,94). Numerous genetic syndromes, such as the Beckwith-Wiedemann and Donahue syndromes, include abnormalities of the female external genitalia abnormalities, such as bicornuate uterus and clitoromegaly (95,96).

Chromosomal rearrangements in patients with Müllerian anomalies provide an opportunity to identify genes required for normal female reproductive tract development. Karyotypic abnormalities are uncommon in women with developmental defects of the genital tract (68,88,97,98). Infants with trisomy of chromosomes 13 and 18 often have bicornuate uterus, along with numerous other developmental defects (95). Because the frequency of cytogenetic abnormalities in patients with Müllerian anomalies is not significantly elevated above the background population frequency, it is not necessary to perform cytogenetic analysis on patients with genital tract abnormalities. However, several isolated CAUV patients with major chromosomal abnormalities have been described (99–101). Investigation of these rare patients using molecular genetic methods may pinpoint genes critical for Müllerian development at the sites of their chromosomal rearrangements. The rearrangement breakpoints in each of these patients are at widely different chromosomal locations, suggesting that defects at several unlinked loci can result in CAUV. Some of these chromosome rearrangement breakpoints are in the same chromosomal regions as genes thought to have a role in normal Müllerian development, such as *WT-1* and *AMHR* (100,101).

Other etiologies for Müllerian anomalies have been proposed. Apoptosis, or programmed cell death, may have a role in the etiology of developmental anomalies of the Müllerian ducts. It is likely that the midline uterine septum is resorbed by a regulated developmental process that includes apoptosis. Bcl-2 protein, an apoptosis inhibitor, is present in the fetus in regions that persist in the adult, such as the endometrium, and absent in the midline septum, which normally undergoes regression (102). An abnormality in the regulation of apoptosis could potentially result in the persistence of a uterine septum. Although not confirmed by other investigators, associations between genital malformations and blood group antigens have been found (89). Others have reported an association between genital anomalies and human lymphocyte antigen (HLA) histocompatibility antigens (103). Linkage data based on analyses of blood cell markers may help identify chromosomal regions that carry genes necessary for normal Müllerian development.

The development of both the renal collecting system and the Müllerian ducts require the proper growth and differentiation of the mesonephric (Wolffian) ducts (104). During early mammalian embryonic development, the renal and reproductive systems develop together from intermediate mesoderm, physically and temporally (105). The Wolffian ducts either induce or act as a template for the development and expansion of the Müllerian ducts. In boys, the Müllerian ducts almost completely disappear, and the Wolffian ducts differentiate into the epididymis, vas deferens, and seminal vesicles. In girls, because of the absence of gonadal androgen production, almost all portions of the Wolffian ducts degenerate, and the Müllerian ducts develop into the fallopian tubes, uterus, and upper vagina. If the Wolffian ducts are disrupted during development before they contact the urogenital sinus, further development of the Müllerian ducts beyond the point of interruption does not occur (104).

Abnormal mesonephric duct development could then result in defects of the derivatives of the Wolffian and Müllerian ducts, including the kidney. Renal abnormalities commonly occur along with Müllerian anomalies (106). Because of the common developmental pathway of the renal system and the female reproductive tract, gene products required for complete renal development may also be needed for early Müllerian duct development. Unicornuate uterus is accompanied by renal abnormalities in approximately 40% of cases (107). Patients with hereditary renal adysplasia, or bilateral renal agenesis (also known as Potter's syndrome), commonly have female genital abnormalities, including vaginal atresia, bicornuate uterus, and didelphic uterus (108,96). In other multiple organ system malformation syndromes that affect both male and female individuals, Müllerian duct developmental defects, including bicornuate uterus and vaginal atresia, have been found (96,109).

Specific Genes That May Have an Essential Role in Female Reproductive System Development

Many malformation syndromes include genital anomalies in males and females. Causative mutations have been identified for only a few of them (Table 1). In most of these syndromes, even when a single causative gene has been identified as etiologic, genital malformations often are a minor and in some cases an uncommon component of the entire spectrum of abnormalities. The Donahue syndrome and Beckwith-Wiedemann syndrome are prominent examples (95,96,110).

HOXA13

Hand-foot-genital syndrome is an autosomal dominant disorder that includes uterine fusion defects and multiple distal skeletal malformations (123). A mouse mutant strain, *hypodactyly,* with a similar spectrum of abnormalities, has a mutation in the

TABLE 1. *Common congenital malformations of the female genital tract, associated syndromes, and causative genes*

Abnormality	Syndromes	Inheritance mode	Causative gene	Ref.
External genitalia				
Clitoromegaly	Beckwith-Wiedemann	Autosomal dominant	*BWR1A*	96
	Donahue's (leprechaunism)	Autosomal recessive	*INSR*	110,111
	Roberts'	Autosomal recessive	Centromere protein	96
Labial fusion	Single family	Unknown		112
Labial/clitoral hypoplasia	Robinow's	Autosomal recessive or dominant		113
	Pterygium	Autosomal recessive		114
Hymen				
Imperforate hymen	Ulnar-mammary	Autosomal recessive	*TBX3* mutation	115,116
	Isolated families	Autosomal recessive		93,94
	Single family	Dominant		92
Vaginal defects				
Transverse septum	McKusick-Kaufman	Autosomal recessive	Chr. 20	117
	Langer-Giedion	Autosomal dominant	Chr. 8	96
Longitudinal septum	Edwards-Gale	Autosomal dominant		118
	Meckel's	Autosomal recessive		95
	Johanson-Blizzard	Autosomal recessive		119
Vaginal atresia	Winter's	Autosomal recessive		95
	Waardenburg type 2	Autosomal dominant	*MITF*	120
Lateral fusion defects	Hand-foot-genital	Autosomal dominant	*HOXA13*	72
	Fraser's	Autosomal recessive		109
	Meckel's	Autosomal recessive		95
	Bardet-Biedl	Autosomal recessive	Several loci	121
	Beckwith-Wiedemann	Autosomal dominant	*BWR1A*	96
	Donohue's (leprechaunism)	Autosomal recessive	*INSR*	110,111
	Roberts'	Autosomal recessive	Centromere protein	96
	Denys-Drash	Sporadic	*WT1*	122
Absence of uterus	Isolated families	Autosomal recessive		69,91,101

Hoxa13 gene (124). As discussed above, a family with HFG syndrome was shown to have a nonsense mutation in the human *Hoxa13* gene (72). This mutation would eliminate normal DNA binding of the Hoxa13 transcription factor. The phenotypic variation in the extent of uterine fusion in female carriers of this mutation suggests that other factors, such as the expression of other genes, have a role in Müllerian development. It is not known if isolated cases of Müllerian anomalies that lack skeletal abnormalities are caused by mutations in the *Hoxa13* gene.

CFTR

Mutations in the *CFTR* gene cause cystic fibrosis, a well-known and common potentially lethal genetic disorder. The numerous diverse *CFTR* gene mutations result in a wide range of disease phenotypes, ranging from no symptoms at all to severe respiratory and pancreatic deficiency. Approximately 80% of men with congenital absence of the vas deferens (CAVD) have mutations in the *CFTR* gene (125,126). Although the vas deferens is a Wolffian duct derivative, it is possible that normal *CFTR* function is necessary for normal development of the Müllerian ducts, since their development is dependent on the presence of the Wolffian ducts. To test the hypothesis that female reproductive tract anomalies are analogous to CAVD in males in having *CFTR* gene mutations as the etiology, a small group of CAUV patients was tested for a panel of the most common *CFTR* gene mutations (127). These patients did not have an increased incidence of common mutations compared to normal subjects. It remains possible that CAUV-specific *CFTR* mutations exist and were not detected by the screening for classic cystic fibrosis–associated mutations.

WT1

The *WT1* gene takes its name from the Wilms' tumor nephroblastoma, the most common intraabdominal solid tumor in children, occurring in 1 in 10,000 newborns. The *WT1* gene is among the genes in the 11p13 chromosomal region that are deleted in patients with Wilms' tumor, aniridia, genitourinary malformation, and mental retardation syndrome (122). Germline *WT1* gene mutations are nearly always present in patients with the Denys-Drash syndrome (DDS). Male DDS patients have urogenital abnormalities, pseudohermaphroditism, and a high incidence of Wilms tumors (128,129). Mutant mice lacking *WT1* gene expression fail to develop kidneys and gonads, suggesting that normal urogenital tract development depends on *WT1* gene expression (130). *WT1* mRNA has been detected in the mammalian embryonic kidney, mesothelium, genital ridge, gonads, and uterus. The requirement for *WT1* gene expression in the earliest events of female urogenital development during the period of Wolffian and paramesonephric duct development has not been demonstrated. Thus, WT1 protein might be required for normal female reproductive development, and mutations of the *WT1* gene might result in the inappropriate activation of the gene encoding Müllerian inhibiting substance (MIS), leading to partial regression of the Müllerian ducts. To test this hypothesis, DNA from 25 CAUV patients was analyzed using denaturing gradient gel electrophoresis; no *WT1* gene mutations were detected (131).

MIS/AMHR

Deficiency of MIS signaling, caused by absence of MIS or its receptor, results in the anomalous persistence of the Müllerian ducts in males (132,133). Conversely, in female development, inappropriate expression of the *MIS* gene, or constitutive activation of its receptor, encoded by the anti-Müllerian hormone receptor *(AMHR)* gene, could potentially result in abnormal regression of the Müllerian ducts (134). However, it seems unlikely that inappropriate expression of MIS in females could cause the partial Müllerian duct regression typically found in CAUV and other less extreme uterine defects (135). Preliminary analysis of the *MIS* and the *AMHR* genes has not revealed mutations in 23 patients with CAUV (136).

Specific Anomalies and Proposed Genetic Influences

External Genitalia

Congenital fusion of the labia minora is an uncommon anomaly in prepubertal girls. Congenital fusion has been reported in several families (112). In addition, disorders of excess androgens, such as in CAH, could produce labioscrotal fusion in some families (137). The majority of cases are caused by abnormal healing in a hypoestrogenic state after infection or trauma. Other abnormalities of the external genitalia have been found in patients with complex genetic syndromes. Patients with the Beckwith-Wiedemann and Donahue syndromes sometimes have clitoral hypertrophy (96,110).

Hymen

Imperforate hymen occurs in approximately 0.1% of female newborns (138). Although most cases are sporadic, three familial clusters have been reported, as mentioned above. In two reports nontwin siblings were affected, suggesting a recessive pattern of inheritance (93,94). The most recent case report includes affected patients in two generations, with a probable dominant mode of inheritance (92). In patients with ulnar-mammary syndrome, abnormal development of the skeleton and apocrine glands is present, as well as imperforate hymen in some girls (115). These patients have mutations in the TBX3 gene; TBX3 protein is a DNA-binding transcription factor (116).

Transverse Vaginal Septum

Transverse vaginal septa usually occur sporadically, with no known etiology. However, several malformation syndromes include vaginal septa in affected females among other abnormal developmental defects. The best known syndrome that includes transverse vaginal septa is the autosomal recessive McKusick-Kaufman syndrome, found in the Old Order Amish ethnic group. This syndrome includes polydactyly and congenital heart disease, in addition to hydrometrocolpos caused by the vaginal septum (117). The genetic locus for this syndrome is on chromosome 20, at the cytogenetic position 20p12. A gene *(JAG1)* responsible for a different developmental disorder, the Alagille syndrome, maps to the same region. Complete DNA sequence analysis of two patients with McKusick-Kaufman syndrome did not reveal any mutations in the *JAG1* gene (117).

Longitudinal Vaginal Septum

Longitudinal vaginal septa result from the incomplete resorption of the vaginal septum formed during Müllerian fusion. Most (87.8%) cases of vaginal septal defects were accompanied by uterine fusion defects (139). It is likely that resorption of the septum in both the vagina and the uterus are controlled by the same mechanism. Others have suggested that rather then being caused by a fusion defect, septa may result from abnormal mesodermal proliferation or the persistence of Müllerian epithelium (140). Two genetic malformation syndromes include longitudinal vaginal septa. The Edwards-Gale syndrome is autosomal dominant; the Johanson-Blizzard syndrome is autosomal recessive (118,119).

Müllerian Fusion Defects

Incomplete Müllerian fusion defects range from a small septate uterus to complete duplication, as in didelphic uterus. The previously mentioned HFG syndrome is the best example of an autosomal dominant disorder producing varying degrees of uterine fusion (72). Only rare examples of familial occurrence of fusion defects have been found, suggesting a multifactorial/polygenic etiology (87). Many malformation syndromes include incomplete Müllerian fusion as one part of a complex phenotype; examples of these syndromes include trisomy 13 and 18; thalidomide toxicity; syndromes described by Meckel, Fraser, Rudiger, and Roberts; and the Bardet-Biedl syndrome (95,121). None of the mutations causing these autosomal recessive syndromes have been identified.

Absence of the Uterus and Vagina

Reviews of CAUV or Müllerian aplasia are difficult to compare because of clinical variability and confusing nomenclature. Patients with complete Müllerian aplasia lack all Müllerian duct derivatives. In contrast, patients with Mayer-Rokitansky-Küster-Hauser syndrome (MRKH) lack the uterus, cervix, and upper vagina, but the fallopian tubes are present, typically attached bilaterally to rudimentary uterine bulbs. Approximately half of MRKH patients have abnormally developed fallopian tubes and/or asymmetric uterine bulbs, with frequent concomitant renal, skeletal, and cardiac abnormalities (106). The remaining half of MRKH patients have normal fallopian tubes, symmetric uterine buds, and only occasional renal, skeletal, and cardiac abnormalities. Familial clusters of complete Müllerian aplasia and MRKH have been described, as mentioned previously. Rare MRKH patients have chromosomal rearrangements. These chromosomal rearrangements may disrupt genes necessary for normal Müllerian development (99). Testing of several candidate genes for mutations in MRKH patients has so far not revealed causative mutations; these genes include *WT-1, PAX-2, MIS, AMHR, GALT,* and *CFTR* (127,131,136,141,142).

CONCLUSIONS

Each step in male sexual differentiation has been described extensively, and the causes of many types of rare developmental defects have been identified. Male sexual differentiation requires both genetic and endocrine components for normal development. In contrast, female sexual differentiation occurs relatively independently of these influences. Unlike male development, none of the major steps in female sexual differentiation or the gene products necessary for normal female genital tract development have been identified. So far, only a single mutant gene (in *Hoxa13*) has been demonstrated to cause abnormalities in female genital tract development. It is likely that the genes necessary for female sexual differentiation are the same as those required for general embryonic development. It would be expected that many of the mutations in such genes would produce lethal effects during embryonic development. With continued genetic analysis of rare patients with reproductive tract abnormalities, it might be possible to describe the developmental genetic pathway for female sexual differentiation.

ACKNOWLEDGMENTS

The authors thank Dr. Megan Karnis for helpful comments on the manuscript and Jennifer Sabbagh for assistance with the manuscript.

REFERENCES

1. Gustafson ML, Donahoe PK. Male sex determination: current concepts of male sexual differentiation. *Annu Rev Med* 1994;45:505–524.
2. Goodfellow PN, Lovell-Badge R. SRY and sex determination in mammals. *Annu Rev Genet* 1993;27:71–92.
3. de la Chappelle A. Nature and origin of males with XX sex chromosomes. *Am J Hum Genet* 1972;24:71–105.
4. Hawkins JR, Taylor A, Goodfellow PN, Migeon CJ, Smith KD, Berkovitz GD. Evidence for increased prevalence of SRY mutations in XY females with complete rather than partial gonadal dysgenesis. *Am J Hum Genet* 1992;51:979–984.
5. Behringer RR, Cate RL, Froelick GJ, Palmiter RD, Brinster RL. Abnormal sexual development in transgenic mice chronically expressing Müllerian inhibiting substance. *Nature* 1990;345:167–170.
6. Mebarki F, Sanchez R, Rheaume E, et al. Non-salt-losing male pseudohermaphroditism due to the novel homozygous N100S mutation in the type II3 beta-hydroxysteroid dehydrogenase gene. *J Clin Endocrinol Metab* 1995;80:2127–2134.
7. Shima H, Kawanaka H, Yabumoto Y, Okamoto E, Ikoma F. A case of 17-alpha-hydroxylase deficiency with chromosomal karyotype 46,XY and high plasma aldosterone concentration. *Int Urol Nephrol* 1991;23:611–618.
8. Can S, Zhu YS, Cai LQ, et al. The identification of 5 alpha-reductase-2 and 17 beta-hydroxysteroid dehydrogenase-3 gene defects in male pseudohermaphrodites from a Turkish kindred. *J Clin Endocrinol Metab* 1998;83:560–569.
9. Imperato-McGinley J. 5 Alpha-reductase-2 deficiency. *Curr Ther Endocrinol Metab* 1997;6:384–387.
10. Brinkmann A, Jenster G, Ris-Stalpers C, van der Korput H, Brüggenwirth H, Boehmer A, Trapman J. Molecular basis of androgen insensitivity. *Steroids* 1996;61:172–175.
11. Jost A. The role of fetal hormones in prenatal development. *Harvey Lect* 1961;55:201.
12. Simón C, Tortajada M, Martinez L, Pellicer A, Pardo F. Müllerian defects in women with normal reproductive outcome. *Fertil Steril* 1991;56:1192–1193.
13. Faiman C, Winter JSD, Reyes FI. Patterns of gonadotropins and gonadal steroids throughout life. *Clin Obstet Gynaecol* 1976;3:467–483.
14. Kaplan SL, Grumbach MM. The ontogenesis of human foetal hormones II. Luteinizing hormone (LH) and follicle stimulating hormone (FSH). *Acta Endocrinol* 1976;81:808–829.
15. Rasmussen DD, Gambacciani M, Swartz W, Tueros VS, Yen SSC. Pulsatile gonadotropin-releasing hormone release from the human mediobasal hypothalamus in vitro: opiate receptor–mediated suppression. *Neuroendocrinology* 1989;49:150–156.

16. Gambacciani M, Liu JH, Swartz WH, Tueros VS, Yen SSC, Rasmussen DD. Intrinsic pulsatility of luteinizing hormone release from the human pituitary in vitro. *Neuroendocrinol* 1987;45:402–406.
17. Beck-Peccoz P, Padmanabhan V, Baggiani AM, et al. Maturation of hypothalamic-pituitary-gonadal function in normal human fetuses: circulating levels of gonadotropins, their common alpha subunit and free testosterone, and discrepancy between immunological and biological activities of circulating follicle-stimulating hormone. *J Clin Endocrinol Metab* 1991;73:525–532.
18. Castillo RH, Matteri RL, Dumesic DA. Luteinizing hormone synthesis in cultured fetal human pituitary cells exposed to gonadotropin-releasing hormone. *J Clin Endocrinol Metab* 1992;75:318–322.
19. Matwijiw I, Faiman C. Control of gonadotropin secretion in the ovine fetus. III. Effect of castration on serum follicle-stimulating hormone levels during the last trimester of gestation. *Endocrinology* 1991;129:1443–1446.
20. Kremer H, Kraaij R, Toledo SPA, et al. Male pseudohermaphroditism due to a homozygous missense mutation of the luteinizing hormone receptor gene. *Nature Genet* 1995;9:160–164.
21. Latronico AC, Anasti J, Arnhold IJP, et al. Brief report: testicular and ovarian resistance to luteinizing hormone caused by inactivating mutations of the luteinizing hormone receptor gene. *N Engl J Med* 1996;334:507–512.
22. Weiss J, Axelrod L, Whitcomb RW, Harris PE, Crowley WF, Jameson LJ. Hypogonadism caused by a single amino acid substitution in the β subunit of luteinizing hormone. *N Engl J Med* 1992;326:179–183.
23. Phillip M, Arbelle JE, Segev Y, Parvari R. Male hypogonadism due to a mutation in the gene for the β-subunit of follicle-stimulating hormone. *N Engl J Med* 1998; 338:1729–1732.
24. Conway GS. Clinical manifestations of genetic defects affecting gonadotropins and their receptors. *Clin Endocrinol* 1996;45:657–663.
25. Liao W-X, Roy AC, Chan C, Arulkumaran S. A new molecular variant of luteinizing hormone associated with female infertility. *Fertil Steril* 1998;69:102–106.
26. Zondek LH, Zondek T. Reproductive organs in anencephaly with special reference to the uterus. *Biol Neonate* 1987;51:346–351.
27. de Roux N, Young J, Misrahi M, Genet R, Chanson P, Schaison G, Milgrom E. A family with hypogonadotropic hypogonadism and mutations in the gonadotropin-releasing hormone receptor. *N Engl J Med* 1997;337:1597–1602.
28. Aittomaki K, Herva R, Stenman UH, et al. Clinical features of primary ovarian failure caused by a point mutation in the follicle-stimulating hormone receptor gene. *J Clin Endocrinol Metab* 1996;81:3722–3726.
29. Chan W-Y. Molecular genetic, biochemical, and clinical implications of gonadotropin receptor mutations. *Molec Genet Metab* 1998;63:75–84.
30. Gulyas BJ, Hodgen GD, Tullner WW, Ross GT. Effects of fetal or maternal hypophysectomy on endocrine organs and body weight in infant Rhesus monkeys *(Macaca mulatta)*: with particular emphasis on oogenesis. *Biol Reprod* 1976;16:216–227.
31. Huhtaniemi IT, Yamamoto M, Ranta T, Jalkanen J, Jaffe RB. Follicle-stimulating hormone receptors appear earlier in the primate fetal testis than in the ovary. *J Clin Endocrinol Metab* 1987;65:1210–1214.
32. Minegishi T, Tano M, Igarashi M, et al. Expression of follicle-stimulating hormone receptor in human ovary. *Eur J Clin Invest* 1987;27:469–474.
33. Nagamani M, McDonough PG, Ellegood JO, Mahesh VB. Maternal and amiotic fluid steroids throughout human pregnancy. *Am J Obstet Gynecol* 1979;134:674–680.
34. Glatstein IZ, Yeh J. Ontogeny of the estrogen receptor in the human fetal uterus. *J Clin Endocrinol Metab* 1995;80:958–964.
35. Kalloo NB, Gearhart JP, Barrack ER. Sexually dimorphic expression of estrogen receptors, but not of androgen receptors in human fetal external genitalia. *J Clin Endocrinol Metab* 1993;77:692–698.
36. Andrews GK, Teng CS. Studies on sex-organ development. Prenatal effect of oestrogenic hormone on tubular-gland cell morphogenesis and ovalbumin-gene expression in the chick Müllerian duct. *Biochem J* 1979;182:271–286.
37. Kaufman RH, Adam E, Binder GL, Gerthoffer E. Upper genital tract changes and pregnancy outcome in offspring exposed in utero to diethylstilbestrol. *Am J Obstet Gynecol* 1980;137:299–308.
38. Senekjian EK, Potkul RK, Frey K, Herbst AL. Infertility among daughters either exposed or not exposed to diethylstilbestrol. *Am J Obstet Gynecol* 1988;158:493–498.
39. Mittendorf R. Teratogen update: carcinogenesis and teratogenesis associated with exposure to diethylstilbestrol (DES) in utero. *Teratology* 1995;51:435–445.
40. Yalcinkaya TM, Siiteri PK, Vigne J-L, Licht P, Pavgi S, Frank LG, Glickman SE. A mechanism for virilization of female spotted hyenas in utero. *Science* 1993;260:1929–1931.

41. Goldsmith O, Solomon DH, Horton R. Hypogonadism and mineralocorticoid excess. The 17-hydroxylase deficiency syndrome. *N Engl J Med* 1967;277:673–677.
42. Morishima A, Grumbach MM, Simpson ER, Fischer C, Qin K. Aromatase deficiency in male and female siblings caused by a novel mutation and the physiological role of estrogens. *J Clin Endocrinol Metab* 1995;80:3689–4698.
43. Korach KS. Insights from the study of animals lacking functional estrogen receptor. *Science* 1994;266:1524–1527.
44. Korach KS, Couse JF, Curtis SW, et al. Estrogen receptor gene distruption: molecular characterization and experimental and clinical phenotypes. *Recent Prog Horm Res* 1996;51:159–186.
45. Newfield RS, New MI. 21-Hydroxylase deficiency. *Ann NY Acad Sci* 1997;816:219–290.
46. Griffin JE. Androgen resistance—the clinical and molecular spectrum. *N Engl J Med* 1992;326:611–618.
47. Winter JSD, Hughes IA, Reyes FI, Faiman C. Pituitary-gonadal relations in infancy: 2. Patterns of serum gonadal steroid concentrations in man from birth to two years of age. *J Clin Endocrinol Metab* 1976;42:679–686.
48. Waldhauser F, Weibenbacher G, Frisch H, Pollak A. Pulsatile secretion of gonadotropins in early infancy. *Eur J Pediatr* 1981;137:71–74.
49. Apter, D. Development of the hypothalamic-pituitary-ovarian axis. *Ann NY Acad Sci* 1997; 816:9–21.
50. Apter D, Cacciatore B, Alfthan H, Stenman, U-H. Serum luteinizing hormone concentrations increase 100-fold in females from 7 years of age to adulthood, as measured by time-resolved immunofluorometric assay. *J Clin Endocrinol Metab* 1989;68:53–57.
51. Conte FA, Grumbach MM, Kaplan SL. A diphasic pattern of gonadotropin secretion in patients with the syndrome of gonadal dysgenesis. *J Clin Endocrinol Metab* 1975;40:670–674.
52. Apter D, Bützow TL, Laughlin GA, Yen SSC. Gonadotropin-releasing hormone pulse generator activity during pubertal transition in girls: pulsatile and diurnal patterns of circulating gonadotropins. *J Clin Endocrinol Metab* 1993;76:940–949.
53. Wu FCW, Butler GE, Kelnar CJH, Stirling HF, Huhtaniemi I. Patterns of pulsatile luteinizing hormone and follicle-stimulating hormone secretion in prepubertal (midchildhood) boys and girls and patients with idiopathic hypogonadotropic hypogonadism (Kallmann's syndrome): a study using an ultrasensitive time-resolved immunofluorometric assay. *J Clin Endocrinol Metab* 1991; 72:1229–1237.
54. Klein KO, Baron J, Colli MJ, McDonnell DP, Cutler GB. Estrogen levels in childhood determined by an ultrasensitive recombinant cell bioassay. *J Clin Invest* 1994;94:2475–2480.
55. Wildt L, Marshall G, Knobil E. Experimental induction of puberty in the infantile female Rhesus monkey. *Science* 1980;207:1373–1375.
56. Sungurtekin U, Fraser IS, Shearman RP. Pregnancy in women with Kallmann's syndrome. *Fertil Steril* 1995;63:494–499.
57. Medhamurthy R, Dichek HL, Plant TM, Bernardini I, Butler GB. Stimulation of gonadotropin secretion in prepubertal monkeys after hypothalamic excitation with aspartate and glutamate. *J Clin Endocrinol Metab* 1990;71:1390–1392.
58. Thorneycroft IH, Mishell DR Jr., Stone SC, Kharma KM, Nakamura RM. The relation of serum 17-hydroxyprogesterone and estradiol-17-beta levels during the human menstrual cycle. *Am J Obstet Gynecol* 1971;111:947–951.
59. Frisch RE. Body fat, puberty, and fertility. *Biol Rev* 1984;59:161–188.
60. de Ridder CM, Bruning PF, Zonderland ML, et al. Body fat mass, body fat distribution, and plasma hormones in early puberty in females. *J Clin Endocrinol Metab* 1990;70:888–893.
61. Flier JS. What's in a name? In search of leptin's physiological role. *J Clin Endocrinol Metab* 1998;83:1407–1413.
62. Kiess W, Blum WF, Aubert ML. Leptin, puberty and reproductive function: lessons from animal studies and observations in humans. *Eur J Endocrinol* 1998;138:26–29.
63. Chehab FF, Lim ME, Lu R. Correction of the sterility defect in homozygous obese female mice by treatment with the human recombinant leptin. *Nature Genet* 1996;12:318–320.
64. Ahima RS, Dushay J, Flier SN, Prabakaran D, Flier JS. Leptin accelerates the onset of puberty in normal female mice. *J Clin Invest* 1997;99:391–395.
65. Strobel A, Issad T, Camoin L, Ozata M, Strosberg AD. A leptin missense mutation associated with hypogonadism and morbid obesity. *Nature Genet* 1998;18:213–215.
66. Mantzoros CS, Flier JS, Rogol AD. A longitudinal assessment of hormonal and physical alterations during normal puberty in boys. V. Rising leptin levels may signal the onset of puberty. *J Clin Endocrinol Metab* 1997;82:1066–1070.

67. Plant TM, Durrant AR. Circulating leptin does not appear to provide a signal for triggering the initiation of puberty in the male Rhesus monkey *(Macaca mulatta)*. *Endocrinology* 1997; 138:4505–4508.
68. Griffin JE, Edwards C, Madden JD, Harrod MJ, Wilson JD. Congenital absence of the vagina. The Mayer-Rokitansky-Küster-Hauser syndrome. *Ann Intern Med* 1976;85:224–236.
69. Sarto GE, Simpson JL. Abnormalities of the Müllerian and Wolffian duct systems. *Birth Defects* 1978;14:37–55.
70. Lischke J, Curtis C, Lamb E. Discordance of vaginal agenesis in monozygotic twins. *Obstet Gynecol* 1973;41:920.
71. Regenstein AC, Berkeley AS. Discordance of Müllerian agenesis in monozygotic twins. *J Reprod Med* 1991;36:396–397.
72. Mortlock DP, Innis JW. Mutations of HOXA13 in hand-foot-genital syndrome. *Nature Genet* 1997;15:179–180.
73. Smith OW, Smith GBS, Hurwitz D. Increased excretion of preganediol in pregnancy from diethylstilbestrol with special reference to the prevention of late pregnancy accidents. *Am J Obstet Gynecol* 1946;51:411–415.
74. Dieckmann W. Does the administration of diethylstilbestrol during pregnancy have any therapeutic value? *Am J Obstet Gynecol* 1953;66:1062–1081.
75. Stumpf WE, Narbaitz R, Sar M. Estrogen receptors in the fetal mouse. *J Steroid Biochem* 1980;12:55–64.
76. Taylor H, Igarashi P, Olive D, Arici A. DES alters *hox* gene expression. 45th Annual Meeting of the Society of Gynecologic Investigation, Atlanta, March 13, 1998.
77. Taylor HS, Vanden Heuvel GB, Igarashi P. A conserved *Hox* axis in the mouse and human female reproductive system: late establishment and persistent adult expression of the *Hoxa* cluster genes. *Biol Reprod* 1997;57:1338–1345.
78. Krumlauf R. *Hox* genes in vertebrate development. *Cell* 1994;78:191–201.
79. Coletta PL, Shimeld SM, Sharpe PT. The molecular anatomy of *Hox* gene expression. *J Anat* 1994;184:15–22.
80. Hoffman W, Grospietsch G, Kuhn W. Thalidomide and female genital malformations? *Lancet* 1976a;ii:794.
81. Hoffman W, Grospietsch G, Kuhn W. Genitalmissbildungen bei thalidomidgeschädigten Mädchen. *Geburtsh Frauenheilk* 1976;56:1066–1069.
82. Mühlenstedt D, Schwarz M. Gynäkologisch-endokrinologische Untersuchungen bei Thalidomidgeschädigten mädchen. *Geburtsh Frauenheilk* 1984;44:243–248.
83. Petrozza JC, Gray MR, Davis AJ, Reindollar RH. Congenital absence of the uterus and vagina is not commonly transmitted as a dominant genetic trait: outcomes of surrogate pregnancies. *Fertil Steril* 1997;67:387–389.
84. Bennett RC, Olds D, Deaton OW, Thrift FA. Nature of white heifer disease (partial genital aplasia) and its mode of inheritance. *Am J Vet Res* 1973;34:13–19.
85. Charlier C, Denys B, Belanche JI, et al. Microsatellite mapping of the bovine roan locus: a major determinant of white heifer disease. *Mamm Genome* 1996;7:138–142.
86. Fleischman RA. From white spots to stem cells: the role of the Kit receptor in mammalian development. *Trends Genet* 1993;9:285–290.
87. Elias S, Simpson JL, Carson SA, Malinak LR, Buttram VC. Genetic studies in incomplete Müllerian fusion. *Obstet Gynecol* 1983;63:276–279.
88. Carson SA, Simpson JL, Malinak LR, et al. Heritable aspects of uterine anomalies. II. Genetic analysis of Müllerian aplasia. *Fertil Steril* 1983;40:86–89.
89. Adamian LV, Murvatov KD, Sorour YA, Kirillova YA, Khashukoyeva AZ. Medicogenetic features and surgical treatment of patients with congenital malformations of the uterus and vagina. *Int J Fertil* 1996;41:293–297.
90. Shokeir MHK. Aplasia of the Müllerian system: evidence for probable sex-limited autosomal dominant inheritance. *Birth Defects* 1978;14:147–165.
91. Jones HW, Mermut S. Familial occurrence of congenital absence of the vagina. *Am J Obstet Gynecol* 1972;114:1100–1101.
92. Stelling JR, Gray MR, Davis AJ, Cowan J, Reindollar RH. Familial transmission of imperforate hymen. 54th Annual Meeting of the American Society of Reproductive Medicine, San Francisco, October 4–9, 1998.
93. Usta IM, Awwad JT, Usta JA, Makarem MM, Karam KS. Imperforate hymen: report of an unusual familial occurrence. *Obstet Gynecol* 1993;82:655–656.

94. McIlroy DL, Ward IV. Three cases of imperforate hymen occurring in one family. *Proc R Soc Med* 1930;23:633–634.

95. Verp MS, Simpson JL, Elias S, Carson SA, Sarto GE, Feingold M. Heritable aspects of uterine anomalies. I. Three familial aggregates with Müllerian fusion anomalies. *Fertil Steril* 1983; 40:80–85.

96. McKusick VA. *Mendelian inheritance in man: a catalog of human genes and genetic disorders*, 12th ed. Baltimore: Johns Hopkins University Press, 1997.

97. Azoury RS, Jones HW. Cytogenetic findings in patients with congenital absence of the vagina. *Am J Obstet Gynecol* 1966;94:178–180.

98. Capraro VJ, Cohen MM. Cytogenetic analysis of patients with developmental anomalies of the Müllerian ducts. *Obstet Gynecol* 1969;33:647–648.

99. van Lingen BL, Gray MR, Davis AJ, Cowan JM, Reindollar RH. Physical mapping of 3p23, a region that includes a translocation breakpoint in a patient with Mayer-Rokitansky-Küster-Hauser (MRKH) syndrome [Abstract]. *Am J Hum Genet* 1997;61:A246.

100. Driscoll DA, van Lingen BL, Gray MR, Reindollar RH. Molecular analysis of the *WT-1* gene in a patient with a balanced translocation and congenital absence of the uterus and vagina [Abstract]. *J Soc Gynecol Invest* 1996;3:135A.

101. Kucheria K, Taneja N, Kinra G. Autosomal translocation of chromosomes 12 q and 14 q in mullerian duct failure. *Ind J Med Res* 1988;87:290–292.

102. Lee DM, Osathanondh R, Yeh J. Localization of Bcl-2 in the human fetal Müllerian tract. *Fertil Steril* 1998;70:135–140.

103. Dabirashrafi H, Mohammad K, Nikbin B, Tabrizi NM, Azari A. Histocompatibility leukocyte antigens in Rokitansky-Küster-Hauser syndrome. *Am J Obstet Gynecol* 1995;172:1504–1505.

104. Gruenwald P. The relation of the growing Müllerian duct to the Wolffian duct and its importance for the genesis of malformations. *Anat Rec* 1941;81:1–19.

105. Gray SW, Skandalakis JE, Broecker B. The female reproductive tract. In: Skandalakis JE, Gray SW, eds. *Embryology for surgeons: the embryological basis for the treatment of congenital defects,* 2nd ed. Baltimore: Williams & Wilkins, 1994:816–847.

106. Strübbe EH, Willemsen WNP, Lemmens JAM, Thijn CJP, Rolland R. Mayer-Rokitansky-Küster-Hauser syndrome: distinction between two forms based on excretory urographic, sonographic, and laparoscopic findings. *AJR* 1993;160:331–334.

107. Fedele L, Bianchi S, Agnoli B, Tozzi L, Vignali M. Urinary tract anomalies associated with unicornuate uterus. *J Urology* 1996;155:847–848.

108. Schimke RN, King CR. Hereditary urogenital adysplasia. *Clin Genet* 1980;18:417–420.

109. Fraser GR. Our genetic load. A review of some aspects of genetical variation. *Ann Hum Genet* 1962;25:387–415.

110. Donohue WL, Uchida IA. Leprechaunism: a euphemism for a rare familial disorder. *J Pediatr* 1954;45:505–519.

111. Psiachou H, Mitton S, Alaghband-Zadeh J, Hone J, Taylor SI, Sinclair L. Leprechaunism and homozygous nonsense mutation in the insulin receptor gene. *Lancet* 1993;342:924.

112. Willman SP, Carr BR, Klein VR. Familial fusion of the labia minora. *Proc Greenwood Genet Center* 1988;7:140.

113. Waddington WB, Tucker VL, Schimke RN. Mesomelic dwarfism with hemivertebrae and small genitalia (the Robinow syndrome). *Am J Dis Child* 1973;126:202–205.

114. Chen H, Chang CH, Misra RP, Peters HA, Grijalva NS, Opitz JM. Multiple pterygium syndrome. *Am J Med Genet* 1980;7:91–102.

115. Bamshad M, Root S, Carey JC. Clinical analysis of a large kindred with the Pallister ulnar-mammary syndrome. *Am J Med Genet* 1996;65:325–331.

116. Bamshad M, Lin RC, Law DJ, et al. Mutations in human *TBX3* alter limb, apocrine and genital development in ulnar-mammary syndrome. *Nature Genet* 1997;16:311–315.

117. Stone DL, Agarwala R, Schäffer AA, et al. Genetic and physical mapping of the McKusick-Kaufman syndrome. *Hum Mol Genet* 1998;7:475–481.

118. Edwards JA, Gale RP. Camptobrachydactyly: a new autosomal dominant trait with two probable homozygotes. *Am J Hum Genet* 1972;24:464.

119. Johanson A, Blizzard R. A syndrome of congenital aplasia of the alae nasi, deafness, hypothyroidism, dwarfism, absent permanent teeth and malabsorption. *J Pediatr* 1971;79:982.

120. Tassabehji M, Newton VE, Read AP. Waardenburg syndrome type 2 caused by mutations in the human microphthalmia *(MITF)* gene. *Nature Genet* 1994;8:251–255.

121. Stoler JM, Herrin JT, Holmes LB. Genital abnormalities in females with Bardet-Biedl syndrome. *Am J Med Genet* 1995;55:276–278.
122. Reddy JC, Licht JD. The *WT1* Wilms' tumor suppressor gene: how much do we really know? *Biochim Biophys Acta* 1996;1287:1–28.
123. Stern AM, Gall JC Jr, Perry BL, Stimson CW, Weitkamp LA, Poznanski AK. The hand-foot-uterus syndrome: a new hereditary disorder characterized by hand and foot dysplasia, dermatoglyphic abnormalities, and partial duplication of the female genital tract. *J Pediatr* 1970;77:109–116.
124. Mortlock DP, Post LC, Innis JW. The molecular basis of hypodactyly *(Hd)*: a deletion in *Hoxa13* leads to arrest of digital arch formation. *Nature Genet* 1996;13:284–289.
125. Dumar V, Gervais R, Rigot J-M, Delomel-Vinner E, Decaestecker B, Lafitte J-J, Roussel P. Congenital bilateral absence of the vas deferens (CBAVD) and cystic fibrosis transmembrane regulator (CFTR): correlation between genotype and phenotype. *Hum Genet* 1996;97:7–10.
126. Dörk T, Dworniczak B, Aulehla-Scholz C, et al. Distinct spectrum of CFTR gene mutations in congenital absence of vas deferens. *Hum Genet* 1997;100:365–377.
127. Reindollar RH, Handelin BL, Alitto B, et al. Cystic fibrosis transmembrane conductance regulator (CFTR) gene mutations in congenital Mullerian aplasia. *Program of the Society for Gynecologic Investigation*, Chicago, 1994:256 [abstract].
128. Pelletier J, Bruening W, Kashtan CE, et al. Germline mutations in the Wilms tumor suppressor gene are associated with abnormal urogenital development in Denys-Drash syndrome. *Cell* 1991;67:437–447.
129. Baird PN, Santos A, Groves N, Jadresic L, Cowell JK. Constitutional mutations in the WT1 gene in patients with Denys-Drash syndrome. *Hum Mol Genet* 1992;1:301–305.
130. Kreidberg JA, Sariola H, Loring JM, et al. WT-1 is required for early kidney development. *Cell* 1993;74:679–691.
131. van Lingen BL, Reindollar RH, Davis AJ, Gray MR. Further evidence that the *WT1* gene does not have a role in the development of the derivatives of the Müllerian duct. *Am J Obstet Gynecol* 1998;179:597–603.
132. Knebelmann B, Boussin L, Guerrier D, et al. Anti-Müllerian hormone Bruxelles: a nonsense mutation associated with the persistent Müllerian duct syndrome. *Proc Natl Acad Sci USA* 1991;88:3767–3771.
133. Imbeaud S, Faure E, Lamarre I, et al. Insensitivity to anti-Müllerian hormone due to a mutation in the human anti-Müllerian hormone receptor. *Nature Genet* 1995;11:382–388.
134. Lindenman E, Shepard MK, Pescovitz OH. Müllerian agenesis: an update. *Obstet Gynecol* 1997;90:30–312.
135. Stelling J, Gray M, Davis A, van Lingen B, Reindollar R. Müllerian agenesis: an update [letter]. *Obstet Gynecol* 1997; 90:1024–1025.
136. van Lingen BL, Sohn SH, Tineo R, Davis AJ, Gray MR, Reindollar RH. Analysis of the role for Müllerian inhibiting substance in congenital absence of the uterus and vagina *(submitted)*.
137. Morel Y, Miller WL. Clinical and molecular genetics of congenital adrenal hyperplasia due to 21-hydroxylase deficiency. In: Harris H, Hirschhorn K, eds. *Advances in human genetics,* vol 20. New York: Plenum Press, 1991:1–57.
138. Kahn R, Ducan B, Bowes W. Spontaneous opening of congenital imperforate hymen. *J Pediatr* 1975;87:768–770.
139. Haddad B, Louis-Sylvestre C, Poitout P, Paniel B-J. Longitudinal vaginal septum: a retrospective study of 202 cases. *Eur J Obstet Gynecol Reprod Biol* 1997;74:197–199.
140. Simpson JL. Gynecologic disorders. In: King RA, Rotter JI, Motulsky AG, eds. *The genetic basis of common disease.* Oxford: Oxford University Press, 1992:564–576.
141. van Lingen BL, Eccles MR, Reindollar RH, Gray MR. Molecular genetic analysis of the *PAX2* gene in patients with congenital absence of the uterus and vagina. 54th Annual Meeting of the American Society of Reproductive Medicine, San Francisco, October 4–9, 1998.
142. Bhagavath B, Stelling JR, van Lingen BL, Davis AJ, Reindollar RH, Gray MR. Congenital absence of the uterus and vagina (CAUV) is not associated with the N314D allele of the galactose-1-phosphate uridyl transferase (GALT) gene. 45th Annual Meeting of the Society of Gynecologic Investigation, Atlanta, March 13, 1998.

Congenital Malformations of the Female Genital Tract: Diagnosis and Management, edited by G. Gidwani and T. Falcone.
Lippincott Williams & Wilkins, Philadelphia © 1999.

3

Examination of the Prepubertal and Adolescent Patient: Tips and Tricks

Ellen S. Rome

Section of Adolescent Medicine, The Cleveland Clinic Foundation, Ohio State University School of Medicine, Cleveland, Ohio 44195

Performing a gynecologic examination on a prepubertal child or adolescent may seem daunting to many clinicians. Societal taboos often inhibit parents from discussing private body parts, and even clinicians may avoid the topic until a problem arises. Pediatricians do not hesitate to evaluate the prepubertal boy for testicular masses or hernias, but many parents still report that no physician has looked at their daughter's bottom since she was out of diapers. Pediatricians, family practice physicians, and gynecologists need to emphasize that the visual inspection of the prepubertal and adolescent child's genitalia is a normal and expected part of every well child exam. Although gynecologic problems in the prepubertal child are relatively rare, inspection of the genitalia gives the clinician the opportunity to diagnose disease and to educate both the parents and the child or adolescent on hygiene, normal development, and other preventive health issues. This chapter will provide tips on how to perform an office examination of the child and adolescent, including positioning for the exam, necessary supplies, and communication with the child and parent. A full discussion of the causes of vulvovaginitis and common sexually transmitted diseases in the adolescent is beyond the scope of this chapter and can be found elsewhere.

OBTAINING A HISTORY

When working with the prepubertal child, the clinician should obtain a history from the parent or care provider while the child plays in the office or exam room. Having child-friendly toys and books available can help keep a child relaxed. The parent should be asked to give a brief review of growth, development, past problems, and current concerns. To put the child at ease, periodic questions can be directed to the child, focusing on toys, school, and other nonthreatening topics first. If the parent has raised a specific gynecologic concern, the child can then be asked if she has pain or itching in her bottom or vagina. If sexual abuse is a concern, she should be asked if anyone has ever touched her girl parts, and whether she or anyone else has ever placed something in her vagina. All questions should be asked while maintaining good eye contact with the child and without stern looks, helping the child to feel that she is an important part of the team and giving her the chance to ask questions.

When a parent mentions vaginal discharge or itching, the clinician should ask about timing and onset of symptoms, color and odor of the discharge, recent antibiotic use, recent infectious exposures at school or home, and perineal hygiene. Recent bubble baths may trigger a chemical vaginitis. Perianal streptococcal infection may present with erythema and itching circumferentially around the anus. A parent may or may not have visualized pinworms, which often come out at night and can be seen with the naked eye. If the parent reports a recent onset of symptoms such as vaginal bleeding, bed wetting, headaches, abdominal pain, or other behavioral change, the possibility of sexual abuse should be raised. With vaginal bleeding, the history should also include use of surreptitious estrogen (e.g., missing birth control pills in mom's packet), use of estrogenic hormone cream (e.g., Premarin) on labial adhesions, recent trauma, signs of puberty, and foreign bodies found previously.

Establishing Confidentiality

With an adolescent, all questions regarding sexual history, vaginal discharge, and vulvar itching should be asked without a parent in the room. After an initial history obtaining information on current concerns, past medical history, family illnesses, and other less personal questions, the parent can be asked if there are any private concerns that he or she wishes to discuss without the child present. The clinician should then clearly and concretely define confidentiality with both parties present, e.g., "Everything I talk about alone with you or your parent will be kept confidential. This means that I am not going to tell you about your parent's private concerns, and I will not tell your parent about your private concerns. The only exception is that if there is something life threatening or dangerous going on, I will tell you, 'Look, we have to tell your family about this'." In addressing parental concerns alone first, the teen can realize that you are not "spilling the beans" by disclosing the parent's confidential issues and likewise are not reporting to the parent the teen's private concerns. This strategy helps to build trust. The clinician can then ask the teen or older child if she wishes to have the parent in the room for the exam or if she prefers to have the parent step out. If the teen chooses to have the parent in the room, the clinician can then get a confidential history by stating, "I will take a few minutes with your daughter alone to address any of her private concerns. Then we will bring you back in for the exam." When the child wishes the parent to leave for the exam, confidential questions may be asked during the performance of the exam.

The HEADS Questions

Risk taking behaviors, depression, family instability, and other psychosocial factors are associated with significant adolescent morbidity. A useful acronym for obtaining a psychosocial history for an adolescent is the HEADS exam (1). *H* is for home, or who lives at home? What happens when there is an argument in the home? *E* is for education, or current grade level and school performance, change in performance over the past year, and age appropriateness of the current grade level. *A* is for activities and attitude. How does the teen spend her time? Is she in a gang? Does she carry a weapon? And if so, can she *not* bring it to your office next time!? *D* is for drugs, including cigarettes, alcohol, and other drugs. Ask about friends' behaviors before asking about the teen's own behaviors; this technique puts the teen at ease and gives the clinician a chance to do an informal role play to help build refusal skills. For instance, if all of the teen's peers smoke but she reports that she does not, the clinician can then ask what she does when her friends ask her to smoke with them. If she cannot think of a response, the clinician can provide several possible replies, encouraging the teen to continue to make healthy choices. Duration of smoking, drinking, and other drug use should also be ascertained, along with how long a pack lasts, number and kind of drinks on a typical night, and similar questions. *D* can also stand for depression and suicidality; all teens should ask if they have ever been depressed. If the answer is yes, they should be asked if they have ever thought about harming or killing themselves and, if so, if they have tried and by what methods. Are they currently suicidal?

Finally, the *S* in the HEADS acronym stands for sex. All teens should be asked if they have ever had sex and, if so, with how many partners over a lifetime? Were condoms used sometimes, most of the time, all of the time, or never? What second method is being used for pregnancy prevention? Asking this question can help educate the teen on the need for dual methods of contraception for disease control plus pregnancy prevention. The teen should be asked if she has a sexual preference for boys, girls, or both, as lesbian concerns may differ from sexuality concerns or disease risk in the heterosexual population. Asking questions nonjudgmentally inspires confidence in the teen and increases the likelihood that she will disclose delicate information that may have an impact on her health. Prior sexually transmitted diseases, vaginal discharge, menstrual history, and other related questions should also be asked confidentially.

THE GYNECOLOGIC EXAM

The Rules

The genital examination should be approached with special verbal acknowledgment to the child (and parent) prior to requesting the patient to unrobe. With the younger child at preventive health care visits, it is useful to state that the doctor will look at your bottom every year to make sure that everything is okay, reminding the child and parent that this part of the exam should be a normal part of every well child exam. It is useful also to state that "it is okay if a doctor looks at your private parts with your mommy here, but it's not okay if anyone else looks at your private parts without your mommy's permission. If anyone ever did that, what would you do?" If the child does not respond, "I would tell my mommy [or the doctor]," give positive feedback for whatever response the child gives but also state that it is very important that the child would also tell her mommy and/or the doctor so that we can keep the child healthy and safe. The exam can also be used to educate on hygiene. For instance, the clinician can state, "I want to talk to you about the rules. One rule is that you don't let poop near your girl parts." A mirror can be used at this point to teach a child how to wipe correctly after elimination.

The clinician should always state clearly what he or she is doing during the exam, as well as describing any findings during the exam. The patient's comfort is foremost, and the patient always should feel in total control over the examination. The clinician should also state that he or she promises not to hurt the child or to cause any pain, and *keep to that promise!*

Before and during the exam, parents may need to hear that the hymen may be variable in size and will not be changed or harmed by your examination. Use of a diagram (Fig. 1) can help educate the parent or older child on normal female anatomy and help clear up any misconceptions. Many parents do not realize that evaluation of the genitalia is a normal part of the exam; helping manage their expectations can educate them on preventive medicine while teaching how to set a tone during a physical examination that will reassure their child rather than raise anxiety. Use of games and tricks may destroy a child's or parent's confidence in the clinician; it is more useful to be straightforward with both parent and child, educating as the exam continues. Tricks such as hiding behind drapes, use of headphones, murals on the ceiling, and other strategies do not allow a child to feel in control of the exam and be an active participant.

Helping the Child Feel in Control

Giving the child choice of a gown color can help establish a sense of control (e.g., "Do you want to put on the red gown or the green gown?" is more useful than ask-

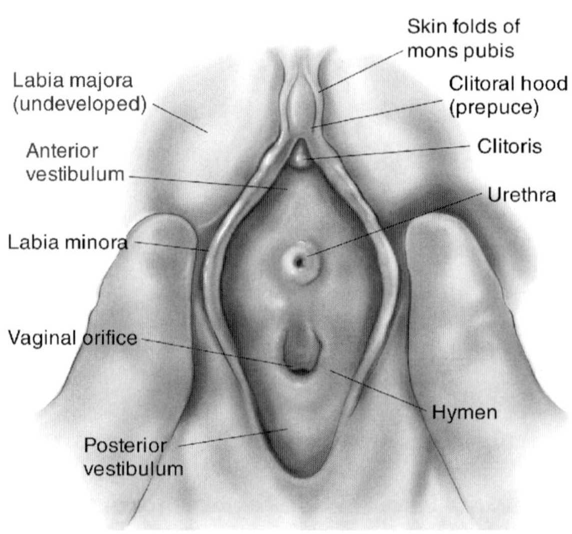

FIG. 1. Normal female anatomy.

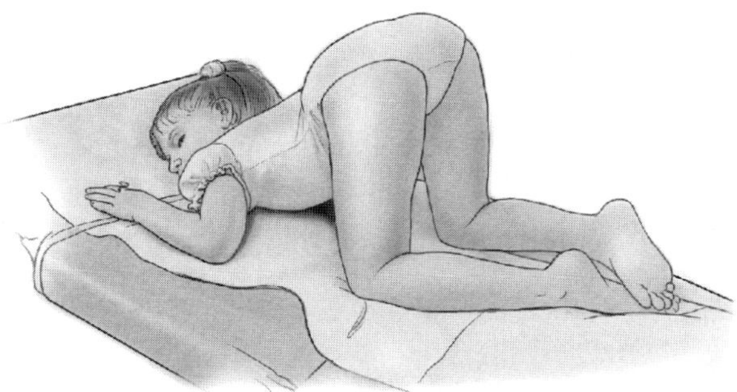

FIG. 2. Knee-chest position used for examining the vagina and cervix in the prepubertal child.

ing, "Will you now put on a gown?"). The otoscope or hand lens can be used for magnification; the child should be allowed to look through the lens to see how it works. If a colposcope will be used, letting the child view jewelry or fingers through the instrument and showing how the light turns on and off can help demystify the exam. As stated earlier, asking the older child if she prefers the parent in or out of the room is another way of helping the patient maintain control.

The Actual Exam

Examination of the child with gynecologic complaints should include measuring weight and height, and doing an evaluation from head to toe, including head and neck, heart, lungs, abdomen, skin (for rashes), breasts (visual inspection and palpation for masses or discharge), and Tanner staging. Gynecologic assessment should include inspection of the external genitalia, palpation of the inguinal area for hernias or masses, and visualization of the vagina. For a complete gynecologic examination, rectoabdominal palpation should be performed and the cervix should also be visualized using knee-chest position if necessary in a younger child (Fig. 2). The child may be told that she should lie on her tummy with her bottom in the air ("just as you may have done while asleep as a baby"). The parent or the child herself can be recruited to spread the buttocks gently. Often foreign bodies such as bits of toilet paper can be visualized in this manner. A butterfly catheter of any size with the needle cut off can be attached to a tuberculin syringe with 1 cm^3 of saline and placed inside a 12-in. red rubber bladder catheter to irrigate or wash off the genitalia (3). This catheter within a catheter is less irritating and less of a surprise during irrigation for many girls (Fig. 3).

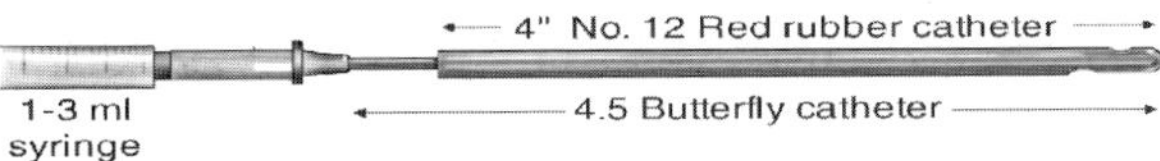

FIG. 3. A catheter in a catheter for irrigation.

During the exam, the clinician should note the presence of pubic hair, the size of the clitoris, hymenal configuration, signs of estrogenization of the vagina and hymen, and perineal hygiene (2). If the hymen is viewed in lithotomy or frog-leg position and likened to the face of a clock, irregular notching or transections of the hymen between 5 and 7 o'clock are suggestive of sexual abuse or forced sexual intercourse. If the hymenal orifice and edges cannot be easily visualized in this position, the labia can be gently gripped and pulled forward with gentle traction. The child can be asked to cough or take a deep breath, allowing the hymen to gape open. In the prepubertal girl, the vaginal mucosa tends to be thin, red, with erythematous perihymenal tissue. In the pubertal girl, the mucosa becomes moist and dull pink under the influence of estrogen. Estrogenized tissues tolerate instrumentation, whereas atrophic tissues are more easily traumatized by the use of instruments.

The pace and extent of the evaluation may vary depending on the clinician's assessment of the likelihood and degree of suspected pathology. Vulvitis is diagnosable on external exam, whereas vaginitis requires culture and/or vaginoscopy. With irritant vulvitis from bubble baths or underlying vulvar skin disorders, superinfection may occur with yeast or other bacteria. Underlying pathology may not be accurately recognized or treated until after the superinfection is treated, providing reason for sequential exams. On the other hand, if a child is found with a large amount of blood in her underwear and is unable or unwilling to provide an adequate explanation of etiology, examination under anesthesia may be indicated if a complete office exam cannot be performed. In this instance, the higher likelihood of intravaginal pathology warrants the more expedient evaluation; if a child were "playing doctor" and had introduced a foreign object with a resultant penetration wound, the risk of sepsis outweighs the risk of anesthesia. Chronicity of symptoms may allow for more leisure in the evaluation. If a child has had a greenish yellow discharge for weeks with occasional spots of blood in the underwear, a hemorrhagic bacterial vaginitis will resolve with no more bloody discharge after antibiotic treatment. A persistent vaginal foreign object or pathologic lesion will continue to be seen, warranting further evaluation.

Positioning the Patient

Most children are comfortable lying on an exam table with a parent close by (Figs. 4 and 5). If a child appears anxious, the parent (mother *or* father) can be placed in a semireclining position on the exam table with the parent's feet in the stirrups and the child's legs straddling the parent's thighs (Fig. 6) If necessary, this position can be tried with the patient clothed before even starting the exam. A hand-held mirror can be used to educate patient (and parent) on normal anatomy while providing a means of allowing the child to be an active participant. The child can also maintain a sense of control by being asked to assist in holding her labia apart. If the clinician acts confident and relaxed, the patient will usually cooperate (2). An anxious clinician or par-

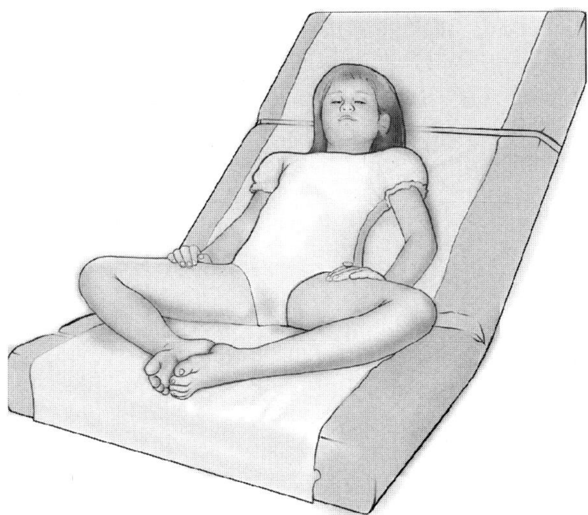

FIG. 4. The prepubertal child can be positioned in the frog leg position, either horizontally or with the head of the examination table raised.

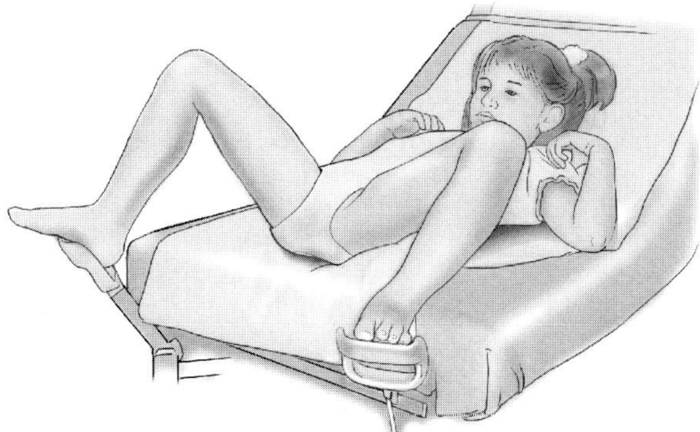

FIG. 5. The prepubertal child can also be examined in lithotomy position.

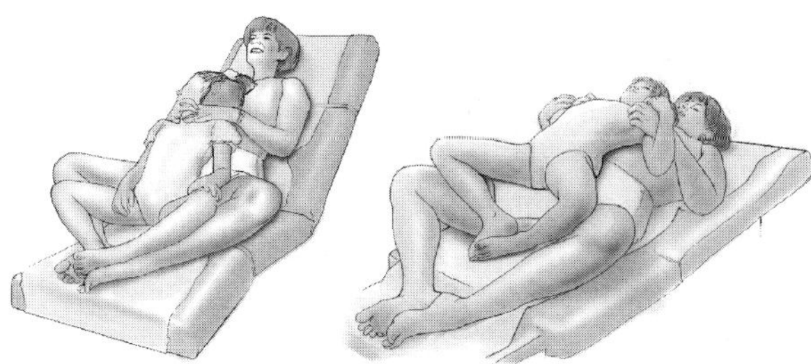

FIG. 6. The child can be examined in the frog-leg or lithotomy position using a parent positioned appropriately.

ent can set the tone for the child, and an abrupt or hurried approach may lead to a child's refusal to continue. If a child needs more time, the examiner can leave the room until the patient feels ready. In a particularly fearful child, it may be necessary to perform the exam in stages over several visits while building confidence that the child will not be hurt. In a child with significant vaginal bleeding, an examination under anesthesia may be necessary if the patient remains extremely fearful or uncooperative.

HYMENAL ANATOMY

Hymenal configuration should be noted and, when an abnormality is found, diagramed in the medical record (Fig. 7). Hymens can be classified as posterior rim or crescentic, annular, or redundant (2,4). Parents are particularly appreciative when an imperforate hymen is diagnosed before puberty, so that anticipatory guidance can be given and an easy procedure can be accomplished before menstrual flow accumulates behind a blocked passageway. Acquired abnormalities of the hymen usually result from sexual abuse and, more rarely, from accidental trauma. Signs of acute trauma with sexual abuse can include hymenal transections, hematomas, abrasions, laceration, and vulvar erythema or irritation. Physical healing after trauma occurs quickly and is often complete at 10 to 14 days (2). Although a hymenal notch, remnant, or scar may be visualized, most girls with a history of substantiated sexual abuse have a completely normal exam (2). Use of sequential drawings in the medical record can prove useful in identifying changes after sexual abuse.

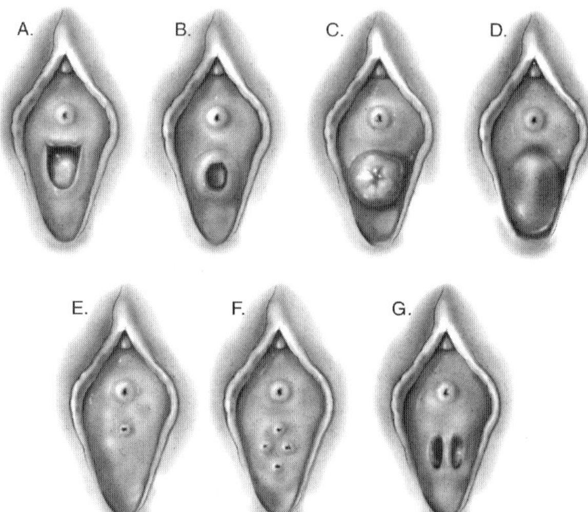

FIG. 7. Hymenal configurations in prepubertal girls. **A:** Posterior rim or crescentic hymen. **B:** Annular hymen. **C:** Fimbriated or redundant hymen. **D:** Imperforate hymen. **E:** Microperforate hymen. **F:** Cribriform hymen. **G:** Septate hymen.

VAGINOSCOPY

If knee-chest or lithotomy position does not provide sufficient visualization, a small vaginoscope, cystoscope, hysteroscope, or flexible fiberoptic scope with water insufflation of the vagina can be used (2). A step-by-step method for insertion of the vaginoscope in a young child was first described by Capraro (5). First, the child is allowed to touch the instrument and told that it feels slippery, funny, and cool. The instrument is then placed against her inner thigh, repeating the same phrase, and then against her labia, with the physician again stating, "This feels slippery, funny, and cool." As the vaginoscope is inserted through the hymen, the clinician repeats the words while firmly pressing the child's buttocks with the other hand to divert her attention (2). Lidocaine jelly or other topical anesthetic may be used at the introitus to ease insertion. A narrow veterinary otoscope speculum or a Killian nasal speculum with an attached fiberoptic light source can also be used; the latter may not be long enough to visualize the upper aspect of the vagina (6).

OTHER NECESSARY SUPPLIES

The clinician should have slides and materials to perform a wet prep using normal saline, 10% potassium hydroxide, and culture media for *Neisseria gonorrhoeae, Chlamydia trachomatis,* and the herpes simplex virus. Newer methods such as DNA probes and ligase chain reaction techniques remain unacceptable evidence in a court of law for cases of sexual abuse. In evaluating the adolescent, nonculture methods may be utilized whenever sexual abuse is not suspected and during the routine pelvic examination. DNA probes for the human papillomavirus are also available and can be used in the adolescent with an abnormal Pap smear. Cotton-tipped applicators and small nasopharyngeal calcium alginate–tipped applicators are used to obtain specimens. The smaller Huffman speculum should be used in the virginal adolescent, whereas the Pedersen (medium-sized) speculum is appropriate for most sexually active adolescents. Only the morbidly obese older adolescent may require the Graves speculum. With obese patients, the tip of a rubber glove can be cut off and placed over the speculum blades of a narrow speculum to prevent the vaginal side walls from obscuring the view of the cervix.

If a vaginal discharge is present, cultures can be obtained in the prepubertal child using a nasopharyngeal Calgiswab moistened with nonbacteriostatic saline. Individual ampules of nebulized saline may be kept for convenient office use (2). In obtaining the sample, care should be taken not to touch the hymenal edges, as the child may be particularly sensitive in this area. The child can be asked to cough during the exam, providing both distraction and a wider opening of the hymen. The catheter-in-a-catheter technique described earlier in this chapter can also be used to sample vaginal secretions.

BRINGING IT ALL TOGETHER

Examination of the prepubertal child and the adolescent may require added time and sensitivity to the needs and fears of the parent and child. The pelvic examination as taught in most settings describes a specific set of procedural techniques that may be surrounded by fear and misperceptions in the parent or child. Both parties need to understand that the examination will be individualized to meet the patient's needs, often with sequential exams used for evaluation while maintaining a patient's comfort and sense of control. The prepubertal and adolescent exam provides an opportunity to educate patient and parents regarding hygiene, the rules of the exam including confidentiality, and our paramount goal to "do no harm."

REFERENCES

1. Goldenring JM, Cohen E. Getting into adolescent heads. *Contemp Pediatr* 1988; July:75–90.
2. Emans SJ, Laufer MR, Goldstein DP. Office evaluation of the child and adolescent. In: *Pediatric and adolescent gynecology*, 4th ed. Philadelphia: Lippincott–Raven Publishers, 1998:1–48.
3. Pokorny SF, Stormer LVN. Atraumatic removal of secretions from the prepubertal vagina. *Am J Obstet Gynecol* 1987;156:581–582.
4. Pokorny SF. Configuration of the prepubertal hymen. *Am J Obstet Gynecol* 1987;157:950–956.
5. Capraro VJ. Gynecologic examination in children and adolescents. *Pediatr Clin North Am* 1972;19:511–528.
6. Hairston L. Physical examination of the prepubertal girl. *Clin Obstet Gynecol* 1997;40:127–134.

*Congenital Malformations of the Female Genital
Tract: Diagnosis and Management,* edited by
G. Gidwani and T. Falcone.
Lippincott Williams & Wilkins, Philadelphia © 1999.

4

Imaging of Müllerian Anomalies

Craig S. Mitchell, Marilyn J. Goske, and Kimberly Applegate

*Section of Pediatric Radiology, Children's Hospital of The Cleveland Clinic Foundation,
Cleveland, Ohio 44195*

IMPORTANCE OF DEFINING ANATOMY

The prevalence of congenital anomalies of the Müllerian system in women has been estimated to be between 0.1% and 3% (1–3). In a selected population of women evaluated for habitual abortion or infertility, the prevalence of uterine anomalies is as high as 8% to 12% (4,5). Women with Müllerian anomalies have fertility rates only slightly lower than the general female population, but their rate of reproductive loss (spontaneous abortion, premature labor) is often elevated (6). It has been estimated that 25% to 67% of female individuals with Müllerian anomalies have some type of reproductive dysfunction including sterility, habitual abortion, low birth weight, premature delivery, and abnormal fetal presentation (3,7,8). In the evaluation of infertility or recurrent abortion, imaging of uterine morphology is important both to detect anomalies and to select treatment options (9). Uterine anomalies have also been reported as being a cause of failed first-trimester pregnancy termination (10). Gilsanz and Cleveland have emphasized that the recognition and description of uterine anomalies are of medical importance for three main reasons (11). The first is that Müllerian anomalies have been associated with problems in sexual function, pregnancy outcome, and difficulties with labor (4,6–8,12–24). Second, there have been reports of an increase in deformities of infants born to mothers with Müllerian duct anomalies (25,26). Many of these abnormalities are attributed to embryonic compression resulting in vascular insult and limb insufficiency. Third, although in general Müllerian anomalies are felt to be isolated and sporadic, there have been reports of involvement of more than one family member (27–29) and of Müllerian anomalies being associated with other anomalies and uncommon syndromes (30–33).

ADVANTAGES OF IMAGING OVER OTHER FORMS OF DIAGNOSIS

The first question one might ask about the topic of this chapter is, "Are there any advantages in evaluating Müllerian anomalies using imaging compared with the more classic modes of diagnosis such as hysterosalpingography (HSG), laparoscopy, hysteroscopy, and physician examination?" Imaging, specifically magnetic resonance imaging (MRI) and ultrasound (US), offers two distinct advantages over most other modes of diagnosis. First, imaging is noninvasive. Patient discomfort and risks of anesthesia and instrumentation are absent. There is no exposure to potentially dangerous ionizing radiation and no exposure to iodinated contrast material. HSG is an invasive technique whose potential complications include exposure to ionizing radiation, iodinated contrast reaction, uterine perforation, and sepsis. Laparoscopy carries the risk of complications associated with general anesthesia as well as visceral injury (34). The second major advantage of imaging is that both the internal and external anatomy of the female genital tract may be evaluated simultaneously. HSG and hysteroscopy allow for evaluation of only the internal anatomy of the genital tract, but both allow for the possibility of therapeutic intervention. Laparotomy and laparoscopy allow for evaluation of the external anatomy of the genital tract only, unless a concomitant hysterotomy is performed. Additionally, HSG and hysteroscopy do not allow evaluation of the proximal aspect of an obstructed system. Imaging also allows for the evaluation of the urinary tract, which is necessary due to the high association between urinary tract and Müllerian anomalies (11,35–41).

Knowledge of the internal and external anatomy of the genital tract is crucial in order to counsel the patient on the potential reproductive consequences associated with her diagnosis and also for potential surgical planning. Müllerian anomalies are grouped according to similarities of clinical manifestations, treatment, and prognosis for fetal salvage. The 1988 American Fertility Society (AFS) classification of Müllerian anomalies (42), or a modification of this classification (43), is widely used for this purpose (Tables 1 and 2). Differentiation between obstructed and nonobstructed

TABLE 1. *American fertility society classification of Müllerian anomalies*

Classification	Anomaly
Class I	Segmental, Müllerian agenesis-hypoplasia
	A. Vaginal
	B. Cervical
	C. Fundal
	D. Tubal
	E. Combined anomalies
Class II	Unicornuate
	A. Communicating
	B. Noncommunicating
	C. No cavity
	D. No horn
Class III	Didelphys
Class IV	Bicornuate
	A. Complete (division down to internal os)
	B. Partial
Class V	Septate
	A. Complete (septum to internal os)
	B. Partial
Class VI	Arcuate
Class VII	Diethylstilbestrol-related

From Ref. 42, with permission.

TABLE 2. *American fertility society classification of uterovaginal anomalies*

Class I	Dysgenesis of the Müllerian ducts
Class II	Disorders of vertical fusion of the Müllerian ducts
	A. Transverse vaginal septum
	1. Obstructed
	2. Unobstructed
	B. Cervical agenesis or dysgenesis
Class III	Disorders of lateral fusion of the Müllerian ducts
	A. Asymmetric-obstructed disorder of uterus or vagina usually associated with ipsilateral renal agenesis
	1. Unicornuate uterus with a noncommunicating rudimentary anlage or horn
	2. Unilateral obstruction of a cavity of a double uterus
	3. Unilateral vaginal obstruction associated with double uterus
	B. Symmetric-unobstructed
	1. Didelphic uterus
	a. Complete longitudinal vaginal septum
	b. Partial longitudinal vaginal septum
	c. No longitudinal vaginal septum
	2. Septate uterus
	a. Complete
	(1) Complete longitudinal vaginal septum
	(2) Partial longitudinal vaginal septum
	(3) No longitudinal vaginal septum
	b. Partial
	(1) Complete longitudinal vaginal septum
	(2) Partial longitudinal vaginal septum
	(3) No longitudinal vaginal septum
	3. Bicornuate uterus
	a. Complete
	(1) Complete longitudinal vaginal septum
	(2) Partial longitudinal vaginal septum
	(3) No longitudinal vaginal septum
	b. Partial
	(1) Complete longitudinal vaginal septum
	(2) Partial longitudinal vaginal septum
	(3) No longitudinal vaginal septum
	4. T-shaped uterine cavity (diethylstilbestrol-related)
	5. Unicornuate uterus
	a. With a rudimentary horn
	(1) With endometrial cavity
	(a) Communicating
	(b) Noncommunicating
	(2) Without endometrial cavity
	b. Without a rudimentary horn
Class IV	Unusual Configurations of Vertical Lateral Fusion Detects

From Ref. 42, with permission.

anomalies is important because obstructive lesions require immediate attention to allow drainage of trapped mucus and/or blood. Distention of obstructed systems may cause urinary retention and obstipation and, in the infant, may cause decreased blood return to the heart secondary to vascular compression and respiratory compromise from restriction of diaphragmatic motion (44–47). Retrograde menstruation secondary to obstruction is associated with an increased incidence of endometriosis and its attendant pain and a decrease in fertility (48–50). Disorders of lateral fusion associated with obstruction are almost invariably associated with absence of the ipsilateral kidney. The level of obstruction is important to note as is the presence or absence of a cervix or the presence of more than one cervix. If there is absence of the uterine cervix, hysterectomy is usually indicated. When no obstruction is present, intervention may not be required immediately but is often required at some point for purposes of increasing fetal salvage or to provide for normal coital function.

Internal and external anatomy of the genital tract must be determined prior to surgery because this information may change the surgical approach. An excellent example is the case of two uterine channels found at HSG. It may be difficult, if not impossible, to distinguish between a septate uterus and a bicornuate uterus without knowing the external appearance of the uterus. The surgical approach to these two anomalies is distinctly different. Lysis of a uterine septum does not require laparotomy but rather is performed transcervically using hysteroscopic scissors or resectoscope. In contrast, unification metroplasty of a bicornuate uterus requires laparotomy.

TECHNICAL ASPECTS OF ULTRASOUND

Medical ultrasound is a safe, noninvasive method used to evaluate the female pelvis. There are basically three approaches to the sonographic interrogation of the female pelvis. The first is transabdominal US. The US transducer is applied to the patient's skin over the bladder and the urine-filled bladder is used as an acoustic window to view the pelvic organs. Typically, a curved array transducer with a large field of view (FOV) is used. A 3-MHz transducer typically provides enough depth for insonation of the pelvis, but in obese patients a 2-MHz transducer may be necessary. Higher frequency transducers offer improved spatial resolution but are limited in their ability to image deeper pelvic structures. High-frequency transducers (5 to 10 MHz) may be of use in interrogating the infant or young child. In disorders of vertical fusion, such as a transverse vaginal septum, an examining finger may be placed within the introitus to aid in determining the position and length of the septum. Transabdominal US has been shown to be a useful method of studying genital tract anomalies in female patients (51–56). In one study of 63 patients, the addition of transabdominal US to HSG increased the accuracy of distinguishing septate versus bicornuate uteri from 55% to 90% (57). In another study of 43 patients, US showed a sensitivity of 92% and a specificity of 100% in those cases where sonographic findings were adequate (91% of cases) (58). Adequate visualization of the uterus may not be possible transabdominally in cases of marked uterine retroflexion or when large leiomyomata are present. Uterine anomalies may be difficult to detect with US and have been confused with a variety of other entities such as cornual leiomyomata, ectopic gestation, placental septations, and uterine scarring (59). US may also be used intraoperatively to help guide the gynecologic surgeon especially in cases of proximally obstructed systems (60).

The second technique used for sonographic interrogation of the pelvis of the female is transvaginal sonography. The US transducer is placed within the vaginal vault, allowing the use of a higher frequency transducer and resulting in greater spatial resolution of the internal genitalia when compared with transabdominal scanning.

Transvaginal sonography is especially useful when transabdominal sonography cannot adequately visualize a retroflexed uterus. Limitations of transvaginal sonography are its relative contraindication in non–sexually active patients and the inability to insert the transducer in patients with a narrow vaginal vault or those with a vaginal septum. Pellerito et al. (61) demonstrated an accuracy of 92% using transvaginal sonography in the evaluation of uterine anomalies.

The third sonography technique used to evaluate the female pelvis is transperineal or translabial scanning. Using this technique, the pelvis is interrogated by a sonographic transducer placed on the perineum or directly on the labia majorum. Scanlan et al. (62) has reported success in evaluating the length of atretic vaginal segments using this technique. Meyer et al. (63) reported using combined transabdominal and transperineal sonography to assist in the diagnosis of a transverse vaginal septum. Using any of these three sonographic techniques, scanning is best performed during the luteal phase of the menstrual cycle in postpubertal patients due to the improved visibility of the relatively thickened and echogenic endometrium.

TECHNICAL ASPECTS OF MAGNETIC RESONANCE IMAGING

Modern magnetic resonance imaging (MRI) is arguably the diagnostic modality of choice for the evaluation of Müllerian anomalies. Advantages include the following: it is noninvasive; it involves no ionizing radiation; imaging can be obtained in any plane; and it demonstrates excellent spatial and tissue contrast. Numerous studies have demonstrated the high level of diagnostic accuracy afforded by MRI in the evaluation of Müllerian anomalies (9,34,39,61,64–68). Sedation is typically not necessary except in young children (e.g., age <6 years) and in cases of significant claustrophobia. MRI is certainly not indicated for the evaluation of every case of suspected Müllerian anomaly. In some cases, US is the only imaging modality necessary, e.g., in cases of imperforate hymen in the neonate or adolescent, or in cases where US and/or HSG clearly delineate the uterine anatomy.

Clinicians should not, however, hesitate to utilize MRI in cases of suspected Müllerian anomalies. There has been some suggestion in the imaging literature that MRI has been underutilized in the evaluation of the female pelvis despite evidence that supports the potential for MRI to minimize costs in working up female pelvic disorders (69–72). Hricak (73) has suggested that a number of factors account for this discrepancy between research data and clinical practice. These factors include (a) a shortage of training and expertise, (b) misconceptions concerning costs, (c) misconceptions about the role of MRI as it relates to other imaging modalities, and (d) the need for education. MRI is best utilized as a problem-solving tool and should be targeted (i.e., planned and executed) to look for specific findings based on clinically suspected conditions (69). Schwartz et al. in 1994 performed a study demonstrating that pelvic MRI may significantly alter treatment, decrease the number of invasive surgical procedures performed, and reduce total health care expenditures (70).

Most modern MR scanners support the use of surface coils, which markedly increases the signal-to-noise ratio (SNR) when compared to the standard body coil. Optimal MRI of the pelvis is performed using a phased-array body coil, except with infants and young children who may be imaged in a head coil. With phased array scanning, coils are placed both anterior and posterior to the patient. The array may be either transversely or longitudinally oriented depending on the coil design. Initial coil design suffered somewhat from increased ghosting artifact and nonuniformity of signal from the surface coils (74). Hayes et al. (75) performed an excellent quantitative assessment of pelvic imaging with phased-array coils. The authors found that the SNR of the transverse array was consistently higher than that of the longitudinal array. The SNR of the transverse and longitudinal array coils exceeded that of the body coil by factors of >3 and at least 2.3, respectively. The advantage of the improved SNR of phased-array coils can be utilized in different ways: (a) the number of excitations (NEX) needed for signal averaging may be reduced resulting in decreased scan time; (b) the spatial resolution may be improved by using a smaller FOV; (c) a full FOV may be retained but higher spatial resolution may be obtained in the frequency and/or phase encoded directions; and (d) thinner sections can be obtained. Increased temporal resolution is also possible with phased-array coils, allowing for faster imaging techniques than possible with a conventional body coil. One or two second ultrafast images (such as gradient-recalled acquisition in the steady state or GRASS, and fast low-angle shot or FLASH) acquired with phased-array coils can have an SNR equivalent to spin echo images obtained with a body coil requiring minutes to acquire.

Two potential shortcomings of phased array coils are as follows: (a) subcutaneous fat creates a much stronger signal than with the standard body coil. This can lead to motion artifacts; however, the use of anterior and posterior saturation pulses usually effectively eliminates the artifact. Motion artifact is typically less of a problem when imaging the pelvis compared with imaging the chest or the abdomen. The phase encoding direction can be aligned parallel with the skin–coil interface, which also decreases motion artifact. (b) The SNR varies markedly with distance from the phased-array coil. This may be problematic with obese or pregnant patients, but this problem can usually be overcome by increasing the FOV and/or decreasing the matrix size.

Most authors seem to agree that fast spin echo (FSE) T2-weighted images are the most useful for evaluating Müllerian anomalies (9,68,69,74–79). Initial coronal breath hold or single-shot FSE images with a large field of view to assess the urinary tract and uterus in a single sequence are often performed initially (68,69). Next, sagittal FSE T2 images are obtained to visualize the long axis of the uterus. Using an FOV of 20 to 26 cm, 4-mm slice thickness, a matrix of 512×256, superior and inferior saturation pulses, and in FOV anterior and posterior saturation pulses, ten high-resolution images in one plane may be obtained in less than 5 minutes (76). Using the sagittal images as a guide, oblique coronal and axial FSE T2-weighted images can then be performed parallel and perpendicular to the long axis of the uterus, respectively (68,80). Oblique coronal images best demonstrate the contour of the uterine fundus, which is necessary to distinguish between a septate and a bicornuate uterus (68). One must be aware that the signal intensity and width of the endometrium vary during the menstrual cycle in menarchal women. The appearance of the endometrium also varies in premenarchal, menarchal, and postmenarchal females. Oral contraceptives and other hormones may affect the appearance of the endometrium, but the endometrium will nearly always clearly be seen as a region of high signal on T2-weighted images in the center of the uterus (81). MRI of uterine anomalies, like sonographic imaging, is best performed during the luteal phase in postmenarchal women due to the relatively thickened and more easily visualized endometrium.

Recently, a comparison of various T2-weighted imaging sequences of the uterus was performed by Gryspeerdt et al. (82). The authors' conclusion was that an optimized T2-weighted FSE imaging sequence that took advantage of partial Fourier reconstruction, reduced echo spacing, and increased echo train length was superior to both conventional FSE and half Fourier acquisition single-shot turbo spin echo (HASTE) images in terms of anatomic sharpness and overall image quality of the normal uterus. The authors did not study any patients with Müllerian anomalies; however, these newer optimized FSE sequences may prove to increase our ability to accurately delineate Müllerian anomalies.

For determining uterine morphology, T1-weighted images are not needed. However, T1-weighted images are acquired faster than FSE T2-weighted images and may be useful in patients who are seriously ill, uncooperative, or claustrophobic. Fat saturation imaging may be quite useful because it tends to make the high-signal endometrium more visible with FSE T2-weighted images. Fat saturation is useful in distinguishing blood from lipid-containing lesions that may appear similar on T1- and T2-weighted images. Small high-signal foci of endometrial implants can blend with pelvic fat and are better seen with fat saturation (83).

In the previous few years, MRI of the pelvis has been described using endovaginal and endorectal-external multicoil arrays. Tan et al. (84) described the use of an endovaginal coil to obtain high-resolution images of the female pelvic floor and urethra. This technique may have future applications in the evaluation of vaginal and uterine malformations. Schnall et al. (85) described a combined endorectal-external multicoil array used to obtain MR images of the pelvis. The authors demonstrated that the endorectal-external multicoil technology allowed for the combination of increased spatial coverage of the external coils with the high SNR of the endorectal coil at the center of the pelvis. This technique may also have future applications in the evaluation of Müllerian anomalies.

A few final technical points about MRI are worth mentioning. Some authors advocate fasting for 8 hours and the use of glucagon to decrease bowel motion during scanning, but we have not found these measures to be necessary. A filled urinary bladder is helpful to displace bowel out of the pelvis but the bladder should not be overfilled. Finally, a tampon may be placed within the vagina prior to scanning. Tampons appear as tubular, very-low-signal regions on MR images and make location of the vagina quite easy in most cases. Vitamin E capsules may be taped to the perineum to mark its location. Figures 1 to 3 demonstrate normal sagittal, coronal, and axial MR anatomy of the uterus and cervix.

COMPUTED TOMOGRAPHY

Computed tomography (CT) probably has no place in the workup of Müllerian anomalies. It is limited by its capability to scan in only the axial plane, its use of ion-

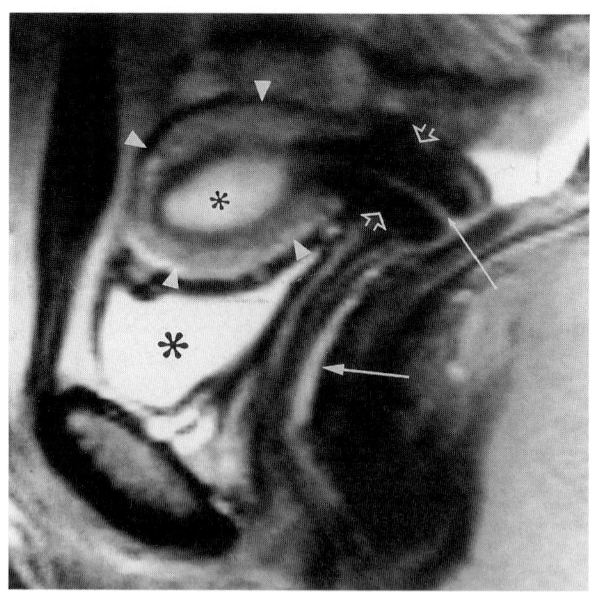

FIG. 1. Normal T2-weighted sagittal MR image of a 21-year-old female pelvis. *Large asterisk,* bladder; *small asterisk,* endometrial cavity; *arrowheads,* uterine body; *open arrows,* uterine cervix; *long thin arrow,* external cervical os; *long thick arrow,* vagina.

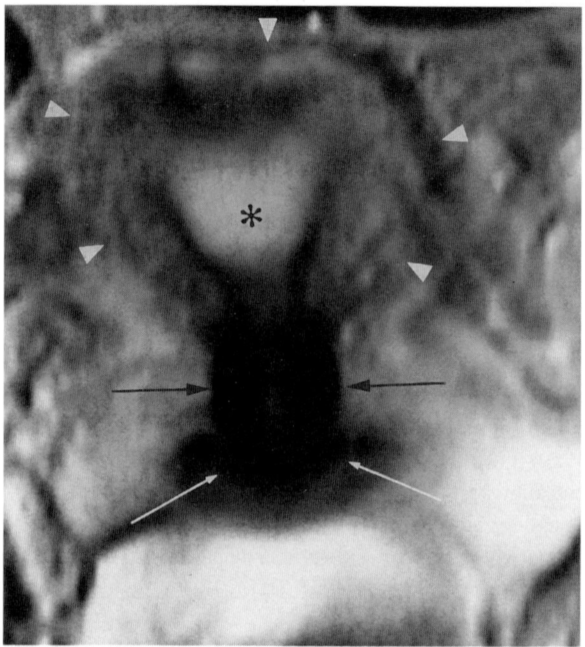

FIG. 2. Normal T2-weighted coronal MR image of a 21-year-old female pelvis. *Asterisk,* endometrial cavity; *black arrows,* uterine cervix; *white arrows,* fornices of vagina; *arrowheads,* uterus.

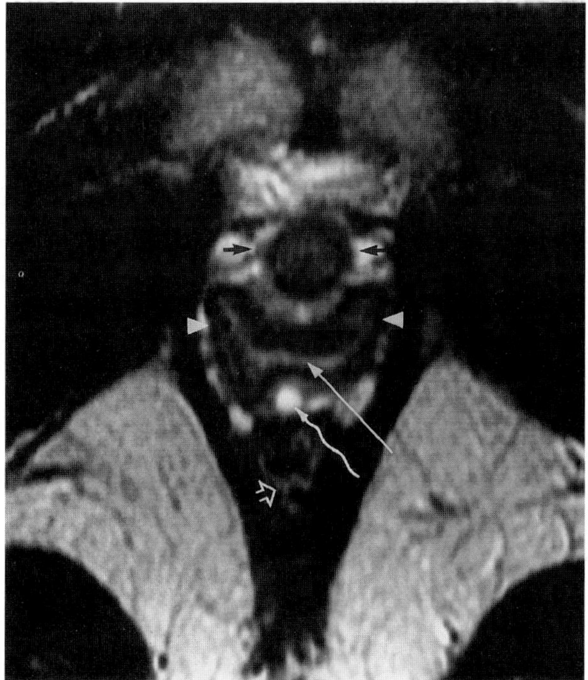

FIG. 3. Normal T2-weighted axial MR image of a 13-year-old female pelvis at the level of the vagina. *Black arrows,* urethra; *arrowheads,* vaginal wall; *white arrow,* vaginal epithelium/luminal secretions; *open arrow,* rectum; *wavy arrow,* probable Nabothian cyst.

izing radiation, and its decreased tissue contrast compared to MRI. Occasionally, however, an unsuspected Müllerian anomaly will be first detected by CT, and so we have included an example in Fig. 4.

GENITOGRAPHY

Genitography, the radiologic evaluation of internal genital structures after the injection of iodinated contrast material through the perineal orifice, may be very helpful in the evaluation of infants with a single urogenital orifice (11,44,83–90). These infants have either a urogenital sinus or cloacal malformation depending on the presence or absence of a patent anus. The majority of cases of hydrometrocolpos in the newborn are due to a urogenital sinus or cloacal malformation. A genitogram demonstrating a urogenital sinus is shown in Fig. 5.

CLASSIFICATION SCHEME AND IMAGING EXAMPLES OF MULLERIAN ANOMALIES

Table 1 outlines the current American Fertility Society (AFS) classification of Müllerian anomalies published in 1988 (42). The classes are categorized according

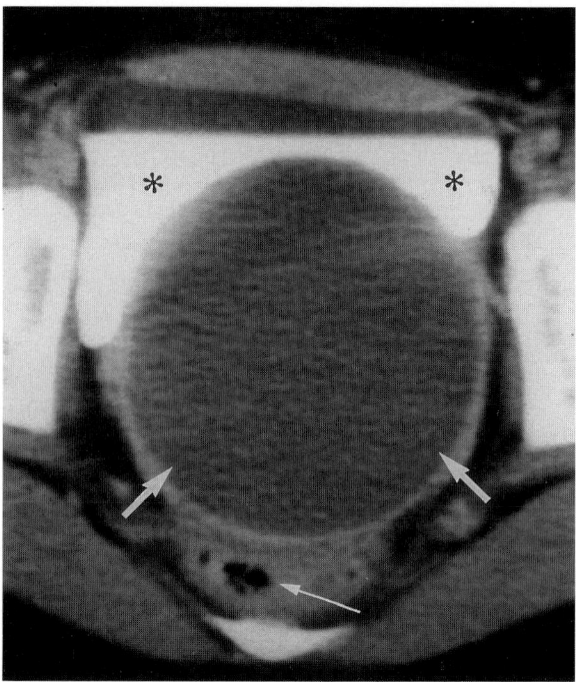

FIG. 4. Axial CT image through the pelvis of an 11-year-old girl with pelvic pain. *Asterisks,* iodinated contrast within urinary bladder; *thick arrows,* hydrocolpos due to low vaginal atresia; *thin arrow,* rectum.

to similarities of clinical manifestation, treatment, and prognosis for fetal salvage. The AFS classification is weighted primarily toward disorders of lateral fusion and does not include associated vaginal anomalies. Rock (43) has proposed that no classification of Müllerian anomalies can focus entirely on the uterus, as the vagina is often involved as well. Rock has developed a modification of the AFS classification of utero-vaginal anomalies (Table 2) that comprises four groups based on embryologic considerations. We will focus on Rock's modification for our discussion and pictorial presentation of the imaging of Müllerian anomalies.

Class I: Dysgenesis (Agenesis) of the Müllerian Ducts (Mayer-Rokitansky-Küster-Hauser Syndrome)

Generally speaking, dysgenesis of the Müllerian ducts is a spectrum of anomalies including agenesis of the uterine corpus, uterine cervix, and upper vagina with ab-

FIG. 5. Genitogram of a 3-day-old girl with a urogenital sinus malformation. **A:** Lateral image with contrast filling vagina *(arrowheads),* bladder *(asterisk),* and urethra ending blindly within labium majorum *(white arrow).* **B:** Same patient showing further contrast filling of the vagina *(large black arrows),* uterus *(large white arrow),* bladder *(asterisk),* and urethra *(small white arrows).* Long black arrow points to catheter with its distal tip within the bladder.

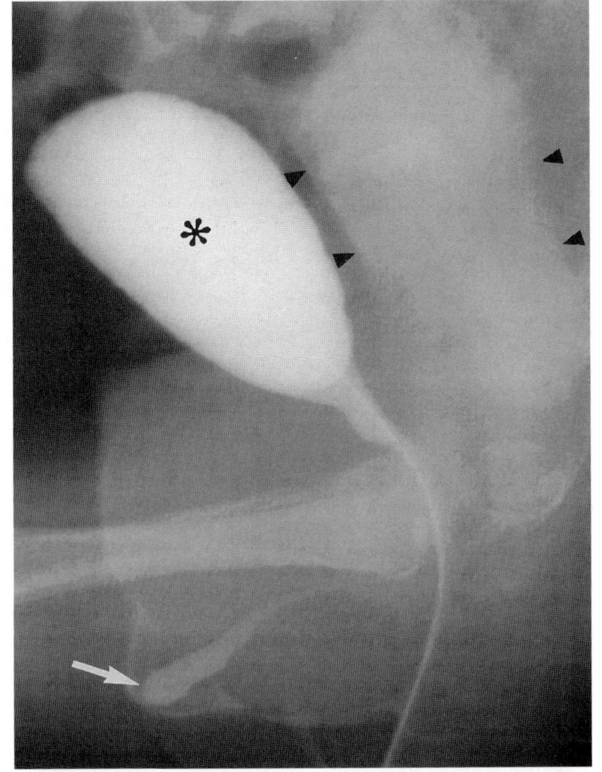

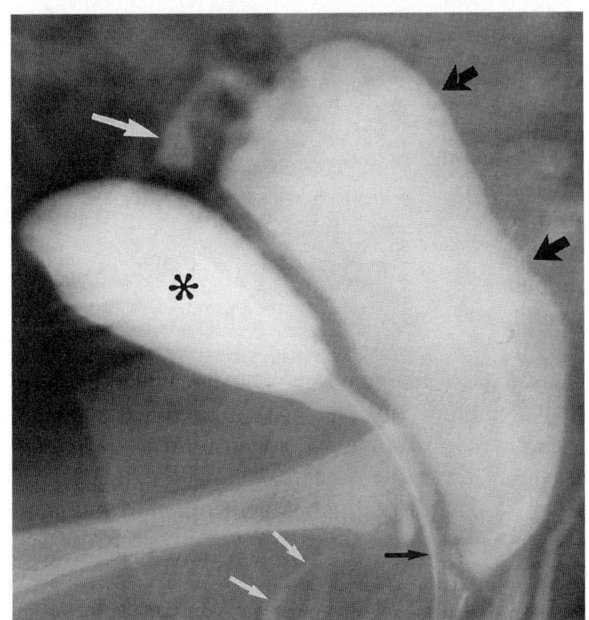

sence or hypoplasia of fallopian tubes in genotypic and phenotypic females who have a normal endocrine status (91). The uterus may vary from anatomically complete to rudimentary bicornuate cords to complete absence. Renal ectopy and agenesis has been reported in 34% and 47% of patients with Müllerian dysgenesis, respectively (40,41). Griffin et al. have also described a 12% incidence of skeletal abnormalities associated with Müllerian dysgenesis as well as a probable increase in cardiac anomalies (40). Specific syndromes associated with Müllerian duct aplasia have been described (33). The overall frequency of vaginal agenesis has been reported to be between 1 in 1,500 to 1 in 80,000 (92,93), but the most widely cited reference is approximately 1 in 5,000 births (94). Remnants of uterine structures may be present and may cause cyclic pelvic pain and require excision. MRI may be of great value in the evaluation of the presence of a vagina and uterus and for the search for endometrium-containing uterine remnants (95).

The Müllerian dysgenesis syndrome is second only to gonodal dysgenesis as a pathologic cause of primary amenorrhea at referral centers (96). Physical examination reveals normal secondary sexual development, normal perineum, and a vaginal dimple/small pouch. The hymenal fringe and small vaginal pouch are usually present as they are both derived from the urogenital sinus and not the Müllerian system.

Both US and MRI should be able to demonstrate the absence of uterus and upper vagina. MRI is probably more accurate than US in finding uterine remnants containing endometrium. Müllerian dysgenesis has been separated into two groups by some authors (97,98). The so-called type A syndrome demonstrates symmetric muscular buds and fallopian tubes. Type B demonstrated asymmetric muscular buds or abnormally developed fallopian tubes. One study found renal and ovarian anomalies in 37% and 15% of patients, respectively, all of whom had the type B syndrome (98).

Three examples of Müllerian dysgenesis are presented, all seen with MRI. The first case is a 16-year-old girl who presented with primary amenorrhea. A sagittal MR image of the pelvis demonstrates absence of the uterus and vagina (Fig. 6). The second example is that of a 15-year-old girl who also presented with primary amenorrhea. MRI of the pelvis in the axial plane revealed absence of the uterus and vagina and bilateral pelvic kidneys (Fig. 7). Figure 8 is a coronal MR image of a girl with absence of vagina and uterus as well as failure of complete descent of the ovaries bilaterally.

Class II: Disorders of Vertical Fusion of the Müllerian Ducts

Transverse Vaginal Septum

This class of disorders includes transverse vaginal septa, both obstructed and nonobstructed, and cervical agenesis or dysgenesis. These disorders can be considered abnormalities of the fusion of the down-growing Müllerian ducts and the up-growing derivatives of the urogenital sinus (43). The transverse vaginal septum is quite rare, with an incidence of 1:2,100 found in one large series (99). The same study reported incidences of septa in the upper, mid-, and lower vagina of 46%, 40%, and 14%, respectively, which is similar to the corresponding incidences of 46%, 35%, and 19% reported by Rock et al. (100). The transverse vaginal septum may vary in thickness and, in general, the thicker septum is more commonly closer to the

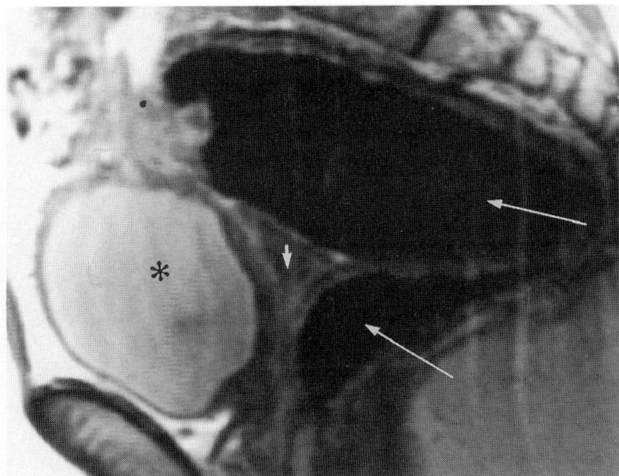

FIG. 6. Mayer-Rokitansky-Küster-Hauser syndrome. Sagittal proton density MR image of the pelvis of a 16-year-old girl presenting with primary amenorrhea. *Asterisk,* bladder; *long arrows,* rectum/sigmoid colon; *short arrow,* expected position of uterus but no uterine tissue present.

cervix. In such patients with thick septa, a considerable segment of the vagina may be underdeveloped. If the segment is sufficiently long that the lower portion of the vagina is involved, this condition is known as congenital absence of the vagina with a uterus and is considered an extreme form of the transverse vaginal septum (101). Patients with transverse vaginal septa have few related anomalies although reported associations include urinary tract anomalies, aortic coarctation, atrial septal defect, and malformations of the lumbar spine (100). An autosomal recessive mode of transmittance of the transverse vaginal septum has been suggested by McKusick et al.

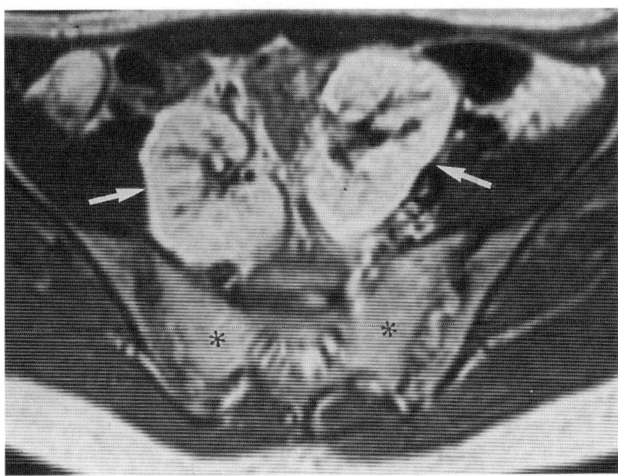

FIG. 7. Axial T1-weighted MR image with intravenous gadolinium of a 15-year-old girl presenting with primary amenorrhea. Image demonstrates bilateral pelvic kidneys *(white arrows).* No uterine or vaginal tissue could be identified. *Asterisk,* sacrum.

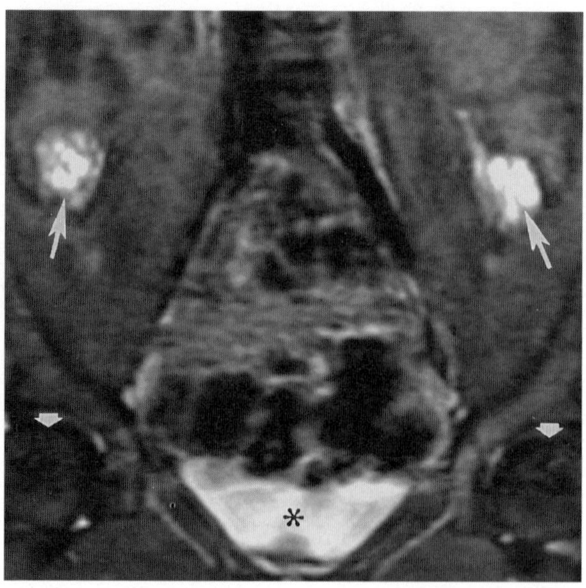

FIG. 8. Mayer-Rokitansky-Küster-Hauser syndrome. Coronal T2-weighted MR image of the pelvis of a 16-year-old girl demonstrating incomplete descent of the ovaries *(large arrows)*. No uterine or vaginal tissue was identified. *Black asterisk,* urinary bladder; *short arrows,* femoral heads.

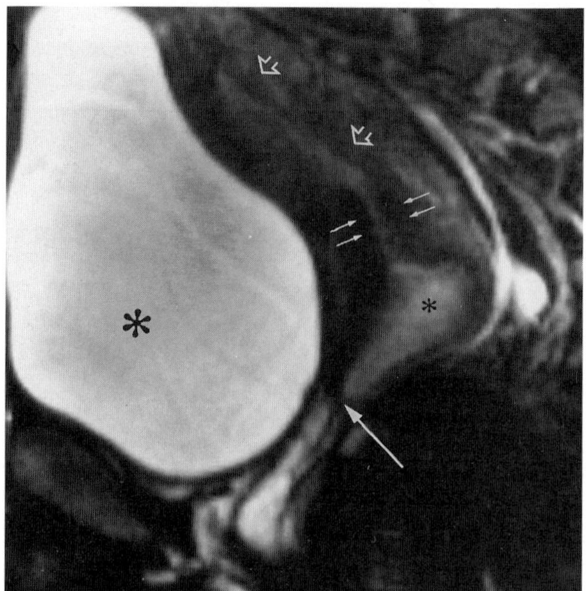

FIG. 9. High transverse vaginal system. Sagittal T2-weighted MR image of the pelvis of a 13-year-old girl presenting with primary amenorrhea. *Large asterisk,* bladder; *open arrows,* endometrial canal; *short white arrows,* uterine cervix; *small asterisk,* dilated proximal vagina; *long white arrows,* transverse vaginal septum.

(102). The incidence of endometriosis in women with transverse vaginal septa is high. MRI has been shown to be of clinical usefulness in the evaluation of disorders of vertical fusion (34,103–105).

Figure 9 is a sagittal T2-weighted MR image of the pelvis of a 13-year-old girl with primary amenorrhea. The image demonstrates a high vaginal atresia with a mildly dilated proximal vagina but essentially normal cervix and uterus. Figure 10 is a T1-weighted image of the pelvis of a 17-year-old girl who also presented with primary

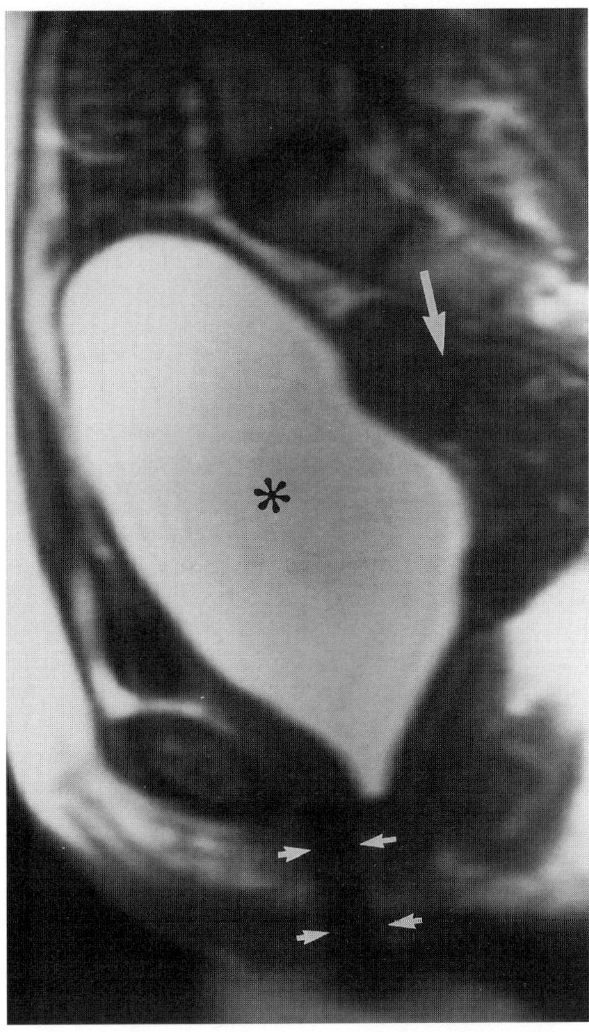

FIG. 10. High transverse vaginal septum. Sagittal T2-weighted MR image of the pelvis of a 17-year-old girl presenting with primary amenorrhea and pelvic pain. *Short arrows,* tampon in lower vagina; *asterisk,* large hematocolpos proximal to vaginal septum; *long arrow,* rectum.

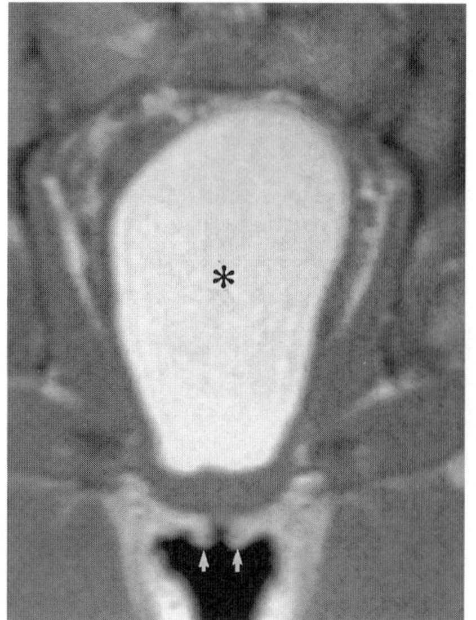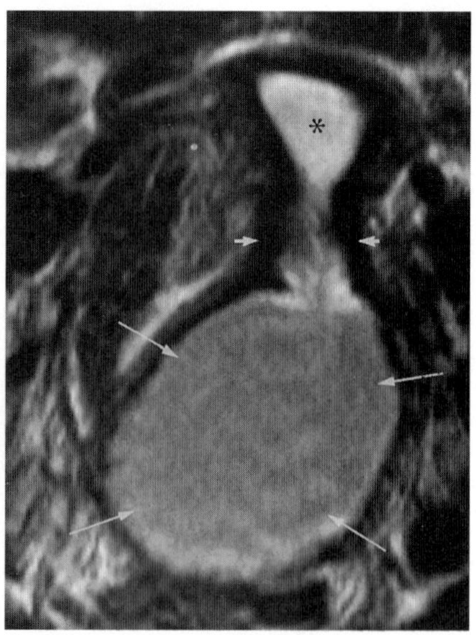

FIG. 11. Low transverse vaginal septum. **A:** Coronal T1-weighted MR image through the pelvis of a 14-year-old girl with primary amenorrhea and several months of pelvic pain. *Asterisk,* large hematocolpos; *white arrows,* labia majora. Note how magnetic resonance imaging can be useful to measure distance from transverse septum to the vestibule. **B:** Axial T2-weighted MR image. *Black asterisk,* uterine cavity; *short white arrows,* uterine cervix; *long white arrows,* hematocolpos.

amenorrhea. This image was taken with a tampon in the vagina and demonstrates a large, blood-filled hydrocolpos exhibiting high signal proximal to the transverse vaginal septum. Figure 11 shows coronal T1-weighted and oblique axial T2-weighted MR images of the pelvis of a 14-year-old girl with amenorrhea and several months of pelvic pain. These images demonstrate a low transverse vaginal septum with moderate hematometrocolpos. The coronal image is useful for estimating the distance from the labia to the obstructing vaginal septum. Figure 12 shows sagittal and transverse transabdominal US images of the pelvis of a 12-year-old girl with pelvic pain. The images demonstrate a low vaginal atresia with a moderately large hematocolpos containing a fluid-debris layer.

Cervical Agenesis or Dysgenesis

Two basic categories of cervical anomalies have been described: (a) cervical aplasia, or lack of a uterine cervix, and (b) cervical dysplasia, which has been further subdivided into four subtypes: (i) intact cervical body with obstruction of the cervical os, (ii) cervical body consisting of a fibrous band of variable length and diameter, (iii) stricture of the midportion of the cervix, and (iv) fragmentation of the cervix (43). Variable portions of the vagina may be atretic but cervical obstruction is usually associated with a vagina of normal length.

Many, if not most, authors have recommended hysterectomy for patients with a functioning uterus and congenital absence of the cervix and vagina (106–110). A hysterectomy will eliminate associated problems such as cryptomenorrhea, sepsis, endometriosis, and multiple operations. If performed early enough, it may be possible to conserve the ovaries and their function. A review of congenital atresia of the uterine cervix in 1986 by Farber (111) revealed that all of the 35 reported cases in the world literature up to that time presented with primary amenorrhea and cyclic or

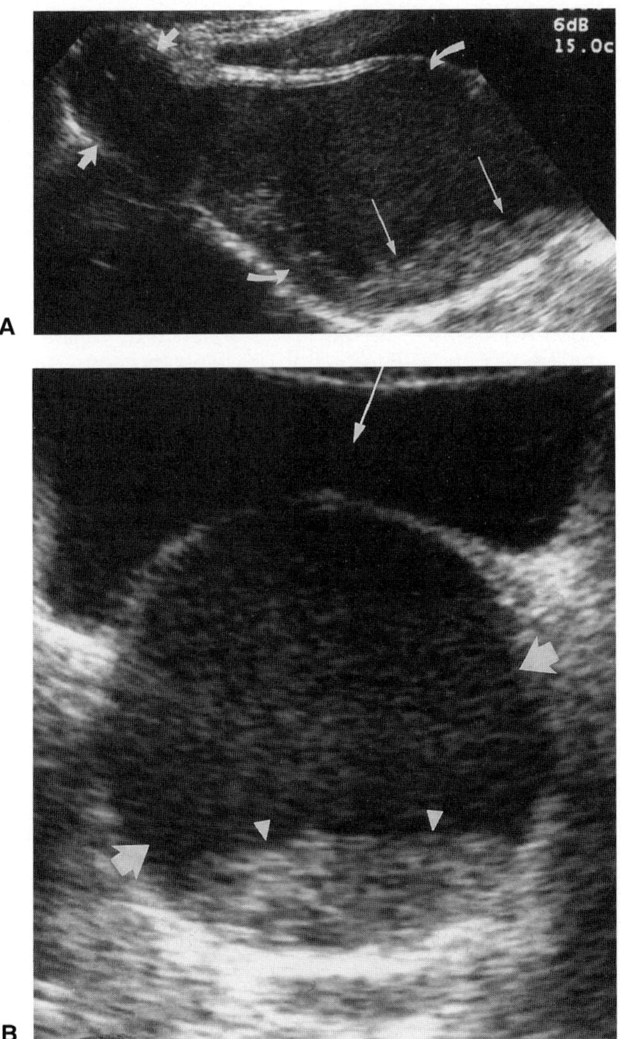

FIG. 12. Low transverse vaginal septum. **A:** Sagittal pelvic ultrasound image of a 12-year-old girl complaining of pelvic pain. *Short straight arrows,* uterus; *curved arrows,* hematocolpos containing mildly echogenic material consistent with blood as well as dependent debris *(long straight arrows)* consistent with clotted blood/sloughed endometrial products. **B:** Axial ultrasound image of pelvis. *Long arrow,* bladder; *short arrows,* hematocolpos; *arrowheads,* dependent debris within hematocolpos.

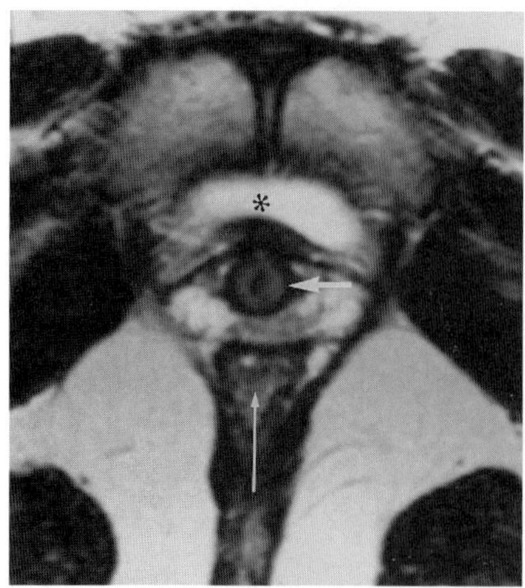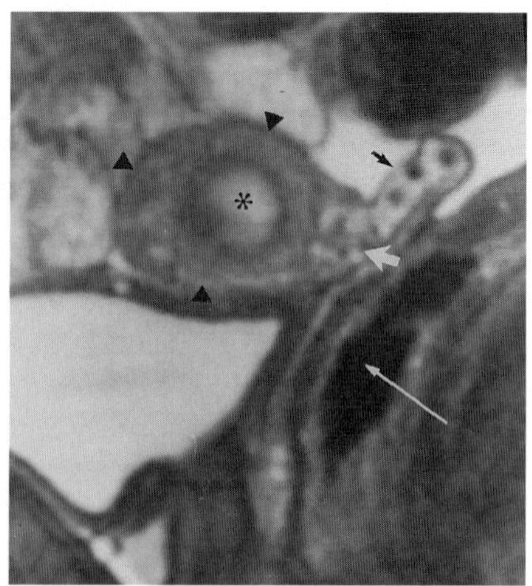

FIG. 13. Cervical dysgenesis with vaginal atresia. **A:** Axial T2-weighted MR image of a 16-year-old girl presenting with primary amenorrhea. *Asterisk,* bladder; *short white arrow,* urethra; *long white arrow,* rectum. Note absence of vagina between urethra and rectum (compare to Fig. 3). **B:** Sagittal T2-weighted image. *Small asterisk,* endometrium; *black arrowheads,* uterus; *short white arrow,* dysgenetic cervix; *black arrow,* ovary; *long white arrow,* rectum; *large asterisk,* bladder. (Courtesy of Andrea B. Magen, M.D.)

chronic pelvic pain. Over 70% of the women suffered from hematometra, hematosalpinx, pelvic endometriosis or adenomyosis, pelvic adhesions, or free intraperitoneal blood. Ten of the 35 women underwent primary hysterectomy. An initial attempt to establish communication between the endometrial cavity and the vagina or neovagina was made in the remaining 25 women using either a stent or direct surgical anastomosis. Of these 25 women, 2 went on to deliver viable fetuses, but hysterectomy was ultimately necessary in many. Farber suggested that abdominal hysterectomy should not be performed primarily in patients with cervical atresia unless the pelvic viscera were determined to be irremediably destroyed by cryptomenorrhea. Figure 13 gives axial and sagittal T2-weighted images of the pelvis of a 16-year-old girl with primary amenorrhea. The images reveal a relatively normal uterus but dysgenesis of the cervix and absence of some or all of the vagina.

Class III: Disorders of Lateral Fusion

Failure of medial fusion of the two Müllerian ducts can be either complete or incomplete and may or may not be associated with obstruction. A true duplication of the uterus is rare. It results from unilateral or bilateral duplication of the Müllerian ducts and may also be associated with duplication of the vulva, bladder, urethra, vagina, and anus (91). Complete failure of fusion of the two Müllerian ducts may lead to complete duplication of the vagina, cervix, and uterus. Partial fusion may result in a single vagina with a single or duplicated cervix and complete or partial duplication of the uterine body. Failure of resorption of the median uterine septum between the fused Müllerian systems results in the persistence of a septum inside the uterus while the external contour of the uterus remains that of a single uterus. The septum typically only separates the upper uterine cavities but may rarely completely divide the uterine cavities and endocervical canal into two equal or unequal components (43). Disorders of lateral fusion may be asymmetric and obstructed or symmetric and unobstructed. Surgical intervention is typically acutely necessary in cases of an obstructed system; however, surgical correction of an unobstructed system is best delayed until reproductive age and then is indicated only if the anomaly is believed to be directly related to pregnancy wastage, infertility, or coital difficulties (112).

Asymmetric-Obstructed Disorder of Uterus or Vagina Usually Associated with Ipsilateral Renal Agenesis

This subclass (see Table 2) contains the following conditions: (a) unicornuate uterus with a noncommunicating rudimentary anlage or horn, (b) unilateral obstruction of a cavity of a double uterus, and (c) unilateral vaginal obstruction associated with double uterus. If one of the Müllerian ducts fails to develop properly, a condition may develop wherein there is a relatively normal unicornuate uterus found on the side of normal Müllerian development but on the opposite side there is absence or hypoplasia of the uterine body, fallopian tube, cervix, ligamentous attachments, and blood supply (43). If a rudimentary uterine horn is present and it contains functioning endometrium, then obstructed menstruation or cryptomenorrhea may begin soon after menarche with its attendant dysmenorrhea and possible retrograde menstruation and endometriosis. In a series of 13 patients with a unicornuate uterus, 11 of 13 had a rudimentary horn and 2 did not (16). Most rudimentary horns (90%) are noncommunicating (113). The fallopian tube associated with a rudimentary horn may be obstructed preventing retrograde menstruation and endometriosis. Figure 14 demon-

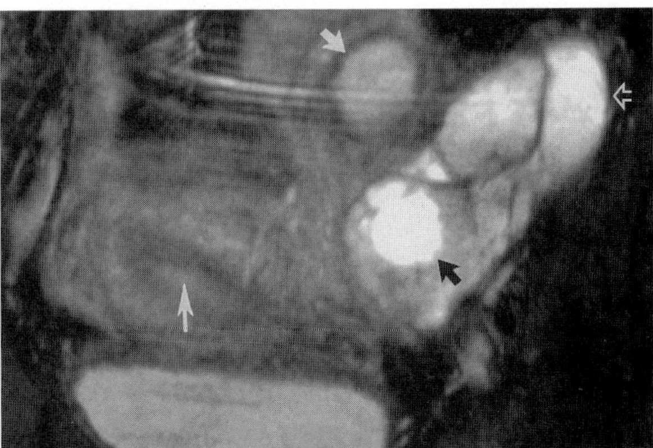

FIG. 14. Unicornuate uterus with noncommunicating rudimentary horn containing endometrium. Coronal T2-weighted MR image. *Long white arrow,* right-sided nonobstructed unicornuate uterus; *short white arrow,* obstructed, noncommunicating rudimentary left uterine horn; *open white arrow,* dilated left fallopian tube associated with rudimentary horn; *black arrow,* left ovary.

strates a coronal T2-weighted MR image of the pelvis of a young woman who suffered from severe dysmenorrhea. The image demonstrates a right unicornuate uterus with a left rudimentary horn containing endometrium, and a left hematosalpinx. MRI has been shown to be useful in the evaluation of unicornuate uteri although it may not be as accurate as laparoscopy in detecting minimal endometriosis and tubal conditions (9,34,65,66,114).

Figure 15 depicts a uterine didelphys with an obstruction of the right hemivagina and resultant hematometrocolpos, hematosalpinx, and blood products in the pelvis in a 15-year-old girl with persistent pelvic pain. This patient also had an absent right kidney (not shown). Figure 16 gives MR examples of a similar case of an 18-year-old female with pelvic pain and a palpable pelvic mass. This patient has a uterinedidelphus with an obstructed left hemivagina and absent left kidney. A tampon was placed in the right hemivagina before the scan. The syndrome of a double uterus, obstruction of the vagina, and ipsilateral kidney has been broken down into three groups by Rock (43). Group 1 patients have complete vaginal obstruction without communication with the uterus resulting in a paravaginal mass and symptoms of severe dysmenorrhea. Group 2 patients have an incomplete vaginal obstruction without uterine communication. The presenting symptoms are lower abdominal pain, severe dysmenorrhea, focal mucopurulent discharge, and, occasionally, intermenstrual bleeding. Group 3 patients have complete vaginal obstruction with communication of the ipsilateral double uterus. These patients typically have a paravaginal mass, lower abdominal pain, and dysmenorrhea. Menses are regular. The patients in Figs. 15 and 16 both belong to group 3 described above.

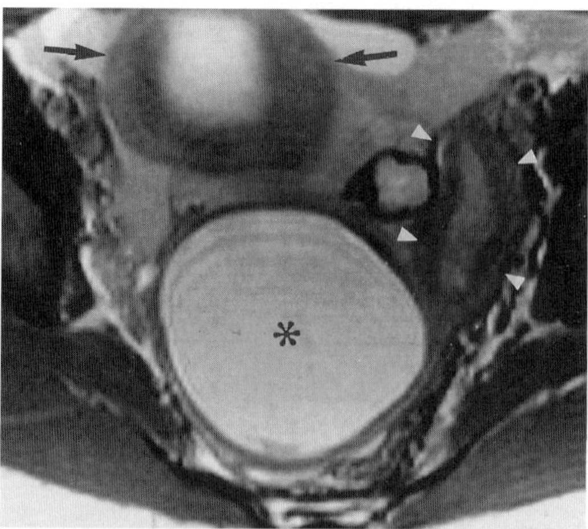

FIG. 15. Didelphic uterus with right-sided hematometrocolpos and absent right kidney in a 15-year-old girl with persistent right pelvic pain. **A:** Axial T2-weighted MR image through pelvis. *Black arrows,* right hematometros; *white arrowheads,* left uterine horn; *asterisk,* right hematocolpos. **B:** Sagittal T2-weighted MR image. *Black arrows,* right hematometros; *arrowheads,* hematocolpos; *small asterisk,* urinary bladder; *large asterisk,* intraperitoneal blood products from retrograde menstruation. **C:** Sagittal ultrasound image. *White arrows,* right hematometros; *black arrowheads,* right hematocolpos. **D:** Coronal T1-weighted MR image. *Large arrows,* right hematosalpinx; *open arrow,* right hematocolpos.

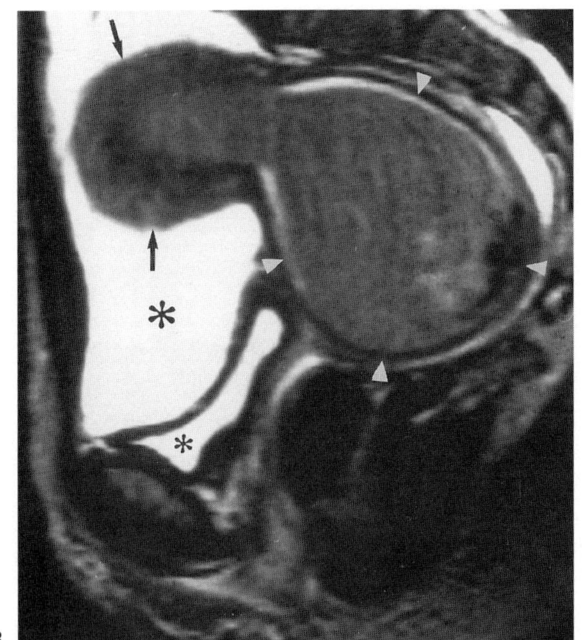

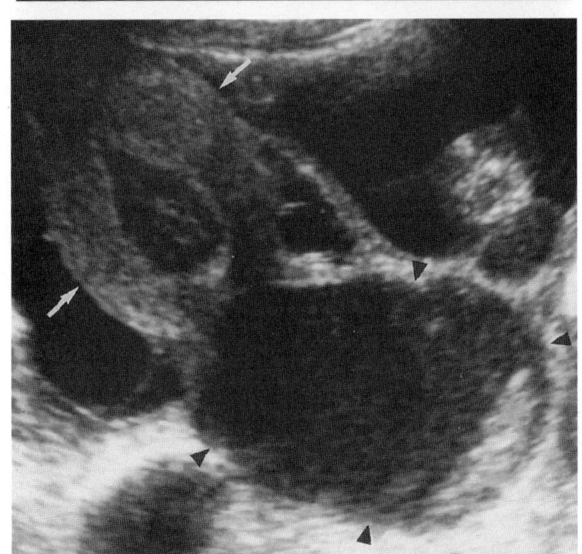

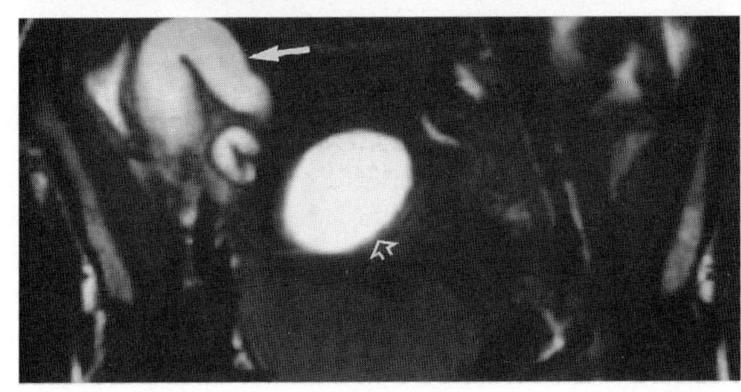

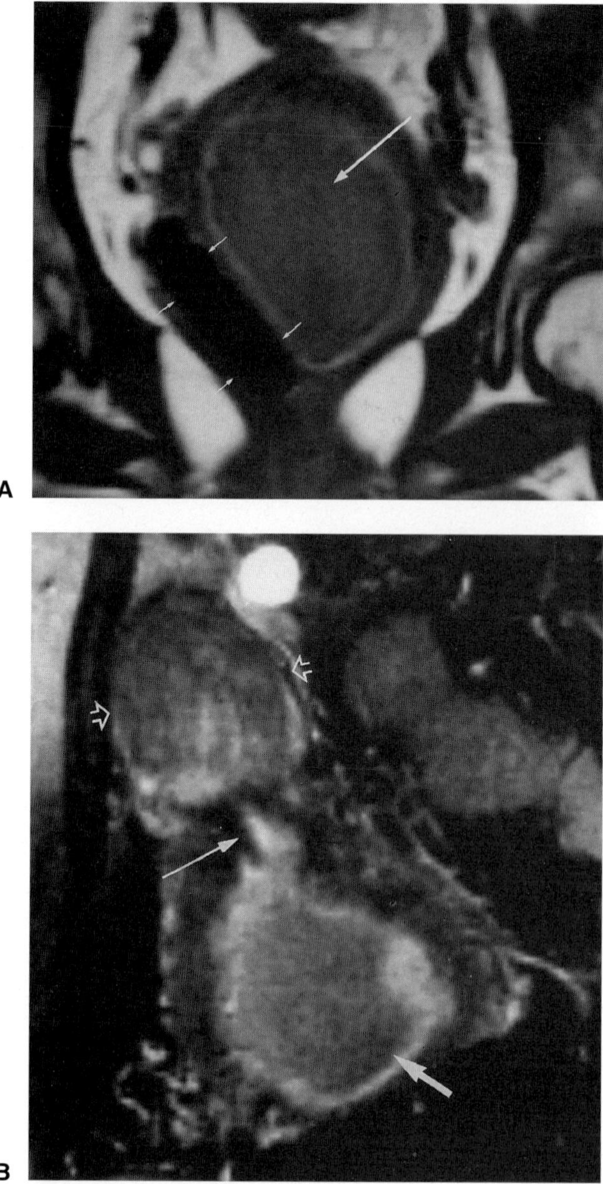

FIG. 16. Uterine didelphys with obstructed left hemivagina in an 18-year-old woman presenting with chronic pelvic pain and a palpable pelvic mass. **A:** Coronal T1-weighted MRI of pelvis. *Short arrows,* tampon in right hemivagina; *long arrow,* left-sided hematocolpos. **B:** Sagittal T2-weighted MR image. *Open arrows,* left-sided uterine horn; *thin white arrow,* left-sided cervix; *thick white arrow,* left-sided hemato-colpos.

Symmetric-Unobstructed

Didelphic Uterus

The didelphic uterus is characterized by two separate uterine bodies, each associated with their own fallopian tube and cervix. The diagnosis is typically easily made when a speculum examination reveals two hemicervices. Most, if not all, patients with uterine didelphus will have a longitudinal vaginal septum (16). Conversely, most patients with a longitudinal vaginal septum will have a didelphic uterus. The didelphic uterus is generally accepted as having the highest rate of successful pregnancy of all the uterine anomalies (with the possible exception of the arcuate uterus). One study reported a fetal survival rate of 64% without metroplasty (16) and another study reported a 57% rate of successful pregnancy (115). However, one study, reported in 1957, considered the didelphic uterus to have the lowest rate of successful pregnancy outcome (116). Yet most current authors believe that most patients with uterine didelphus have adequate reproductive outcomes and that unification metroplasty is contraindicated or at least infrequently indicated (43,91). The unification metroplasty can be very technically difficult with disappointing results, especially when cervical unification is attempted, which may result in cervical incompetence or cervical stenosis. Surgical intervention is typically not warranted except in cases where the longitudinal vaginal septum leads to dyspareunia (101).

MRI has been demonstrated to be quite accurate in discriminating between the various types of double uteri. Fedele et al. (67) reported a sensitivity of 100% and a specificity of 79% when using MRI to differentiate between bicornuate, didelphic, and septate uteri. When only the technically adequate images were considered, both sensitivity and specificity rose to 100%. Bicornuate and didelphic uteri were differentiated from septate uteri based on the presence of a fundal indentation more than 10 mm deep with an angle between the medial margins of the hemicavities of not less than 60 degrees. These criteria were found to be reliable in a previous sonographic study of double uteri (117). The depth of the myometrial spur separating the two hemicervices and the level of its lower apex were also helpful in differentiating types of double uteri. Using a classification scheme based on identifying three points on US and MRI of double uteri, Fedele et al. (118) demonstrated that they could increase the number of hysteroscopic metroplasties, as opposed to abdominal metroplasties, by 21% compared to using laparoscopic indications alone.

Ultrasound has also proven accurate in the differential diagnosis of double uteri. In a study of 39 patients with adequate sonographic visualization of the uterus, transabdominal US demonstrated a sensitivity of 92% and a specificity of 100% in the correct diagnosis of double uteri (58).

Figure 17 is an example of a didelphic uterus imaged by HSG. Figures 18 demonstrates an axial MR image revealing two cervices and an oblique coronal image revealing two separate uterine bodies, respectively. Figure 19 is a vaginogram of a 17-year-old girl who uses two tampons at a time during her menstrual period. The vaginogram demonstrates two separate vaginas. Figure 20 is an US example of a 16-year-old girl with hand-foot-uterus syndrome. The US demonstrates two separate endometrial canals. Figure 21 shows coronal and transverse images through the pelvis of a 30-year-old woman demonstrating uterine didelphys and bicollis with complete vagina septum.

Septate Uterus

When midline fusion of the two Müllerian ducts occurs but the midline tissue is not resorbed, a septate uterus results. Septate uteri are generally considered to be a Müllerian anomaly with poor reproductive prognosis (6). Mahgoub (119) has postulated that the increase in pregnancy loss associated with the septate uterus is due either to decreased intrauterine space for fetal growth or to placental implantation on a poorly vascularized septum. However, a study of 182 women with uterine anomalies published in 1982 reported a fetal survival rate of 86% with complete septate uteri, 50% with complete bicornuate uteri and 40% with unicornuate uteri (16). Jones and Jones considered septate uteri to be associated with the highest reproductive loss

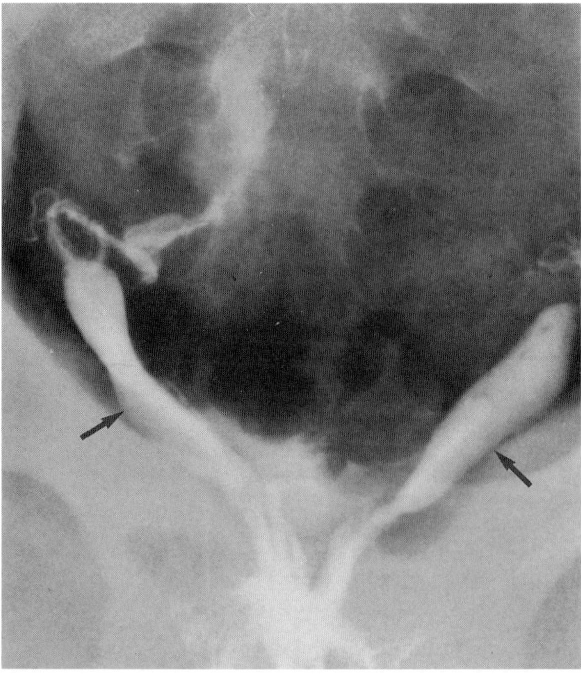

FIG. 17. Hysterosalpingogram of a young woman with a didelphic uterus. *Arrows,* bilateral uterine horns.

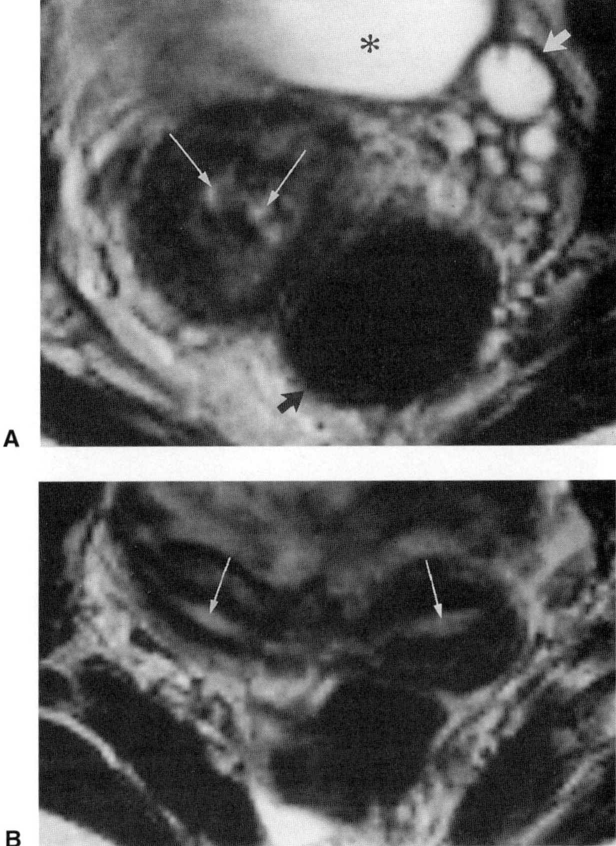

FIG. 18. A 31-year-old woman with didelphic uterus who is status post trocar drainage of obstructed left vagina at the age of 26 years. **A:** Axial T2-weighted MR image of the pelvis. *Long white arrows,* two uterine cervices; *small white arrow,* left ovary with multiple follicles; *black arrow,* rectum; *asterisk,* urinary bladder. **B:** Axial T2-weighted MR image superior to A. *White arrows,* two uterine horns of didelphic uterus.

among the Müllerian anomalies (120). In 1980, Jewelewicz et al. estimated the spontaneous abortion rate to be 34% in women with a bicornuate uterus, 22% in those with a septate uterus, and 35% in women with a unicornuate uterus (18). Capraro et al. reported a preoperative fetal salvage rate of 33% for septate uteri, 10% for bicornuate uteri, and 0% for didelphic uteri (121). Postoperatively the salvage rate was 100% for the bicornuate uteri, 80% for the septate uteri, and 66% for the didelphic uteri. Rock has stated that most patients evaluated for repeated abortion who are found to have a uterine anomaly will have a septate uterus, but that fetal survival rates are higher after septate uterus repair than after repairs of other uterine anomalies (43).

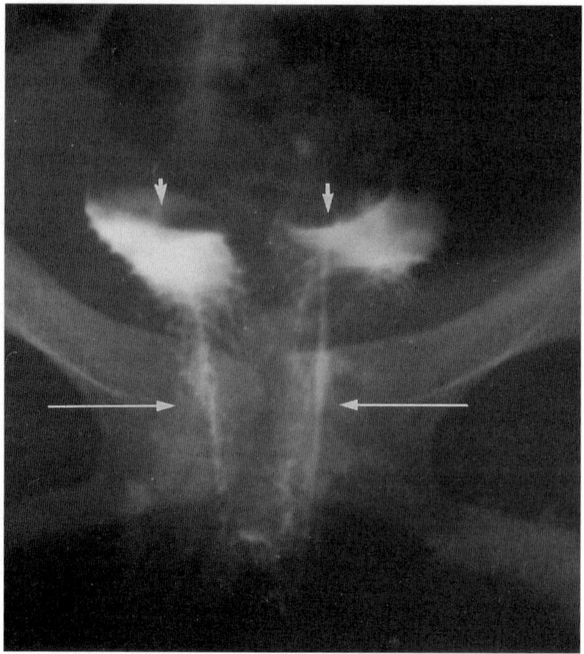

FIG. 19. Didelphic uterus with complete longitudinal vaginal septum in a 17-year-old girl who uses two tampons during menses. *Long arrows,* two hemivaginas; *short arrows,* filling defects from two uterine cervices.

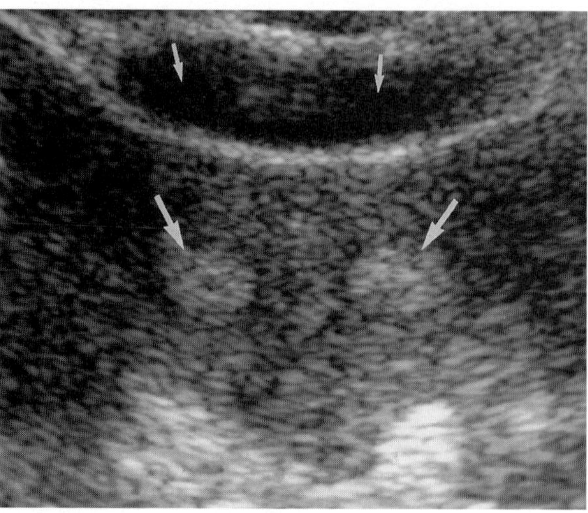

FIG. 20. Transverse ultrasound image through lower pelvis of a 16-year-old girl with hand-foot-uterus syndrome and a didelphic uterus. *Long arrow,* two echogenic endometrial canals; *short arrows,* urinary bladder.

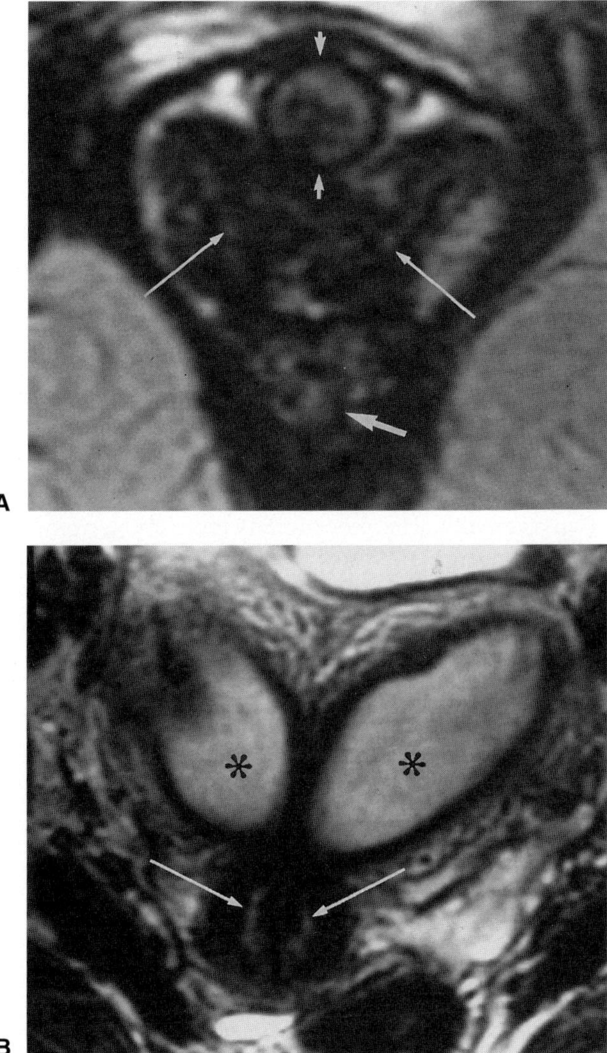

FIG. 21. A 30-year-old woman with didelphic uterus bicollis and complete longitudinal vaginal septum. **A:** Axial T2-weighted MR image through the lower pelvis. *Short arrows,* urethra; *long thin arrows,* two hemivaginas; *wide white arrow,* rectum. **B:** Axial T2-weighted MR image superior to A. *Asterisks,* two uterine horns; *long arrows,* two cervices.

Rock and Jones reported 43 patients with septate uteri treated with Jones metroplasty (122). Ninety-five percent of the 43 patients became pregnant postoperatively, 73% carried to term, and 77% delivered a live-born child.

Transcervical lysis of uterine septa using a hysteroscope or resectoscopic excision has been shown to compare favorably with the more traditional transabdominal approach with term pregnancy rates approaching 80% to 85% after these procedures (123–127). Fedele et al. have suggested that US may be useful to determine where the implantation has occurred in a septate uterus and that this information may have significant prognostic implications for pregnancy outcome (13).

Until the early 1980s, both septate and bicornuate uteri were treated by transabdominal procedures. However, more recently the transcervical approach has been shown to be comparable to the transabdominal approach for lysing a uterine septum. The transcervical approach, which is not appropriate for the repair of a bicornuate uterus, takes less time to perform than the transabdominal approach, requires less convalescent time, patients are allowed to conceive much earlier, and many patients deliver transvaginally. The procedure is typically performed under simultaneous laparoscopy to decrease the risk of uterine perforation. These different approaches to the treatment of septate and bicornuate uteri make their preoperative distinctions of great importance. Reuter et al. (57) demonstrated with 63 patients that HSG findings alone had an accuracy of 55% in distinguishing septate from bicornuate uteri but when US examination was added to the HSG the diagnostic accuracy improved to 90%. Numerous other studies have reported the increased accuracy of US and MRI over HSG in distinguishing between septate and bicornuate uteri (34,51,52, 58,61,66,68). Figure 22 demonstrates a coronal MR image of a septate uterus.

Bicornuate Uterus

A bicornuate uterus results from the partial nonfusion of the two Müllerian ducts, as opposed to the complete nonfusion associated with uterine didelphus. The septum separating the two horns is composed of myometrium and may extend to the level of the internal cervical os (uterus bicornuate unicollis) or the external cervical os (uterus bicornuate bicollis).

The imaging diagnoses of the various types of double uteri and their reproductive potential have been described in the previous two sections. As previously mentioned, patients with bicornuate uteri are not candidates for transcervical lysis because of the nearly certain occurrence of perforation. Nonuterine causes of infertility must be ruled out before metroplasty is considered as a last resort. Strassman (128) has stated that primary infertility could be cured in 60% of patients with uterine anomalies if all other potential causes of infertility were excluded. Heinonen and Pystynen (17) stressed that uterine anomalies are rarely the cause for infertility. Rock (43) has stated that even when no other cause for infertility is

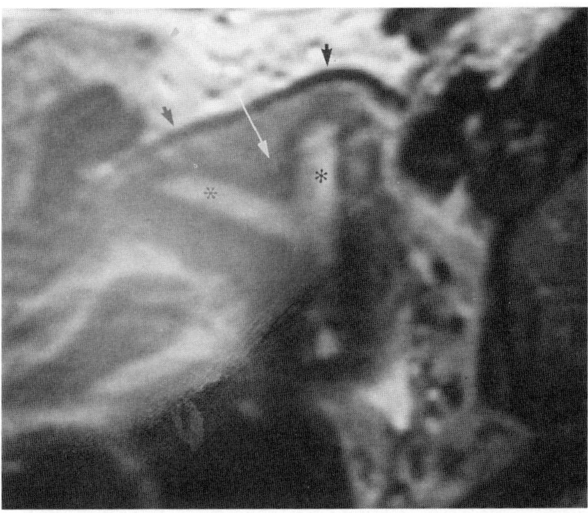

FIG. 22. Septate uterus in a 28-year-old woman. Axial T2-weighted MR image through pelvis. *Asterisks,* two uterine canals separated by incomplete septum; *white arrow,* uterine septum; *black arrows,* external uterine contour. Note there is no indentation as would be seen with bicornuate uterus. Also note that the septum is partial (uterus subseptum).

found, there still may not be a proper indication for metroplasty if the uterus is septate or bicornuate. The question of when to perform a metroplasty has not yet been answered, according to Rock. An example of a bicornuate uterus imaged with MR is shown in Fig. 23.

Diethylstilbestrol-Related Uterine Anomalies

Exposure of the female fetus to diethylstilbestrol (DES) can cause significant anomalous development of the uterus with the T-shaped uterine variant most commonly seen (129,130). The T-shaped uterus is associated with increases in spontaneous abortion, ectopic pregnancy, and preterm delivery. Additional uterine anomalies associated with DES exposure include T-shaped uterus with dilated horns and T-shaped variation (91). Nagel and Malo (131) reported a group of eight women with DES-exposed uteri and similar nonfusion anomalies. Their results suggest that hysteroscopic metroplasty may decrease pregnancy loss in these patients but may not enhance fertility. Figure 24 is an example of a T-shaped uterus evaluated by HSG.

Unicornuate Uterus

The unicornuate uterus has been discussed previously in this chapter (see pages 69–70). As previously mentioned, most patients with a unicornuate uterus have a rudi-

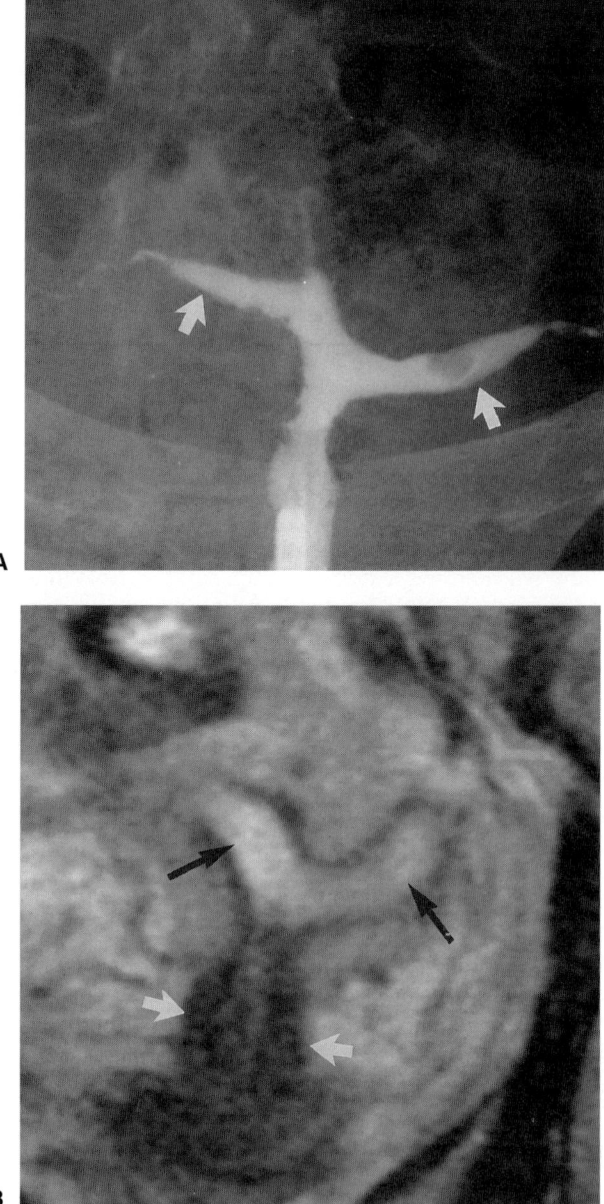

FIG. 23. Bicornuate uterus in a 34-year-old woman. **A:** Hysterosalpingography demonstrates two uterine channels *(arrows)*. **B:** Coronal T2-weighted image demonstrates two uterine horns *(black arrows)*. *White arrows,* cervix.

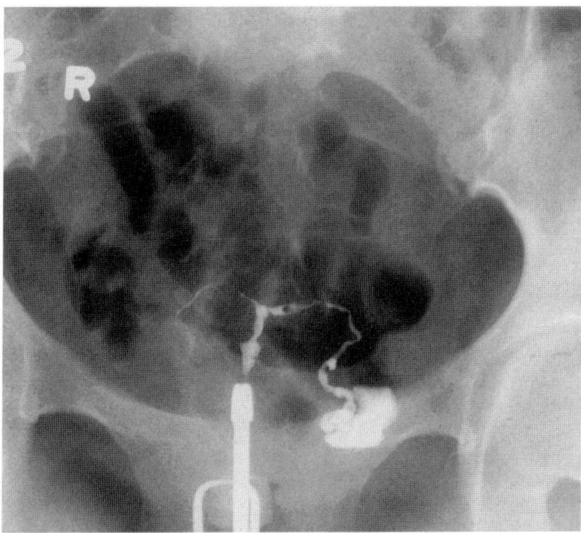

FIG. 24. T-shaped uterus.

mentary horn (16) and most rudimentary horns are noncommunicating (113). The rudimentary horn may or may not contain endometrium. Figure 14 is an example of a unicornuate uterus associated with an endometrium containing rudimentary horn imaged with MR. Figure 25 demonstrates a unicornuate uterus with no rudimentary horn.

Class IV: Unusual Configuration of Vertical Lateral Fusion Defects

Müllerian duct anomalies can occur in association with a number of other congenital anomalies. Stanton (132) reported that 43% of patients with bladder extrophy exhibited gynecologic abnormalities including vaginal narrowing, absent vagina, septate vagina, bicornuate uterus, and uterine didelphys. Jones (133) reported that approximately two thirds of female patients with bladder extrophy have a nonfunctioning vagina. Blakely and Mills (134) described 18 girls with bladder extrophy or epispadias, 15 of whom had genital anomalies ranging from vaginal stenosis (most common) to bicornuate uterus, septate vagina, and hematometros.

Occasionally, vertical and lateral fusion defects can be seen in a single patient. Bakri et al. (135) reported a case of a 16-year-old girl having bicornuate nonfused rudimentary uterine horns with functioning endometrium and cervical and vaginal agenesis diagnosed with MRI.

ACKNOWLEDGMENTS

The authors thank Andrea B. Magen, M.D. for her contributions and suggestions.

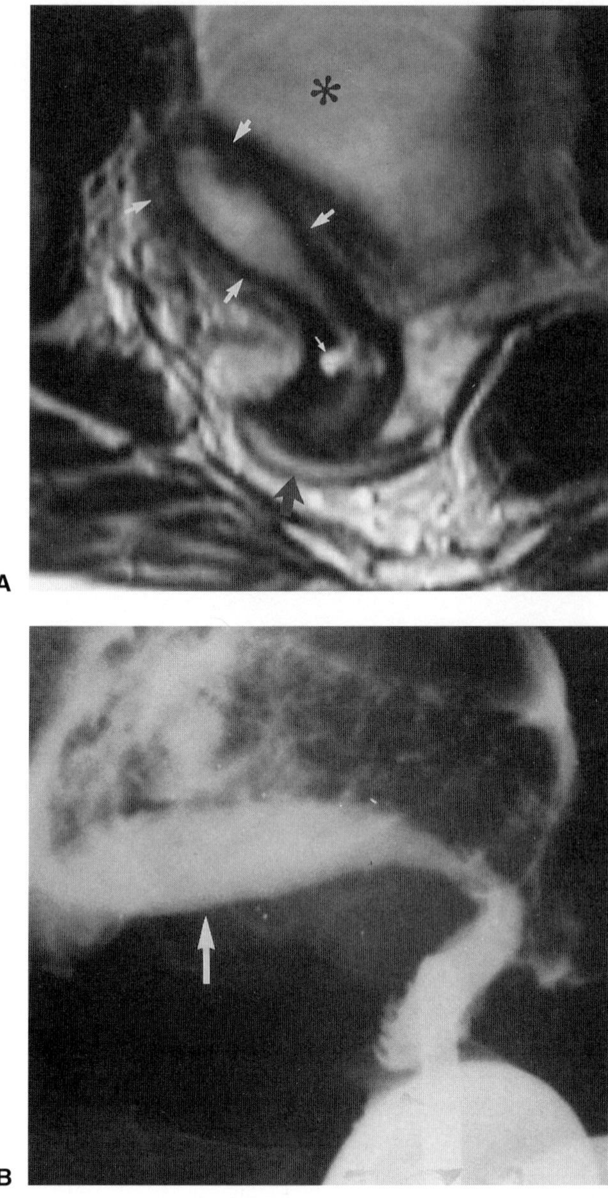

FIG. 25. A 31-year-old infertile woman with a unicornuate uterus without a rudimentary horn. **A:** Axial T2-weighted MR image of the pelvis. *Small white arrow,* Nabothian cyst; *large white arrows,* unicornuate uterus; *black arrow,* vagina; *asterisk,* bladder. **B:** Hysterosalpingography. Arrow points to unicornuate uterus.

REFERENCES

1. Pinsonneault O, Goldstein DP. Obstructing malformations of the uterus and vagina. *Fertil Steril* 1985;44:241–247.
2. Sanfilippo JS, Wakim NG, Schikler KN, Yussman MA. Endometriosis in association with uterine anomaly. *Am J Obstet Gynecol* 1986;154:39–43.
3. Golan A, Langer R, Bukovsky I, Caspi E. Congenital anomalies of the Müllerian system. *Fertil Steril* 1989;51:747–755.
4. Zanetti E, Ferrari LR, Rossi G. Classification and radiographic features of uterine malformations: hysterosalpingogram study. *Br J Radiol* 1978;51:161–170.
5. Hay D. Uterus unicollis and its relationship to pregnancy. *J Obstet Gynaecol Br Commonw* 1961;68:361–377.
6. Buttram VC, Gibbons WE. Müllerian anomalies: a proposed classification (an analysis of 144 cases). *Fertil Steril* 1979;32:40–48.
7. Green LK, Harris RE. Uterine anomalies: frequency of diagnosis and associated obstetric complications. *Obstet Gynecol* 1976;47:427–429.
8. Buttram VC Jr. Müllerian anomalies and their management. *Fertil Steril* 1983;40:159–165.
9. Wagner BJ, Woodward PJ. Magnetic resonance evaluation of congenital uterine anomalies. *Semin Ultrasound Comput Tomogr Magn Reson Imaging* 1994;15(1):4–17.
10. Pennes DR, Bowerman RA, Silver TM, Smith SJ. Failed first trimester pregnancy termination: uterine anomaly as etiologic factor. *J Clin Ultrasound* 1987;15:165–170.
11. Gilsanz V, Cleveland RH. Duplication of the Müllerian ducts and genitourinary malformation. *Radiology* 1982;144(4):793–796.
12. Jones HW. Reproductive impairment and the malformed uterus. *Fertil Steril* 1981;36(2):137–148.
13. Fedele L, Dorta M, Brisochi D, Giudici MN, Candiani GB. Pregnancies in septate uteri: outcome in relation to site of uterine implantation as determined by sonography. *Am J Roentgenol* 1989;152:781–784.
14. Fedele L, Zamberletti D, Vercellini P, Dorta M, Candiani GB. Reproductive performance of women with unicornuate uterus. *Fertil Steril* 1987;47:416–419.
15. Stray-Petersen B, Stray-Peterson S. Etiologic factors and subsequent reproductive performance in 195 couples with a prior history of habitual abortion. *Am J Obstet Gynecol* 1984;148:140–146.
16. Heinonen PK, Saarikoski S, Pystynen P. Reproductive performance of women with uterine anomalies. *Acta Obstet Gynecol Scand* 1982;61:157–162.
17. Heinonen PK, Pystynen P. Primary infertility and uterine anomalies. *Fertil Steril* 1983;40:311–316.
18. Jewelewicz R, Husami N, Wallach EE. When uterine factors cause infertility. *Contemp Obstet Gynecol* 1980;16:95–108.
19. Rock JA, Schlaff WD. The obstetrical consequences of uterovaginal anomalies. *Fertil Steril* 1985;43:681–692.
20. Ludmir J, Samuels P, Brooks S, Mennuti MT. Pregnancy outcome of patients with uncorrected uterine anomalies managed in a high-risk obstetric setting. *Obstet Gynecol* 1990;75:906–909.
21. Bennett MJ, Berry JVJ. Preterm labor and congenital malformations of the uterus. *Ultrasound Med Biol* 1979;5:83–85.
22. Stein AL, March CM. Pregnancy outcome in women with uterine malformations. *J Reprod Med* 1990;35:411–414.
23. Greiss FC Jr, Mauzy CH. Genital anomalies in women: an evaluation of diagnosis, incidence, and obstetric performance. *Am J Obstet Gynecol* 1961;82:330–339.
24. Fedele L, Zamberletti D, D'Alberton A, Vercellini P, Candiani GB. Gestational aspects of uterus didelphys. *J Reprod Med* 1988;33:353–356.
25. Miller ME, Dunn PM, Smith DW. Uterine malformation and fetal deformation. *J Pediatr* 1979;94(3):387–390.
26. Graham JM, Miller ME, Stephan MJ, Smith DW. Limb reduction anomalies and early in utero limb compression. *J Pediatr* 1980;96(6):1052–1056.
27. Tyler GT. Didelphis in sisters. *Am J Surg* 1939;45:337–338.
28. Drescher H. Sur frage gehaufsen familiaren vorkommens von uterus-missbildungen. *Zentralbl Gynaeko* 1966;88:1673–1675.
29. Polishuk WZ, Ron MA. Familial bicornuate and double uterus. *Am J Obstet Gynecol* 1974;119:982–987.
30. Stern AM, Gall AC, Perry BL, Stinson CW, Weitkamp LR, Poznanski AK. The hand-foot-uterus syndrome. *J Pediatr* 1970;77:109–116.

31. Poznanski AK, Kuhns LR, Lapides J, Stern AM. A new family with the hand-foot-uterus-genital syndrome: a wider spectrum of the hand-foot-uterus syndrome. In: Bergama D, ed. *Genetic forms of hypogonadism.* Miami Symposia Specialists for the National Foundation, March of Dimes, Bd: OAS XI, 1975;4:127–135.
32. Pinsky L. A community of human malformation syndromes involving the Müllerian ducts, distal extremities, urinary tract, and ears. *Teratology* 1973;9:65–80.
33. Duncan PA, Shapiro LR, Stangel JJ, Klein RM, Addonizio JC. The MURCS association: Müllerian duct aplasia, renal aplasia, and cervicothoracic somite dysplasia. *J Pediatr* 1979;95(3):399–402.
34. Carrington BM, Hricak H, Nurudden RN, Secaf E, Laros RK Jr, Hill EC. Müllerian duct anomalies: MR imaging evaluation. *Radiology* 1990;176:715–720.
35. Fielding C. Obstetric studies in women with congenital solitary kidneys. *Acta Obstet Gynecol Scand* 1965;44:555–562.
36. Thompson DP, Lynn HB. Genital anomalies associated with solitary kidney. *Mayo Clin Proc* 1966;41:538–549.
37. Erdogan E, Okan G, Daragenli O. Uterus didelphis with unilateral obstructed hemivagina and renal agenesis on the same side. *Acta Obstet Gynecol Scand* 1992;71:76–77.
38. Banner EA. The ectopic kidney in obstetrics and gynecology. *Surg Gynecol Obstet* 1965;121:32–36.
39. Li YW, Sheik CP, Chen WJ. Unilateral occlusion of duplicated uterus with ipsilateral renal anomaly in young girls: a study with MRI. *Pediatr Radiol* 1995;25:S54–S59.
40. Griffin JE, Edwards C, Madden JD, Harrod MJ, Wilson JD. Congenital absence of the vagina: the Mayer-Rokitansky-Kuster-Hauser syndrome. *Ann Int Med* 1976;85:224–236.
41. Fore SR, Hammond CB, Parker RT, Anderson EE. Urologic and genital anomalies in patients with congenital absence of the vagina. *Obstet Gynecol* 1975;46(4):410–416.
42. The American Fertility Society. The American Fertility Society classifications of adnexal adhesions, distal tubal occlusion, tubal occlusion secondary to tubal ligation, tubal pregnancies, Müllerian anomalies, and intrauterine adhesions. *Fertil Steril* 1988;49(6):944–955.
43. Rock JA. Surgery for anomalies of the Müllerian ducts. In: Rock JA, Thompson JD, eds. *Te Linde's operative gynecology,* 8th ed. Philadelphia: Lippincott–Raven Publishers, 1997; 687–727.
44. Reed MH, Griscom NT. Hydrometrocolpos in infancy. *AJR* 1973;118:1–13.
45. Pansini L, Torricelli M, Gomarasca A, Brambilla C, Beolchi S, Sideri M. Acute urinary retention due to didelphys uterus associated with an obstructed hemivagina in a 5 month old infant. *J Pediatr Surg* 1988;23(10):984–985.
46. Cook GT, Marshall VF. Hydrocolpos causing urinary obstruction. *J Urol* 1964;92:127–132.
47. Wilson DA, Stacy TM, Smith EI. Ultrasound diagnosis of hydrocolpos and hydrometrocolpos. *Radiology* 1978;128:451–454.
48. Olive DL, Henderson DY. Endometriosis and müllerian anomalies. *Obstet Gynecol* 1987;69(3):412–415.
49. Hanton EM, Malkasian GD Jr, Dockerty MB, Pratt JH. Endometriosis associated with complete or partial obstruction of menstrual egress. Report of 7 cases. *Obstet Gynecol* 1966;28:626–629.
50. Fedele L, Bianchi S, DiNola G, Franchi D, Candiani GB. Endometriosis and nonobstructive Müllerian anomalies. *Obstet Gynecol* 1992;79(4):515–517.
51. Valdes C, Malini S, Malenak LR. Ultrasound evaluation of female genital tract anomalies: a review of 64 cases. *Am J Obstet Gynecol* 1984;149:285–290.
52. Malini S, Valdes C, Malinak LR. Sonographic diagnosis and classification of anomalies of the female genital tract. *J Ultrasound Med* 1984;3:394–404.
53. Nussbaum AR, Sanders RC, Gearhart JP. Obstructed uterovaginal anomalies: demonstration with sonography. Part I. Neonates and infants. *Pediatr Radiol* 1991;179:79–83.
54. Nussbaum AR, Sanders RC, Rock RA. Obstructed uterovaginal anomalies: demonstration with sonography. Part II. Teenagers. *Pediatr Radiol* 1991;179:84–88.
55. Jones TB, Fleischer AC, Daniell JF, Lindsay AM, James AE. Sonographic characteristics of congenital uterine anomalies and associated pregnancy. *J Clin Ultrasound* 1980;8:435–437.
56. Sailer JF. Hematometra and hematocolpos: ultrasound findings. *AJR* 1979;132:1010–1011.
57. Reuter KL, Daly DC, Cohen SM. Septate versus bicornuate uteri: errors in diagnostic imaging. *Radiology* 1989;172:749–752.
58. Fedele L, Ferrazzi E, Dorta M, Vercellini P, Candiani GB. Ultrasonography in the differential diagnosis of double uteri. *Fertil Steril* 1988;50(2):361–364.
59. Pennes DR, Bowerman RA, Silver TM. Congenital uterine anomalies and associated pregnancies: findings and pitfalls of sonographic diagnosis. *J Ultrasound Med* 1985;4:531–538.

60. Edwards-Freeman C, Amin HK, Abiri M, Giustino PBS. The use of intraoperative ultrasonography in the surgical correction of a transverse vaginal septum. *J Clin Ultrasound* 1991;19:48–50.
61. Pellerito JS, McCarthy SM, Boyle MB, Glickman MG, DeCherney AH. Diagnosis of uterine anomalies: relative accuracy of MR imaging, endovaginal sonography, and hysterosalpingography. *Radiology* 1992; 183:795–800.
62. Scanlan KA, Pozniak MA, Fagerholm M, Shapiro S. Value of transperineal sonography in the assessment of vaginal atresia. *AJR* 1990;154:545–548.
63. Meyer WR, McCoy MC, Fritz MA. Combined abdominal-perineal sonography to assist in diagnosis of transverse vaginal septum. *Obstet Gynecol* 1995;85:882–884.
64. Mintz MC, Grumbach K. Imaging of uterine anomalies. *Semin Ultrasound Comput Tomogr Magn Reson Imaging* 1988;9(2):167–174.
65. Mintz MC, Thickman DI, Gussman D, Kressel HY. MR evaluation of uterine anomalies. *AJR* 1987;148:287–290.
66. Woodward PJ, Wagner BJ, Farley TE. MR imaging in the evaluation of female infertility. *Radiographics* 1993;13:293–310.
67. Fedele L, Dorta M, Brioschi D, Massari C, Candiani GB. Magnetic resonance evaluation of double uteri. *Obstet Gynecol* 1989;74(6):844–847.
68. Fielding JR. MR imaging of Müllerian anomalies: impact on therapy. *AJR* 1996;167:1491–1495.
69. Ascher SM. MR imaging of the female pelvis: the time has come. *Radiographics* 1998;18:931–945.
70. Schwartz LB, Panageas EP, Lange R, Rizzo J, Comite F, McCarthy S. Female pelvis: impact of MR imaging on treatment decisions and net cost analysis. *Radiology* 1994;192:55–60.
71. Doughty A, Nash SI, Gift DA. Deployment and utilization of MR imaging in Michigan: observations of a statewide data base. *Radiology* 1992;185:53–61.
72. Yu KK, Hricak H. Can MRI of the pelvis be cost effective? *Abdom Imaging* 1997;22:597–601.
73. Hricak H. Widespread use of MRI in gynecology: a myth or reality? *Abdom Imaging* 1997;22:579–588.
74. McCauley TR, McCarthy S, Lange R. Pelvic phased array coil: image quality assessment for spin-echo MR imaging. *Magn Reson Imaging* 1992;10:513–522.
75. Hayes CE, Dietz MJ, King BF, Ehman RL. Pelvic imaging with phased-array coils: quantitative assessment of signal to noise ratio improvement. *J Magn Reson Imaging* 1992;2:321–326.
76. Smith RC, Reinhold C, McCauley TR, Lange RC, Constable RT, Kier R, McCarthy S. Multicoil high-resolution fast spin echo MR imaging of the female pelvis. *Radiology* 1992;184:671–675.
77. Smith RC, Reinhold C, Lange RC, McCauley TR, Kier R, McCarthy S. Fast spin echo MR imaging of the female pelvis. 1. Use of a whole-volume coil. *Radiology* 1992;184:665–669.
78. Nghiem HV, Herfkens RJ, Frances IR, et al. The pelvis: T2-weighted fast spin echo MR imaging. *Radiology* 1992;185:213–217.
79. Outwater EK, Mitchell DG. Magnetic resonance imaging techniques in the pelvis. *MRI Clin N Am* 1994;2(2):161–188.
80. Baumgartner BR, Bernadino ME. MR imaging of the cervix: off axis scan to improve visualization of zonal anatomy. *AJR* 1989;153:1001–1002.
81. Demas BE, Hricak H, Jaffe RB. Uterine MR imaging: effects of hormonal stimulation. *Radiology* 1986;159:123–126.
82. Gryspeerdt S, Van Hoe L, Bosmans H, Baert AL, Vergote I, Marchal G. T2-weighted MR imaging of the uterus: comparison of optimized fast spin-echo and HASTE sequences with conventional fast spin echo sequences. *AJR* 1998;171:211–215.
83. Sugimara K, Okizuka H, Imauka I, Kayi Y, Takahashi K, Kitao M, Ishida T. Pelvic endometriosis: detection and diagnosis with chemical shift imaging. *Radiology* 1993;188:435–438.
84. Tan IL, Stoker J, Zwamborn AW, Entius KAC, Calame JJ, Lameris JS. Female pelvic floor: endovaginal MR imaging of normal anatomy. *Radiology* 1998;206:777–783.
85. Schnall MD, Connick T, Hayes CE, Lenkinski RE, Krensel HY. MR iamging of the pelvis with an endorectal-external multicoil array. *J Magn Reson Imaging* 1992;2:229–232.
86. Williams DI, Bloomberg S. Urogenital sinus in the female child. *J Pediatr Surg* 1976;11:51–57.
87. Hahn-Pederson J, Kvist N, Nielsen OH. Hydrometrocolopos: current views on pathogenesis and management. *J Urol* 1984;132:537–540.
88. Bartholemew TH, Gonzales ET. Urologic management in cloacal dysgenesis. *Urology* 1978;11:549–557.
89. Marshall FF, Jeffs RD, Sarafyan WK. Urogenital sinus abnormalities in the female patient. *J Urol* 1979;122:568–572.

90. Shatzkes DR, Haller JO, Velcek Francesca T. Imaging of uterovaginal anomalies in the pediatric patient. *Urol Radiol* 1991;13:58–66.

91. Laufer MR, Goldstein DP. Structural abnormalities of the female reproductive tract. In: Emans SJ, Laufer MR, Goldstein DP, eds. *Pediatric and adolescent gynecology*, 4th ed. Philadelphia: Lippincott-Raven Publishers, 1998:303–362.

92. Currie JL. Asymptomatic Müllerian anomalies. *Med Ann Dist Columbia* 1974;43:18–21.

93. Baird PA, Lowry RB. Absent vagina and the Kleppel-Feil anomaly. *Am J Obstet Gynecol* 1974;118:290–291.

94. Evans TN, Poland ML, Boving RL. Vaginal malformations. *Am J Obstet Gynecol* 1981;141:910–920.

95. Fedele L, Dorta M, Broschi D, Gindici MN, Candiani GB. Magnetic resonance imaging in Mayer-Rokitansky-Küster-Hauser syndrome. *Obstet Gynecol* 1990;76:593–596.

96. Carr BR. Disorders of the ovary and female reproductive tract. In: Wilson JD, Foster DW, eds. *Williams textbook of endocrinology*, 8th ed. Philadelphia: WB Saunders, 1992:733–798.

97. Schmed-Tannwald I, Hauser G. Deuting der "atypischen" formen des Mayer-Rokitansky-Küster syndrome. *Geburt-Shilfe Frauenheilkd* 1977;37:386–392.

98. Strübbe EH, Willemsen WNP, Lemmens JAM, Thijn CJP, Rolland R. Mayer-Rokitansky-Küster-Hauser syndrome: distinction between two forms based on excretory urographic, sonographic, and laparoscopic findings. *AJR* 1993;160:331–334.

99. Lodi A. Contribuo clinico statistico sulle malformazione alla vagina osservate nella. Clinica Obstetricia e Gynecologia di Milano dal 1906 al 1950. *Ann Obstet Gynecol Med Perinatal* 1951;73:1246–1251.

100. Rock JA, Zacur HA, Dlugi AM. Pregnancy success following surgical correction of imperforate hymen and complete transverse vaginal septum. *Obstet Gynecol* 1982;59:448–451.

101. Rock JA. Anomalous development of the vagina. *Semin Reprod Endocrinol* 1986;4:13–31.

102. McKusick VA, Bauer L, Koop CE, Scott RB. Hydrometrocolpos as a simply inherited malformation. *JAMA* 1964;189:813–816.

103. Barach B, Falces E, Benzian SR. Magnetic resonance imaging for diagnosis and preoperative planning in agenesis of the distal vagina. *Ann Plastic Surg* 1987;19:192–194.

104. Hugosson C, Jorulf H, Bakri Y. MRI in distal vaginal atresia. *Pediatr Radiol* 1991;21:281–283.

105. Siegelman ES, Outroater EK, Banner MP, Ramchandani P, Anderson TL, Schnall MD. High resolution MR imaging of the vagina. *Radiographics* 1997;17:1183–1203.

106. Geary WL, Weed JC. Congenital atresia of the uterine cervix. *Obstet Gynecol* 1973;42:213–217.

107. Maciulla GJ, Heine MW, Christian CD. Functional endometrial tissue with vaginal agenesis. *J Reprod Med* 1978;21:373–375.

108. Dillon WP, Mudalian NA, Wingate NB. Congenital atresia of the cervix. *Obstet Gynecol* 1979;54:126–129.

109. Niver DH, Barrette G, Jewelewicz R. Congenital atresia of the uterine cervix and vagina—three cases. *Fertil Steril* 1980;33:25–29.

110. Jones HW, Rock JA, eds. *Reparative and constructive surgery of the female generative tract*. Baltimore: Williams & Wilkins, 1983.

111. Farber M. Congenital atresia of the uterine cervix. *Semin Reprod Endocrinol* 1986;4:33–38.

112. Markham SM, Waterhouse TB. Structural anomalies of the reproductive tract. *Curr Opin Obstet Gynecol* 1992;4:867–873.

113. O'Leary JL, O'Leary JA, Rudimentary horn pregnancy. *Obstet Gynecol* 1963;22:371–375.

114. Fedele L, Dorta M, Brisochi D, Giudic MN, Villa L. Magnetic resonance imaging of unicornuate uterus. *Acta Obstet Gynecol Scand* 1990;69:511–513.

115. Musich JR, Behrman SJ. Obstetric outcome before and after metroplasty in women with uterine anomalies. *Obstet Gynecol* 1978;52:63–66.

116. Jones WS. Obstetric significance of female genital anomalies. *Obstet Gynecol* 1957;10:113–127.

117. Candiani GB, Ferrazzi E, Fedele L, Vercellini P, Dorta M. Sonographic evaluation of uterine morphology: a new scanning technique. *Acta Eur Fertil* 1986;17:345–349.

118. Fedele L, Dorta M, Broschi D, Villa L, Arcaina L, Bianchi S. Re-examination of the anatomic indications for hysteroscope metroplasty. *Eur J Obstet Gynecol Rep Biol* 1991;39:127–131.

119. Mahgoub SE. Unification of a septate uterus: Mahgoub's operation. *Int J Gynecol Obstet* 1978;15:400–404.

120. Jones HW, Jones GE. Double uterus as an etiologic factor in repeated abortion: indications for surgical repair. *Am J Obstet Gynecol* 1953;65:325–339.

121. Capraro VJ, Chuang JT, Randall CL. Improved fetal salvage after metroplasty. *Obstet Gynecol* 1968;31:97–103.
122. Rock JA, Jones HW. The clinical management of the double uterus. *Fertil Steril* 1977;28:798–805.
123. Valle RF, Sciarra JJ. Hysteroscopic treatment of the septate uterus. *Obstet Gynecol* 1986;67:253–257.
124. Daly DC, Walters CA, Soto-Albors CE, Riddick DH. Hysteroscopic metroplasty: surgical technique and obstetric outcome. *Fertil Steril* 1983;39:623–628.
125. Chevenak FA, Newirth RS. Hysteroscopic resection of the uterine septum. *Am J Obstet Gynecol* 1981;141:351–353.
126. DeCherney AH, Russel JB, Graebe RA, Polan ML. Resectoscopic management of Müllerian fusion defects. *Fertil Steril* 1986;45:726–728.
127. Israel R, March CM. Hysteroscopic incision of the septate uterus. *Am J Obstet Gynecol* 1984; 149:66–73.
128. Strassman EO. Operations for double uterus and endometrial atresia. *Clin Obstet Gynecol* 1961;4:240–255.
129. Kaufman RH, Bender GL, Gray PM, Adam E. Upper genital tract changes associated with exposure in utero to diethylstilbestrol. *Am J Obstet Gynecol* 1977;128:51–59.
130. Haney AF, Hammond CB, Soules MR, Creasman WT. Diethylstilbestrol induced upper genital tract abnormalities. *Fertil Steril* 1979;31:142–146.
131. Nagel TC, Malo JW. Hysteroscopic metroplasty in the diethylstilbestrol-exposed uterus and similar nonfusion anomalies: effects on subsequent reproductive performance; a preliminary report. *Fertil Steril* 1993;59:502–506.
132. Stanton S. Gynecologic complications of epispadius and bladder extrophy. *Am J Obstet Gynecol* 1974;199:749–754.
133. Jones HW. An anomaly of the external genitalia in female patients with extrophy of the bladder. *Am J Obstet Gynecol* 1973;117:748–756.
134. Blakely CR, Mills WG. The obstetric and gynecologic complications of bladder extrophy and epispadius. *Br J Obstet Gynecol* 1981;88:167–173.
135. Bakri YN, AL-Sugair A, Hugosson C. Bicornuate nonfused rudimentary uterine horns with functioning endometria and complete cervical-vaginal agenesis: magnetic resonance diagnosis. *Fertil Steril* 1992;58:620–621.

Congenital Malformations of the Female Genital Tract: Diagnosis and Management, edited by G. Gidwani and T. Falcone.
Lippincott Williams & Wilkins, Philadelphia © 1999.

5

Management of Emergencies Associated with Congenital Malformations of the Female Genital Tract

Betsy Schroeder and *Joseph Salvatore Sanfilippo

*Department of Obstetrics and Gynecology, University of Louisville, Louisville, Kentucky 40292, and *Department of Obstetrics and Gynecology, Allegheny University of the Health Sciences, Pittsburgh, Pennsylvania 15212*

The paramesonephric system is responsible for Müllerian tract development. Failure of lateral fusion or lack of resorption of the vertical midline septum results in a Müllerian anomaly. Due to the intimate anatomic and embryologic development of the urinary and genital systems, the urinary tract is often also affected; skeletal defects, including spina bifida occulta, occur as well.

The classification of Müllerian anomalies is an effort to meet the challenges of succinctly placing the frequently varied findings into clear categories. The American Fertility Society, now called the American Society for Reproductive Medicine, classification (1) (Fig. 1) is perhaps the most commonly utilized system; however, clinicians should also be aware of the classification described by Toaff et al. (2) (Fig. 2).

The typical scenario for presentation of a Müllerian anomaly is often variegated with respect to signs and symptoms and may prove to be a clinical challenge. They may escape detection or be incidental findings as manifested by a case report of a 27-year-old woman, gravida 4, para 2, who presented for tubal ligation, at which time her unicornuate uterus and rudimentary horn were first recognized (3). Oftentimes the patient may be totally asymptomatic until there is evidence of repeat pregnancy wastage, and appropriate consideration to the presence of a communicating or noncommunicating rudimentary horn must be in the differential diagnosis. There may be a pelvic mass, which may or may not be associated with symptoms. A vaginal bulging mass or hemivagina is indicative of complete or partial outflow tract obstruction. One must be cognizant that when an adolescent presents with pelvic pain, either in association with primary amenorrhea or several months following the onset of menarche, consideration should be given to a Müllerian anomaly. When presentation is symptomatic, emergent management might be required.

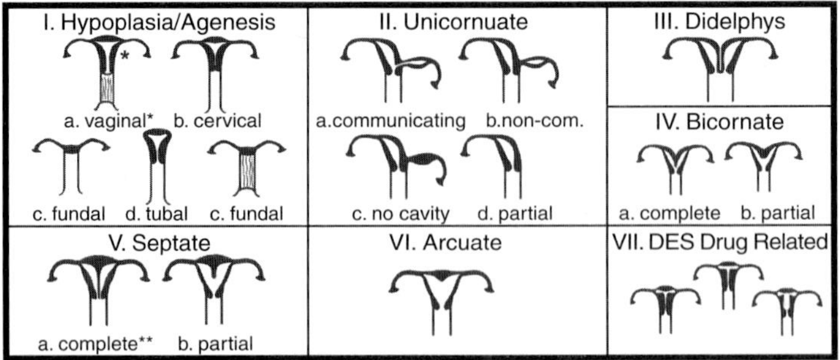

FIG. 1. The American Fertility Society classification of Müllerian anomalies. (From ref. 1, with permission.)

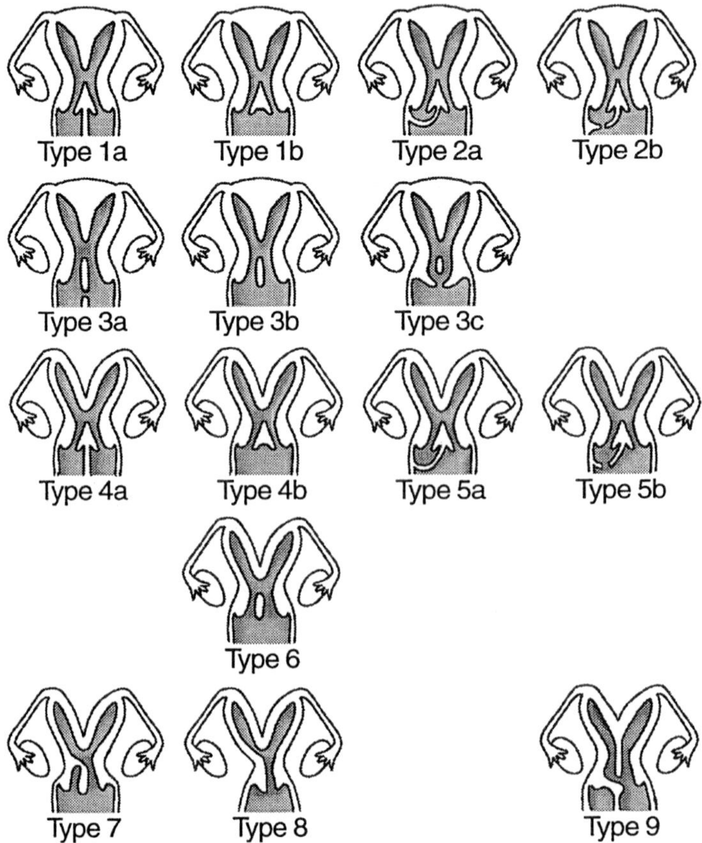

FIG. 2. Morphologic classification of communicating uteri. (From ref. 2, with permission.)

OUTFLOW TRACT OBSTRUCTION

Outflow tract obstruction can result from a number of distinct anomalies including the imperforate hymen, transverse vaginal septum, and noncommunicating rudimentary horn. As menstrual fluid accumulates proximal to the obstruction, the resulting hematocolpos, hematometra, or hematocolpometra causes cyclic pain and/or a pelvic mass. These obstructions are best divided according to the location of the obstruction.

Distal Vagina/Imperforate Hymen

Distal vagina/imperforate hymen is perhaps the most common obstructive anomaly, and familial occurrences have been reported (4). In the newborn period and early infancy, this may be diagnosed by a bulging membrane due to a mucocolpos from maternal estrogen stimulation. If it is not noted at this time, it is often not diagnosed until puberty, when menstrual fluid accumulates. The clinical presentation is often that of a bulging blue-black membrane, primary amenorrhea, and normal secondary sex characteristics. Depending on the circumstance, the patient may have cyclic abdominal pain and/or a pelvic mass. This problem requires incision/resection of the membrane, thus relieving the outflow tract obstruction (5) (Fig. 3). Repair should occur at the time of diagnosis if the patient is symptomatic. While repair may be accomplished anytime during infancy, childhood, or adolescence, it is facilitated by estrogen stimulation and thus ideally performed in adolescence.

Proximal or Midvaginal Transverse Septum

Vertical fusion defects can result in a transverse septum that may be imperforate and associated with a hematocolpos or hematometra in adolescents or a mucocolpos in children, or it may have a small, pinpoint aperture and cyclic menses. Patients frequently become symptomatic as fluid accumulates in the vagina. As with the imperforate hymen, a mass may be present, and the vagina will appear short or blind-ended. The approach to resection of the septum depends on the presence or absence of an opening. In the presence of such, cannulation should be attempted with resection of the septum. Postoperatively, use of a vaginal stent may be necessary.

Rudimentary Horns

Clinical emergency with respect to rudimentary horns in the non-pregnant patient results from the presence of a horn with a functional endometrium and outflow tract obstruction. As with other types of outflow tract obstruction, severe lower abdominal pain with a pelvic mass is the primary presentation for a blind rudimentary horn. In contrast to other forms of outflow tract obstruction, however, primary amenorrhea is usually not present since the opposite horn is unlikely to be obstructed.

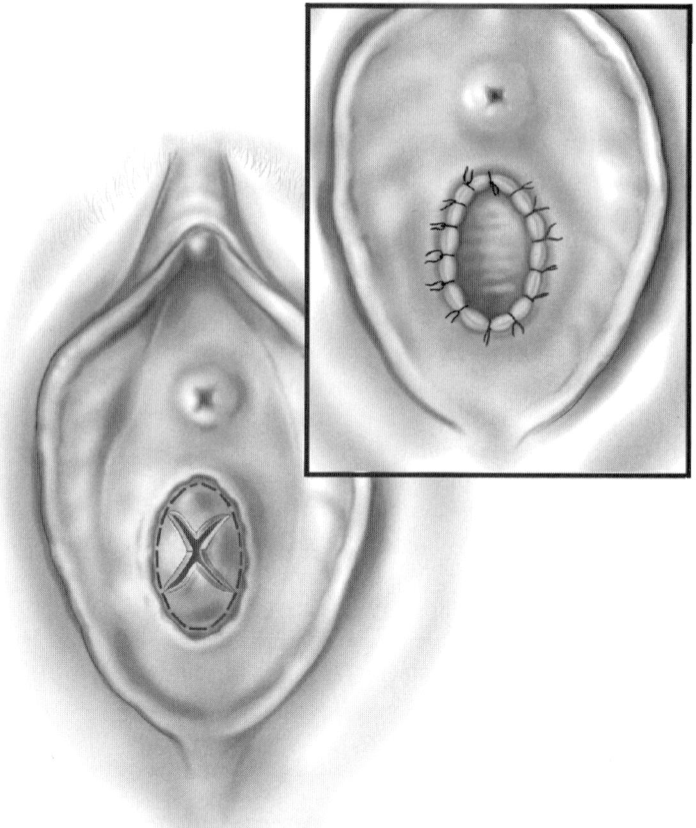

FIG. 3. Hymenectomy of an imperforate hymen with a stellate incision. (Adapted from ref. 5, with permission.)

Ultrasonography is instrumental in identifying and differentiating various aspects of the rudimentary horn. An intravenous pyelogram or renal ultrasound should be obtained with all Müllerian anomalies. If there is evidence of a functional endometrium, the primary recommendation is to proceed with surgical extirpation. This can be accomplished either via laparotomy or laparoscopy.

Asymptomatic rupture of a rudimentary horn was reported by Muram and co-workers in a 41-year-old woman who was admitted for a right adnexal mass (5 cm in diameter). Ultrasound identified a normal main body of the uterus and an ovoid solid anterior mass on the right side contiguous to the uterus. The patient was felt to have had a "chronic ectopic pregnancy." At the time of laparotomy, a bicornuate uterus was identified with the right horn being rudimentary, attached to the left horn with a wide band of fibrous tissue. A hemihysterectomy was performed, resulting in preservation of fertility (6).

RUDIMENTARY HORN PREGNANCY

Pregnancy in a rudimentary horn is extremely rare, occurring in an estimated 1/40,000 to 1/400,000 (7–9) pregnancies and in 1/5,000 to 1/15,000 ectopic pregnancies (10,11). This may occur as a result of a fibromuscular or fibrous band connecting the unicornuate uterus and the rudimentary horn, but 80% to 85% of cases are noncommunicating (11). In this situation, the pregnancy is the result of transperitoneal migration of either sperm or the fertilized ovum (12). This is supported by the fact that the corpus luteum is found on the contralateral side in 10% of reported cases (8,13).

In contrast to tubal pregnancies, rudimentary horn pregnancies are often not detected until the second trimester. The duration of the pregnancy is related to the thickness of the rudimentary horn's musculature as well as the ability of the myometrium to hypertrophy and dilate (11). Due to the greater muscle wall thickness of most horns, rupture typically occurs later than in tubal gestation (14). The average gestational age is 21 weeks, but it may occur as early as 5 weeks or as late as 35 weeks (11,13).

Most patients are diagnosed only after rupture occurs. They have acute abdominal pain with peritoneal signs, and they are often in shock. When rupture does occur, the intraperitoneal hemorrhage that is present may be so massive as to be life threatening and require immediate surgical intervention (15–17). Maternal mortality is quoted at 5%, with 90% of this occurring within 10 to 15 minutes after rupture (18). While fetal salvage has been described (16,17,19–21), fetal demise occurs in 98% (13).

Prior to rupture, diagnosis of a rudimentary horn pregnancy may be quite difficult. It should be suspected in any gravida with a known rudimentary horn, and these patients should be followed closely until an intrauterine pregnancy has been documented. In those who have not been previously diagnosed with a rudimentary horn, findings on early pelvic exam may raise the possibility and are similar to findings of tubal ectopic pregnancy. These include deviation of the cervix to one side with an adnexal mass on the opposite side. Findings prior to rupture include an extrauterine gestational sac next to a slightly enlarged uterus. The confines of the rudimentary horn delineate the placenta and gestational sac within it, and this differentiates it from a tubal or cornual pregnancy (10,22,23).

Management is surgical resection of the rudimentary horn. If the diagnosis is made prior to rupture in early gestation, this may be accomplished laparoscopically (24). In the majority of cases, however, as the diagnosis is not made until rupture with excessive intraperitoneal hemorrhage or the pregnancy is too large to be removed via laparoscopy, laparotomy is required.

ACUTE URINARY RETENTION

In children and adolescents, acute urinary retention most commonly occurs as a result of dysuria due to a urinary tract infection (25). In women, it is most frequently associated with a pelvic mass, occurring in one third of cases excluding those who are postoperative or postpartum (26). Not surprising, then, is the association between Müllerian anomalies with outflow tract obstruction and urinary retention (27–32). While some authors believe it to be quite a rare condition (33,34), others cite the incidence of acute urinary retention in patients with an imperforate hymen and hematocolpometra to be as high as 37% to 60% (31,32).

Any outflow tract obstruction resulting in accumulation of fluid in the vagina and/or uterus may cause urinary retention. Several theories may explain the development of urinary retention as a result of mucocolpos in the first years of life or hematocolpos, hematometra, or hematocolpometra during the pubertal years. The retained fluid in the vagina compresses the urethra, and this is aggravated by the fluid-filled uterus applying pressure on the posterior wall of the bladder and changing the angle of the urethra (32). Pressure on the sacral plexus from the distended vagina has also been offered as an explanation (35).

Patients typically present as adolescents with lower abdominal pain and the inability to void. They may have other urinary symptoms such as hesitancy and incomplete voiding for several days prior to presentation. They also generally have primary amenorrhea, a history of cyclic lower abdominal pain, and a pelvic mass. However, if the obstruction is unilateral, as with a noncommunicating rudimentary horn or an obstructed hemivagina, the patient may have normal menses.

Temporary but immediate relief can be provided by urethral catheterization. If resistance occurs with an appropriately sized rubber catheter, a pediatric feeding tube may be used, or, if necessary, a spinal needle may be passed suprapubically to empty the bladder. Urine should be sent for urinalysis and culture as urinary stasis promotes infection. Once the acute condition has been addressed, the underlying problem should be evaluated appropriately and treated to evacuate the obstructing mass.

While not as severe as acute urinary retention, urinary tract infections have also been associated with Müllerian anomalies. This may result from renal anomalies with vesicourethral reflux, or it may precede retention as a result of vaginal outflow obstruction. This has been described by Brevetti et al. (36) in a 7-week-old girl with a pyocolpos due to an imperforate hymen, as well as by Capraro et al. (37) who described the microperforate hymen after studying 25 girls with recurrent urinary tract infections or vulvovaginitis. Müllerian anomalies should be part of the differential diagnosis in all prepubertal girls with two or more urinary tract infections or a single case of pyelonephritis.

CONCLUSION

When an adolescent presents with pelvic pain soon after menarche, think "Müllerian anomaly." Prompt diagnosis and surgical intervention is especially important with pregnancy in a rudimentary horn. In the nonpregnant state, outflow tract obstruction and acute urinary retention might also require emergent attention. Clinicians should always entertain the possibility of a Müllerian tract defect and evaluate appropriately.

REFERENCES

1. American Fertility Society. The American Fertility Society classifications of adnexal adhesions, distal tubal occlusion, tubal occlusion secondary to tubal ligation, tubal pregnancies, Müllerian anomalies, and intrauterine adhesions. *Fertil Steril* 1988;49(6):944.

2. Toaff ME, Lev-Toaff AS, Toaff R. Communicating uteri: review and classification with introduction of two previously unreported types. *Fertil Steril* 1984;41:661.
3. Robischon K, Baram D, Phipps WR. Presentation of a Müllerian anomaly with outflow obstruction after tubal ligation. *Fertil Steril* 1996;65(4):866.
4. Usta IM, Awwad JT, et al. Imperforate hymen: report of an unusual familial occurrence. *Obstet Gynecol* 1993;82:655.
5. Rock JA, Horowitz IR. Surgical conditions of the vagina and urethra. In: Rock JA, Thompson JD, eds. *Te Linde's operative gynecology,* 8th ed. Philadelphia: Lippincott-Raven Publishers, 1997;913.
6. Muram D, McAlister MS, Winer-Muram HT, Smith WC. Asymptomatic rupture of a rudimentary horn. *Obstet Gynecol* 1987;69:486.
7. Sfar E, Zina S, Bourghida S, Bettaieb A, Chelli H. Pregnancy in a rudimentary horn: main clinical forms. *Rev Fr Gynecol Obstet* 1994;89(1):21.
8. Johansen K. Pregnancy in a rudimentary horn. *Obstet Gynecol* 1983;61:565.
9. Seoud MA, Khalil AM, Abdel-Karim FW, Suidan JS. Pregnancy in a non-communicating rudimentary horn. *Int J Gynaecol Obstet* 1989;28(3): 275–278.
10. Holden R, Hart P. First trimester rudimentary horn pregnancy: prerupture ultrasound diagnosis. *Obstet Gynecol* 1983;61:56S.
11. O'Leary J, O'Leary J. Rudimentary horn pregnancy. *Obstet Gyncol* 1963;22:371.
12. Aydemit V, Ulusoy M, Bozkaya H. Pregnancy in a noncommunicating rudimentary horn. *Isr J Med Sci* 1993;29:314.
13. Rolen A, Choquette A, Semmens J. Rudimentary uterine horn: obstetric and gynecologic implications. *Obstet Gynecol* 1966;27:806.
14. Wahlen T. Pregnancy in a noncommunicating rudimentary uterine horn. *Acta Obstet Gynecol Scand* 1972;51:155.
15. Virkud A, Rajwade A, Deshmukh M. Rupture of rudimentary horn pregnancy (case report). *J Postgrad Med* 1988;34:57.
16. Nagele F, Langle R, Stolzlechner J, Taschner R. Noncommunicating rudimentary horn—obstetric and gynecologic implications. *Acta Obstet Gynecol Scand* 1995;74:566.
17. Zaidi J, Carr J. Rupture of rudimentary uterine horn with fetal salvage. *Acta Obstet Gynecol Scand* 1994;73:359.
18. DeNicola R, Peterson M. Pregnancy in rudimentary horn of uterus. *Am J Surg* 1947;73:382.
19. Larsen P, Hahn-Pederson J, Lange A. Pregnancy in a noncommunicating rudimentary horn with a successful outcome. *Acta Obstet Gynecol Scand* 1983;62:93.
20. Heinonen P, Aro P. Rupture of pregnant noncommunicating horn with fetal salvage. *Eur J Obstet Gynecol Reprod Biol* 1988;27(3):261.
21. O'Grady J, Salem F. Rudimentary horn pregnancy with neonatal and fetal survival. *J Natl Med Assoc* 1978;70:863.
22. Chang W, Lin H, Ho H, Sheu B, Huang S, Lee T. Ultrasound diagnosis of rudimentary horn pregnancy in fourteen weeks of gestation: a case report. *Asia Oceana J Obstet Gynaecol* 1994;20(3): 279.
23. Achiron R, Tadmor O, Kamar R. Prerupture ultrasound diagnosis of interstitial and rudimentary horn pregnancy in the second trimester. *Int J Reprod Med* 1992;37:89.
24. Dulemba J, Medgett W, Freeman M. Laparoscopic management of a rudimentary horn pregnancy. *J Am Assoc Gynecol Laparosc* 1996;3(4): 627.
25. Peter J, Steinhardt G. Acute urinary retention in children. *Pediatr Emerg Care* 1993;9(4):205.
26. Doran J, Roberts M. Acute urinary retention in the female. *Br J Urol* 1976;47:793.
27. Yu T, Lin M. Acute urinary retention in two patients with imperforate hymen. *Scand J Urol Nephrol* 1993;27:543.
28. Loong E, Yuen P. Acute urinary retention caused by a unilateral hematometra. *Arch Gynecol Obstet* 1990;247:211.
29. Nisanian A. Hematocolpometra presenting as urinary retention: a case report. *J Reprod Med* 1993;38:57.
30. Wort S, Heman-Ackah C, Davies A. Acute urinary retention in the young female. *Br J Urol* 1995;76:659.
31. Calvin J, Nichamin S. Hematocolpos due to imperforate hymen. *Am J Dis Child* 1936;51:832.
32. Tompkins P. The treatment of imperforate hymen with hematocolpos: a review of 113 cases in the literature and the report of five additional cases. *JAMA* 1939;113:913.
33. Sondgrass M. Acute urinary retention in females: report of a case due to hematocolpometra. *JAMA* 1931;97:777.

34. Lazarus J. Two cases of urinary retention from vaginal occlusion. *NY State Med J* 1932;32:339.
35. Bejanga I. Hematocolpos with imperforate hymen. *Int Surg* 1978;63:97.
36. Brevetti L, Brevetti G, Lawrence J, Soper R. Pyocolpos: diagnosis and treatment. *J Pediatr Surg* 1997;32(1):110.
37. Capraro V, Dillon W, Gallego M. Microperforate hymen, a distinct clinical entity. *Obstet Gynecol* 1974;44:903.

Congenital Malformations of the Female Genital Tract: Diagnosis and Management, edited by G. Gidwani and T. Falcone.
Lippincott Williams & Wilkins, Philadelphia © 1999.

6

Management of Disorders of the External Genitalia

Robert Kay and Jonathan H. Ross

Section of Pediatric Urology, The Cleveland Clinic Foundation, Cleveland, Ohio 44195

Children with abnormal external genitalia pose a medical, surgical, and psychological challenge to the pediatric health care team responsible for patient management. A rational, unbiased approach to the patient, with decision and treatment performed early in life, will lead to the best possible outcome of an unfortunate embryologic developmental abnormality. As a better understanding of embryologic development evolves coupled with increasing surgical sophistication and better functional and cosmetic outcomes, the child born with abnormal external genitalia can be helped to live a productive, fulfilling, and psychologically stable life. The embryologic development, diagnosis, and management of children with abnormal external genitalia can fall under a much larger subject of intersexual abnormalities. This includes genetic and gonadal abnormalities, with external genitalia abnormalities presenting as a manifestation of this broader context. The purpose of this chapter is to focus on the normal embryologic development of the genitalia, their abnormal development, and the manifestation of the external genitalia in these children with a specific treatment approach when it has been decided to rear the patient as a female infant.

NORMAL DEVELOPMENT OF EXTERNAL GENITALIA

The external genitalia of the fetus is unique in the developing embryo as it has the ability to become either that which is normally associated with male development or that which is normally associated with female development. This universal tissue, which is modulated by the external hormonal milieu, gives us great understanding in both the development of the normal and abnormal genitalia. The embryologic tissues of the internal and external genitalia, i.e., the Wolffian and Müllerian structures, are present in all children and are dependent on the hormonal milieu to either reach maximal development or regress to vestigial remnants. The external genitalia possess the same potential in that there is a single, generic tissue that may develop and grow or regress and present clinically as male or female, depending on the functional level of hormones to which the child is exposed.

As described in more detail elsewhere in this book, the genital development of the female is a more passive process than that of the male. In the absence of sex steroid hormones or other factors, the internal and external genitalia will develop along a female line. On the opposite end of the spectrum is the fully developed male. This is dependent on two separate and distinct hormones: androgens in the form of testosterone and a Müllerian-inhibiting substance (1). These two hormones are produced by the developing testis.

By the eighth week of gestation, the developing testis begins to have an endocrine function (2). Because the fetal circulation is poor at this point, most actions are local rather than systemic. Testosterone is produced by the Leydig cells and stimulates the Wolffian ducts to develop into the epididymis, vas, and the seminal vesicle. The concentration of testosterone reaches a maximum at 12 weeks, at which time all of the external genitalia have differentiated (3). The masculinization of the external genitalia is dependent on the conversion of testosterone to its more powerful androgenic analog, 5-dihydrotestosterone. This conversion is dependent on the presence of the enzyme 5α-reductase. In the absence of this enzyme, the external genitalia will not develop and the female phenotype will ensue. 5-Dihydrotestosterone induces the genital tubercle to enlarge. In addition, the urogenital groove will close, forming the urethra. Mesoderm will expand and form the scrotum, and later in gestation the testis will descend. The development of the male genitalia is then complete by the third month, with growth of the penis occurring shortly before birth.

The female development, in contrast, is hormonally independent and an autonomous process. In the classic experiments by Jost in 1947, experiments on fetal rabbits clearly delineated the effects of androgen and Müllerian-inhibiting substances (4). In those fetal rabbits that had been castrated early in gestation, the female phenotype was seen. In those in which there was a unilateral castration, the local process dictated that on the side on which there was no gonad, female internal genitalia developed, but if there was a testis on the other side, the Wolffian structure developed on the ipsilateral side. When testosterone crystals were applied locally, the Wolffian structures developed as if they had a normal testis but the Müllerian structures developed as if there was no Müllerian-inhibiting substance. The development of the external genitalia depended on the circulation of androgens.

CLASSIFICATION

There are several classification schemes for intersexual disorders that are based on the etiology of the intersexual abnormalities or on gonadal histology. Although either is acceptable, both reflect intersex as a discrepancy between genetic sex, gonadal sex, and phenotypic sex, and attempt to create a framework in which the specific disease may be identified and understood within the context of normal sexual development (Table 1) (5).

TABLE 1. *Classification of intersex states*

Disorders of genetic sex
    Turner's syndrome
    Mixed gonadal dysgenesis
    Kleinfelter's syndrome
    46,XX male
Disorders of gonadal sex
    True hermaphroditism
    Pure gonadal dysgenesis
    Vanishing testis syndrome
Disorders of phenotypic sex
    Female pseudohermaphroditism
      Congenital adrenal hyperplasia
      Nonadrenal
        Maternal progestational agents
        Virilizing tumors of mother
    Male pseudohermaphroditism
      Abnormalities in androgen synthesis
      Abnormalities in androgen action
        Complete testicular feminization
        Incomplete testicular feminization
          Type 1. Reifenstein's, Lubs' syndromes
          Type 2. 5α-Reductase deficiency
    Persistent Müllerian duct syndrome

DIAGNOSIS AND EVALUATION

Evaluation of intersexual patients should include a complete family history, a physical examination, biochemical evaluation, karyotype, and an assessment of internal genitalia by genitogram, ultrasound, and, if needed, laparoscopy and gonadal biopsy (Table 2) (5).

TABLE 2. *Evaluation of ambiguous genitalia*

History
    Family history
    Pregnancy (drugs, illness)
Physical examination
    Phallus size
    Location of urethra
    Labioscrotal folds
    Palpable gonads
    Excessive pigmentation
    Rectal (presence of cervix)
Genetic determination
    Karyotype
Biochemical
    Plasma 17-OH progesterone
Genitogram
Ultrasound of pelvis
Endoscopy
Laparoscopy or laparotomy
Gonadal biopsy

The infant with any abnormal external genitalia should raise an immediate index of suspicion as a possible intersexual anomaly. The length of the phallus should be measured and compared to norms (6). At any time that there is an abnormality in the penile length, a suspicion of intersex should be entertained. In addition, the location of the urethra should be identified. Although the majority of these patients will have isolated, classic hypospadias, further evaluation should occur if the infant also has a unilateral impalpable gonad or a very small phallus.

Labial scrotal folds should be observed and characterized. Again, an index of suspicion for intersexual abnormality should be raised. A palpable gonad usually represents a testis. Rare situations may occur in which a hernia with an ovary could be present, but again, in the overwhelming majority of cases a palpable gonad is a testis. A rectal exam should also be included to attempt to palpate a cervix.

MANAGEMENT

Male Rearing

Sex assignment may depend on many factors including the child's potential to successfully develop and function in an assigned sex. If the child is to be reared as a boy, hormones will be required. Exogenous androgen may be started in the immediate newborn period. In most cases we use testosterone 25 mg IM every 3 weeks, measuring hormonal levels and the growth of the phallus. When the phallus reaches an acceptable size, the child is monitored and hormonal supplements are used as necessary. Although some treating physicians use topical testosterone cream, parenteral administration controls the systemic amount and avoids any psychological bonding issues that may arise from the parents' rubbing cream onto the genitals hoping for growth. This may be repeated at any point during the child's infancy and childhood life to ensure adequate age-specific growth of the phallus. Before 1 year of age all abnormalities should be surgically repaired including chordee, hypospadias, and orchidopexy, if necessary.

Female Rearing

Timing

Once the decision has been reached to rear the child as a girl, surgical correction should be done as soon as possible. In the setting of congenital adrenal hyperplasia that means as soon as the child's medication is tolerated and the child is medically stable and can undergo surgery. If the child has no hormonal abnormalities, this may be done in the newborn period.

Surgery of the Clitoris

Clitoromegaly

It is very clear that the historical surgical treatment of clitorectomy for clitoromegaly is contraindicated and has no place in the modern management of these children. The sensation of the glans clitoris has been shown to be important for adult function and should be retained. This may be done by either clitoral recession or reduction clitoroplasty.

Recession clitoroplasty can only be used for the very small clitoris. Popularized by Lattimer and later by Randolph and Hung, this effectively involves recessing the clitoris under the symphysis so that it is covered and not seen (7,8). Late problems such as growth of the corpus cavernosa with painful erections and unsightly external genitalia have rendered this operation obsolete except in very rare cases.

Reduction clitoroplasty is the procedure of choice (9–11) (Fig. 1). This allows preservation of the neurovascular bundle with normal sensation and excellent cosmetic appearance. The operation consists of excising all corpus cavernosa, reduction of the size of the glans, creation of the labia majora and labia minora, and recession of the glans clitoris.

Procedure

Vaginoplasty. Vaginoplasty must be performed in many of these patients. Congenital adrenal hyperplasia will serve as the prototype for this discussion but vaginoplasty may have to be done in more complex patients such as those with mixed gonadal dysgenesis.

Timing

The question of timing of vaginoplasty remains controversial. The proponents of early vaginoplasty argue that the child should appear as a normal girl as soon as possible, which is important both in terms of psychological bonding from the family and the child's self-image. Reconstruction of hypospadias in boys is now successfully done as early as 6 months in order to minimize psychological trauma to both parents and child (11,12). The same principles may be applied to the genital reconstruction in girls. The disadvantage, however, is a higher incidence of introital stenosis, which may lead to secondary operations later in life (13). These issues must be considered on a case-by-case basis with no universal approach for all children with these abnormalities.

Late repair in adolescence or early adulthood, immediately prior to sexual activity, is done to try to prevent introital stenosis. This could be done with cooperation of the patient using dilatation, obturation, or even sexual activity to ensure introital patency. Although the results may obviate the need for further surgery, it commits the patient to a childhood devoid of a vagina.

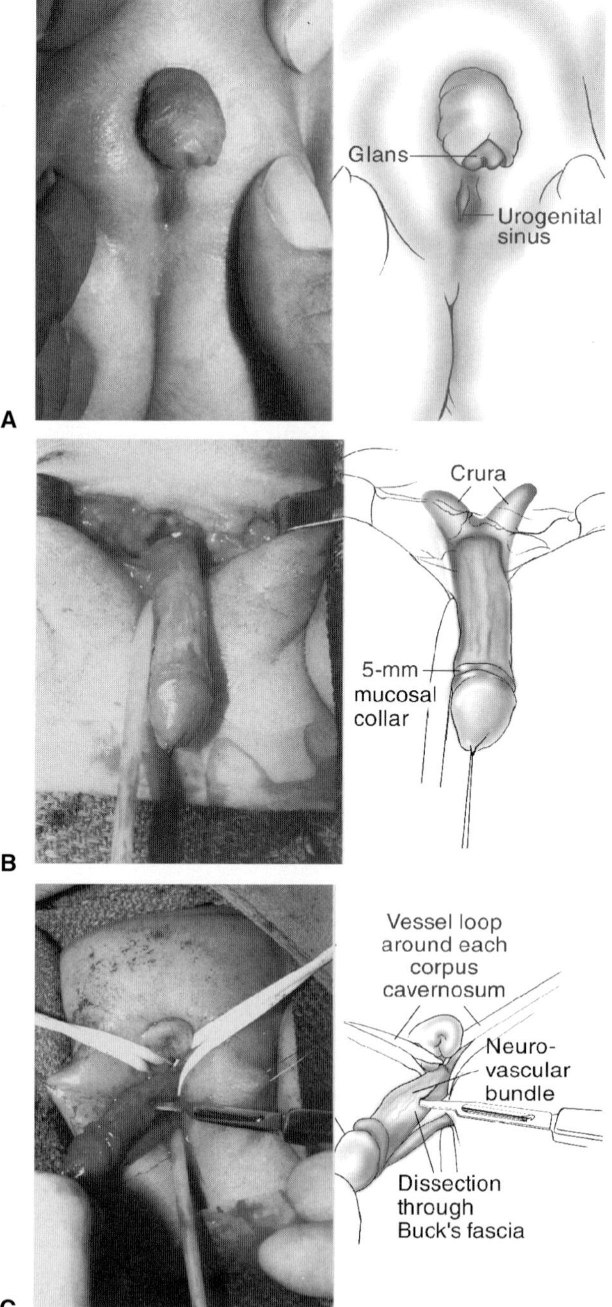

FIG. 1. A: A reduction clitoroplasty is demonstrated. Preoperative appearance of the infant with congenital adrenal hyperplasia with an enlarged phallus and a solitary urogenital sinus. **B:** The phallus is degloved with a 5-mm mucosa collar. The dissection is extended to beyond the symphysis pubis and the bifurcation of the corpora cavernosum. **C:** After degloving of the phallus and control of each corpus cavernosum, an incision is made through Buck's fascia and into the tunica albuginea. This incision will allow the neurovascular bundle to be separated from the corpora cavernosum without injury.

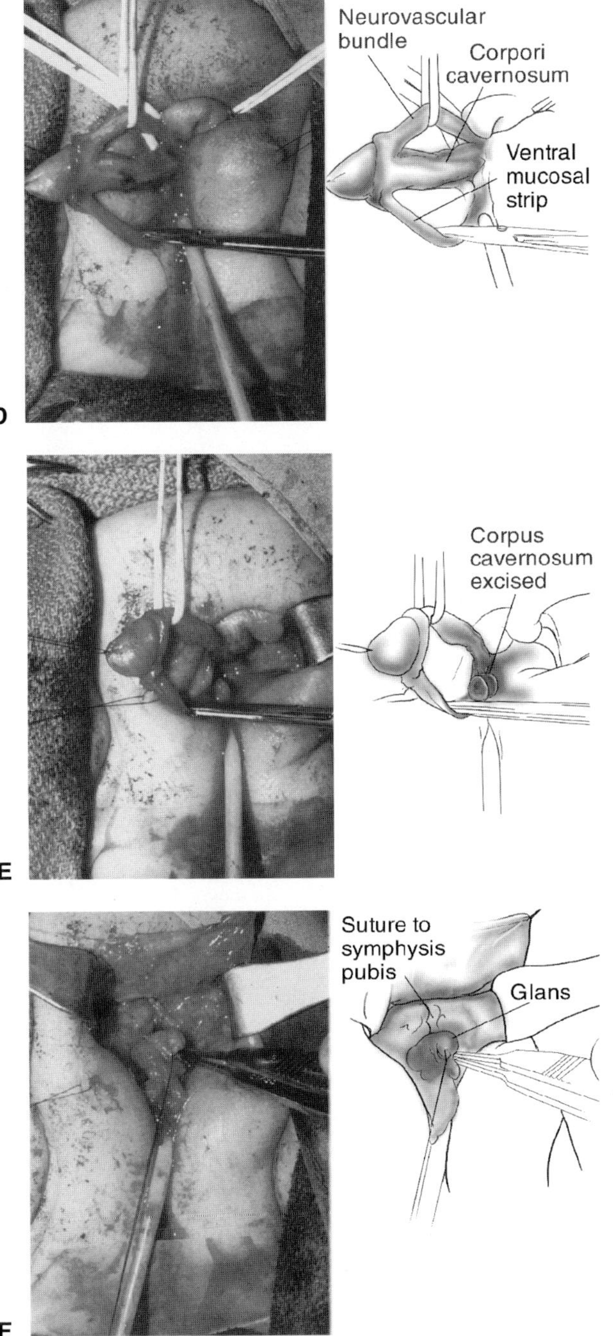

FIG. 1. *Continued.* **D:** The neurovascular bundle has now been separated from the corpora cavernosum. The ventral mucosa strip is also dissected free from the corpora cavernosum. **E:** Each corpus cavernosum is then suture-ligated at its respective proximal and distal ends. They are then removed, leaving only the neurovascular bundle and ventral strip of mucosa. **F:** The glans is now recessed. The corpora cavernosum is sutured to the symphysis pubis, pulling the glans back for purposes of concealment.

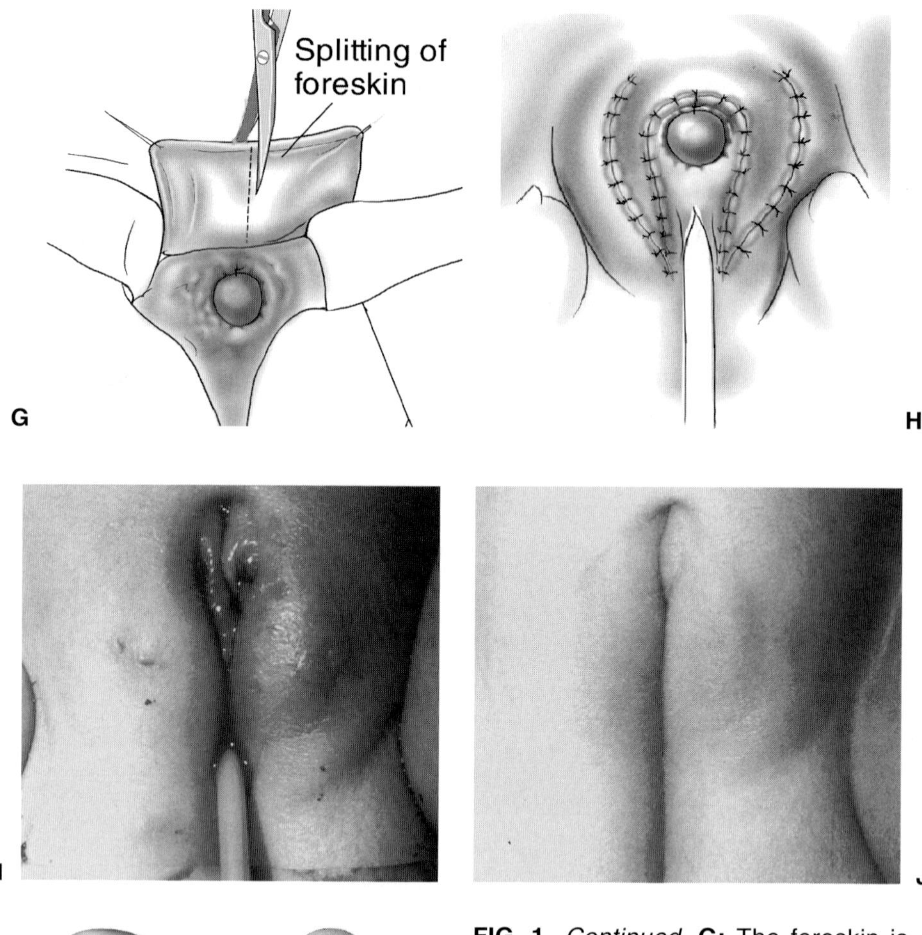

FIG. 1. *Continued.* **G:** The foreskin is then split in its midline and will be rotated ventrally to create labia minora. **H:** The completed operation with the creation of new labia minora and the concealment of the glans. **I:** Immediate postoperative appearance with the newly created labia minora and the concealed glans. **J:** Appearance one month after surgery. **K:** The glans may be quite large and may need to be reduced. This may be done through a series of ventral incisions or a single dorsal incision. This demonstrates the excision of glandular tissue. The incisions are then closed using interrupted 5-0 Vicryl.

SURGICAL PROCEDURE

The type of vaginoplasty depends on the location of the vagina. If the vagina is beneath the levator ani and is close to the perineum, a perineal-based flap vaginoplasty may be done (Fig. 2A–E). It is convenient to perform it at the same time as the reduction clitoroplasty. A vertical incision in the posterior fourchette with a flap ad-

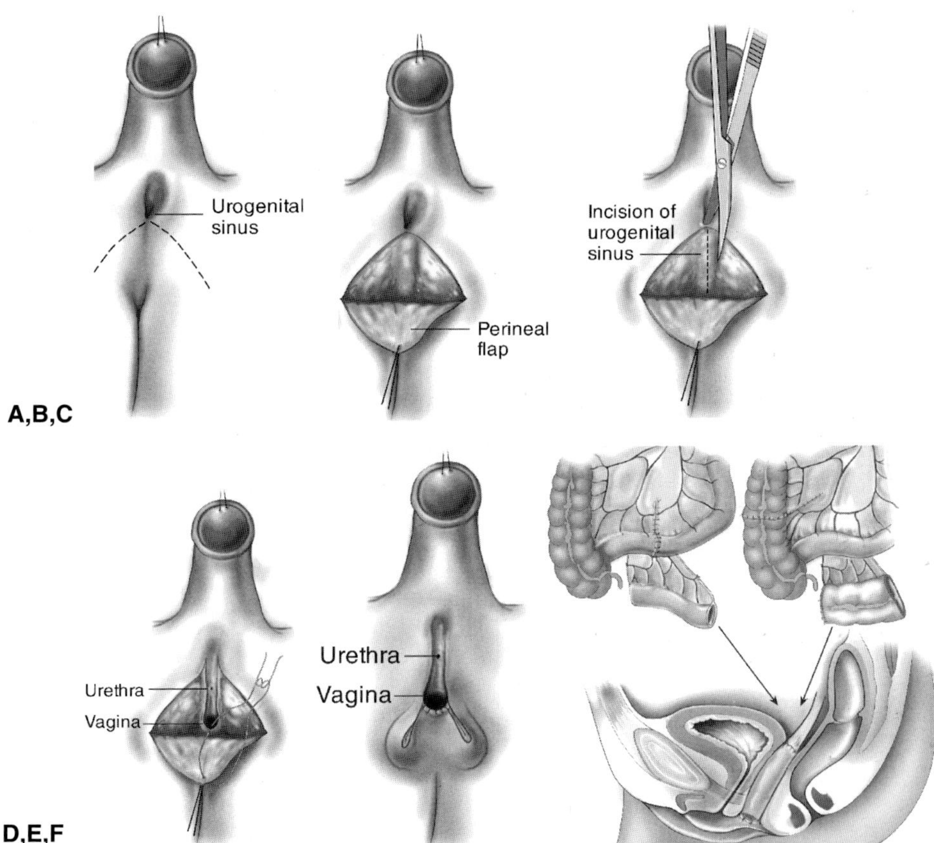

FIG. 2. A: A perineal based flap is outlined immediately beneath the solitary urogenital sinus. **B:** A full-thickness perineal flap is raised, guaranteeing vascular viability. **C:** An incision is made through the common channel of the urogenital sinus to the area where the urethra and vagina may be clearly visualized. **D:** The vagina is then opened along its posterior wall to create a satisfactory orifice. The perineal flap is then sutured in place with 4-0 Vicryl. **E:** The completion of the vaginoplasty with the perineal flap sutured into the vaginal orifice. **F:** A segment of ileum or sigmoid colon may be used for creation of the vagina. The segment of intestine is mobilized on its mesentery and gastrointestinal continuity is restored. The ileum or sigmoid is then rotated to reach the perineum and is sutured to a newly created perineal orifice.

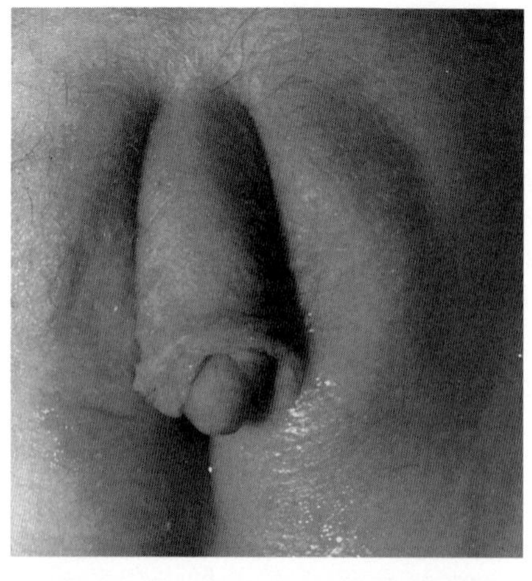
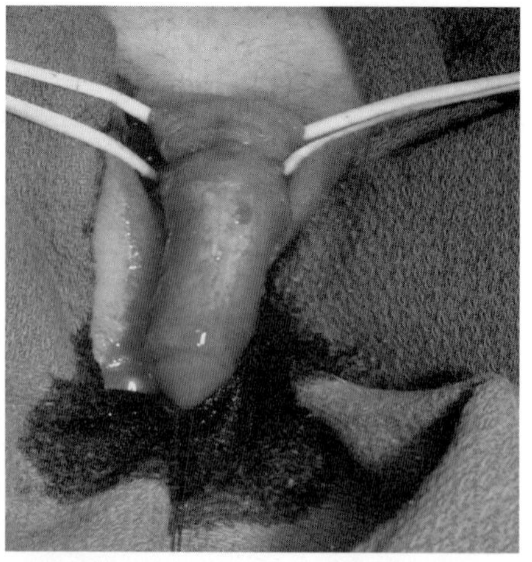
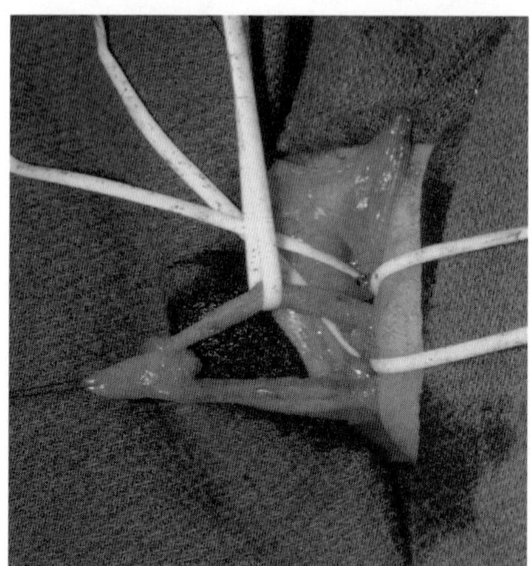
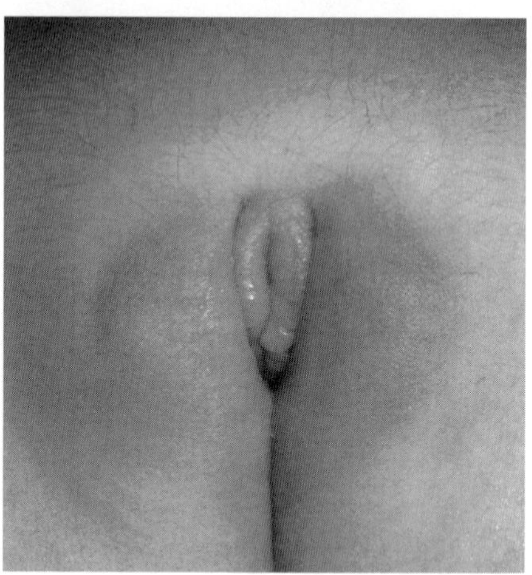
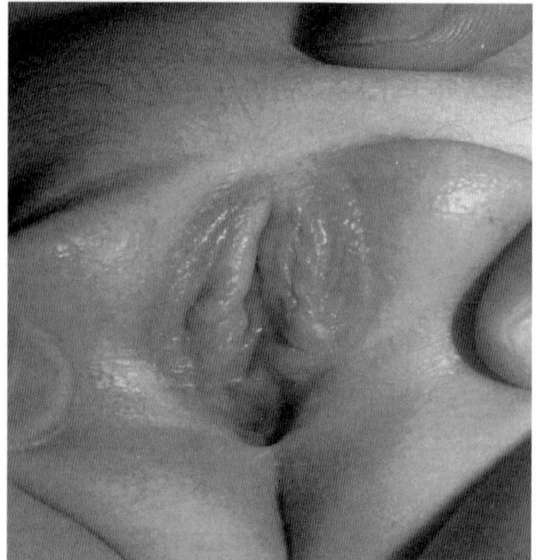

FIG. 3. A 2-year-old girl presented with signs of virilization including pubic hair and body odor. She was discovered to have a non-salt-losing congenital adrenal hyperplasia. She was placed on appropriate medication and subsequently underwent surgery. **A:** The enlarged clitoris is noted with sparse pubic hair in this 2-year-old child. **B:** The phallus has been degloved and vessel loops are placed around each corpora body after its divergence beyond the level of the symphysis pubis. **C:** The corpora bodies have been excised. The superior vessel loop is around the intact neurovascular bundle and the mucosal strip is noted to be intact. **D:** Postoperative appearance. **E:** Postoperative appearance shows that the small glans clitoris is hidden by the labia minora and external genitalia appear normal.

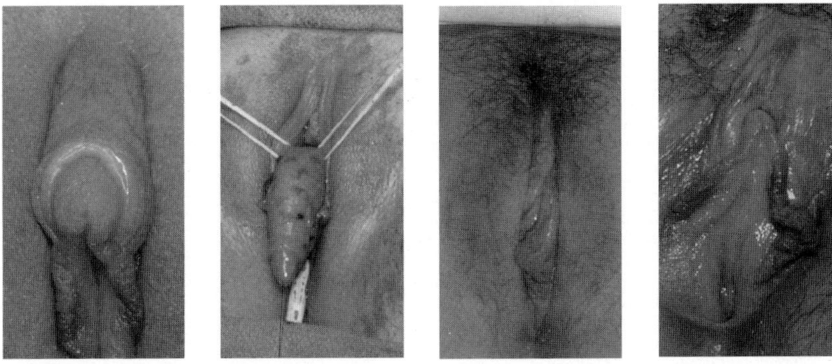

FIG. 4. A 15-year-old girl presented with abdominal pain and underwent an exploratory laparotomy for a presumed appendicitis. She was discovered to have a testicular tumor. Subsequent evaluation revealed a 46,XY phenotypic female. The only sign of virilization was a slightly enlarged clitoris (which had not been noted prior to surgery). **A:** The external genitalia demonstrates a slightly enlarged clitoris. **B:** This intraoperative photograph demonstrates the enlarged clitoris. Vessel loops are around each corpora body that has been dissected, diverging to beyond the symphysis pubis. **C:** Postoperatively the external genitalia appear normal. **D:** A viable and intact glans clitoris is demonstrated.

vancement allows normal external genitalia. The advantages of doing this early in life include better cosmesis and reassurance to the parents that there is a vagina and a normal female child. The growth of the vagina may occur and introital stenosis, if present, can be corrected in adolescence. There is no need for an interposition graft with bowel or other tissues.

The disadvantage clearly involves stenosis. It would be unfair to the child and the family to require dilatation and obturator support throughout early childhood. This may be done in the young, mature girl when there is an incentive by the patient herself to participate with all techniques to avoid stenosis. If introital stenosis develops, revision may be more difficult than a primary repair in a young woman with severe scarring.

The high vagina or vaginal agenesis is a much more complicated problem. In severe congenital adrenal hyperplasia or congenital absence of a vagina, the interposition of bowel or other tissues may be required (Fig. 2F). Although there are alternative procedures such as free skin grafts or large pudendal base skin flaps, bowel substitution has gained the most popularity (15–18). The use of bowel is very attractive in that it is a viable, vascular tissue on its own blood supply, which allows it to grow with time. In addition, the normal mucus may serve as a lubrication for sexual relations. Disadvantages include excessive mucus, an additional abdominal operation with interposition and operative reestablishment of gastrointestinal continuity, and the passing of this bowel through the genitourinary diaphragm. The cosmetic appearance, however, may be outstanding and may allow patients to have normal external genitalia.

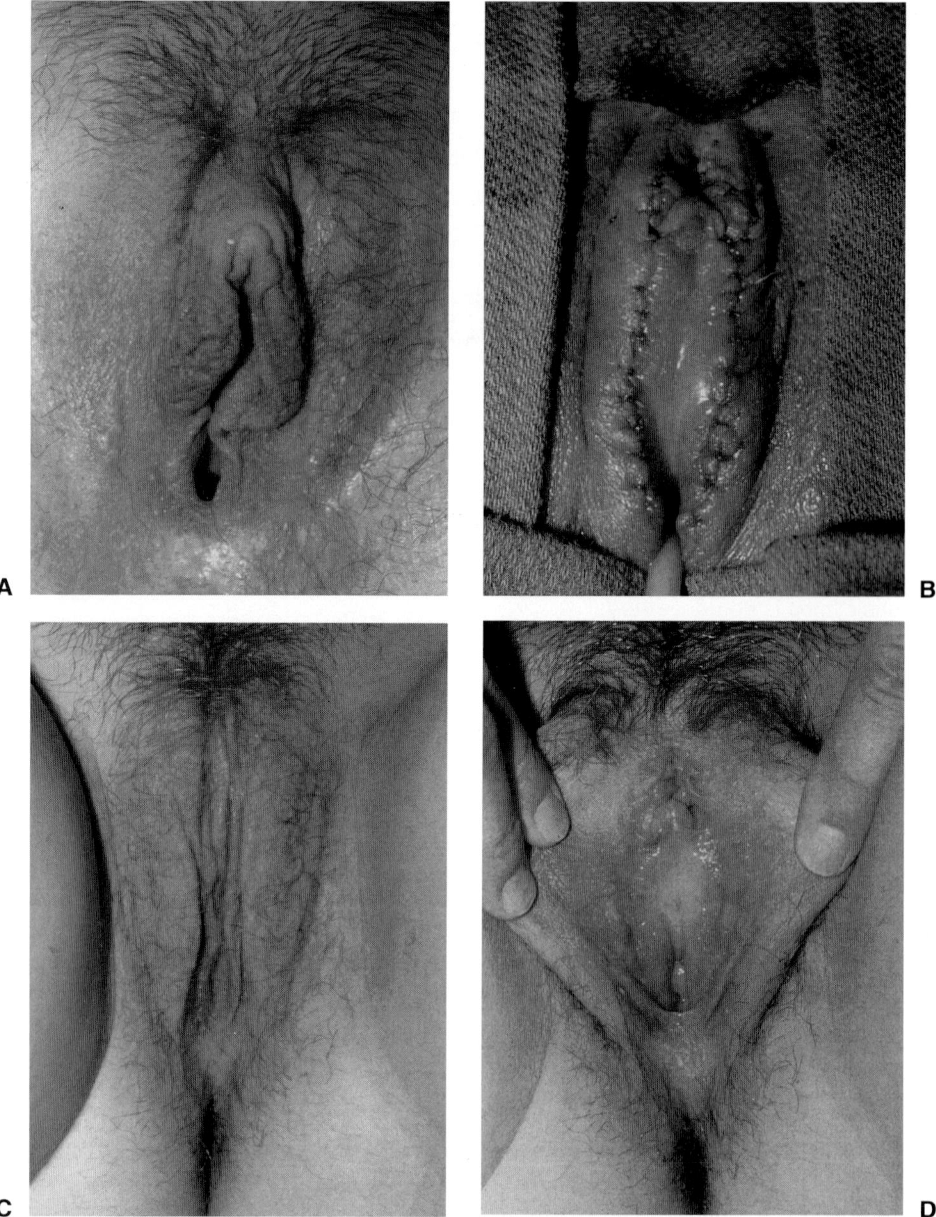

FIG. 5. An 11-year-old girl presented because of concerns about her external genitalia and cosmesis, particularly when wearing a swimsuit. Biochemical evaluation revealed a non-salt-losing form of congenital adrenal hyperplasia. **A:** The external genitalia upon presentation demonstrates an enlarged clitoris and prominent labia. **B:** At the completion of the reduction clitoroplasty, the external genitalia have been reconstructed. **C:** One month post operation. The external genitalia appear normal. **D:** The viable clitoris is recessed and hidden.

REFERENCES

1. Federman D, Donahoe P. Ambiguous genitalia: etiology, diagnosis, and therapy. In: Mazzeferri EL, ed., *Advances in endocrinology and metabolism,* vol. 6. St. Louis: Mosby-Year Book, 1995:91–117.
2. Gillman J. The development of the gonads in man, with a consideration of the role of fetal endocrines and the histogenesis of ovarian tumors. *Carnegie Contrib Embryol* 1948;210(32):83.
3. Molsberry RL, Carr BR, Mendelson CR. Human chorionic gonadotropin binding to human fetal testes as a function of gestational age. *J Clin Endocrinol Metab* 1982;55:791.
4. Jost A. Recherches sur la differenciation sexuelle de l'embryon du lapin. *Arch Anat Microsc Morphol Exp* 1947;36:271.
5. Kay R. Ambiguous genitalia. In: Resnick M, Novick A, eds. *Urology secrets.* Philadelphia: Hanley and Belfus, 1995:175–178.
6. Feldman KW, Smith DW. Fetal phallic growth and penile standards for newborn male infants. *J Pediatr* 1975;86:395–398.
7. Lattimer JK. Relocation and recession of the enlarged clitoris with the preservation of the glans; an alternative to amputation. *J Urol* 1961;86:113–116.
8. Randolph JG, Hung W. Reduction clitoroplasty in females with hypertrophy clitoris. *J Pediatr Surg* 1970;5:224–231.
9. Spence HM, Allen TD. Genital reconstruction in the female with the adrenal genital syndrome. *Br J Urol* 1973;45:126–130.
10. Kay R. Clitoral surgery. In: Stewart BH, ed. *Operative urology.* Baltimore: Williams & Wilkins, 1982.
11. Kogan SJ, Smey P, Levitt SB. Subtunical total reduction clitoroplasty: a safe modification of existing techniques. *J Urol* 1983;130:746.
12. Manley CB, Epstein ES. Early hypospadias repair. *J Urol* 1981;125:698.
13. Belman AB, Kass EJ. Hypospadias repair in children under one year of age. *J Urol* 1982;128:1273.
14. Allen LE, Hardy BE, Churchill BM. The surgical management of the enlarged clitoris. *J Urol* 1982;128:351.
15. Freundt UM, Toolenaar TA, Huikeshoven FJ, Drogendijk AC, Jeekel H. A modified technique to create a neovagina with an isolated segment of sigmoid colon. *Surg Gynecol Obstet* 1992;174:11–16.
16. Lenaghan R, Wilson N, Lucas CE, Ledgerwood AM. The role of rectosigmoid neocolporrhaphy. *Surgery* 1997;122(4):856–860.
17. Wesley JR, Coran AG. Intestinal vaginoplasty for congenital absence of the vagina. *J Pediatr Surg* 1992;27:885–889.
18. Hensle TW, Seaman EK. Vaginal reconstruction in children and adults. *Tech Urol* 1995;1:174–180.

Congenital Malformations of the Female Genital Tract: Diagnosis and Management, edited by G. Gidwani and T. Falcone.
Lippincott Williams & Wilkins, Philadelphia © 1999.

7

Persistent Cloaca and Associated Vaginal Anomalies

Frederick Alexander

Department of Pediatric Surgery, The Cleveland Clinic Foundation, Cleveland, Ohio 44195

Cloacal anomalies are rare, occurring in an estimated 1 per 50,000 live births annually, and represent one of the more complex forms of vaginal atresia. They result from a mesenchymal defect that leads to a failure of separation of the primitive allantois, vagina, and hindgut in the developing female embryo. Patients typically present with a blank perineum and subclitoral urogenital sinus that communicates with the bladder, vagina, and rectum. The plain external appearance gives little indication of the complexity of the internal defect. Vaginal repair is best performed in a single-stage reconstructive procedure in conjunction with anorectal pull-through (1,2). Successful repair requires knowledge of the frequent variations of pelvic anatomy as well as the variety of reconstructive techniques available for repair.

EMBRYOLOGY

Between 4 and 6 weeks of gestation in a female embryo, the primitive allantois, vagina, and rectum all communicate with a single chamber (cloaca) that drains out to the perineum through a tubular urogenital sinus. Subsequent caudal growth of two mesenchymal ridges separates and defines these structures: the sinovaginal plate divides the bladder and vagina, and the urogenital ridge divides the vagina and rectum. At the same time, a muscular sling develops between the pubis and coccyx, which forms a sphincter complex that surrounds and supports the bladder neck, distal vagina, and anorectal canal. Isolated growth failure of the sinovaginal plate results in vaginal atresia wherein the distal vagina remains fused to the urinary tract in a Y configuration draining out to the perineum via a persistent urogenital sinus. Similarly, isolated growth failure of the urogenital ridge results in anorectal atresia wherein the distal rectum remains fused to the dorsal vagina, usually in conjunction with a persistent rectovaginal fistula. The more complex persistent cloaca occurs when there is growth failure of both mesenchymal ridges and all three structures remain fused, draining into a solitary persistent urogenital sinus. The development of the sphincter complex that normally envelopes these tubular structures is interrupted in each case, and the sphincter complex fuses in the midline caudal to each involved atretic structure. The inherent variability of these anomalies relates to the timing of growth arrest during these first weeks of gestational development. Growth arrest at a relatively early gestational age results in suprasphincteric confluence with a poorly formed bladder neck and relatively elongated urogenital sinus, whereas at a late gestational age the confluence may be infrasphincteric with a well-formed bladder neck and short urogenital sinus. Each case is unique and slightly different; yet all cases follow this same general pattern of development.

ASSOCIATED ANOMALIES

All children with cloacal anomalies are at risk for other malformations associated with the VACTERL syndrome (vertebral, anal atresia, cardiac, tracheoesophageal, renal, and lung). Approximately 60% of children with cloacal anomalies have associated upper urinary tract malformations and a similar percentage have associated hydrocolpos caused by partial or complete obstruction of the vaginal outlet (3). Urinary anomalies include vesicoureteral reflux, ureteropelvic or ureterovesical junction obstruction, and ureteroectopia. Hydrocolpos may contribute to bladder outlet and/or ureteral obstruction with urinary stasis and sepsis. In rare cases, there may be congenital absence of the vagina, referred to as the Mayer-Rokitansky-Küster-Hauser syndrome (4). Finally, an estimated 30% to 75% of patients might exhibit lumbosacral spinal anomalies that are highly correlated with urinary and fecal incontinence.

DIAGNOSIS

Cloacal anomalies are readily diagnosed in female patients by the characteristic findings of a blank perineum and subclitoral sinus tract (Fig. 1). In some settings, they have been confused with intersex anomalies; however, the presence of anorectal atresia should indicate an underlying mesenchymal defect rather than a germ cell or adrenal enzymatic defect. In virtually all cases, there is no evidence of clitoral hypertrophy or labial scrotalization. Associated chromosomal anomalies are rare, but not impossible, and thus chromosomal analysis should be undertaken in each case.

Because of the inherent variability of cloacal anomalies, it is extremely important to define the pelvic anatomy as precisely as possible before attempting surgical repair. Initially, a hydrocolpos may be diagnosed upon physical examination by palpation of a pelvic mass. Ultrasonography, renal scan, and intravenous pyelography (after 2 weeks of age) may be used to define upper urinary tract malformations as well as to confirm the presence of hydrocolpos. Sinography and sinoscopy are essential to delineate the course of the urogenital sinus and its relationship to the vagina and rectum. Plain radiographs of the lumbosacral spine are important to rule out spinal anomalies and, if present, should be followed by spinal ultrasound or magnetic resonance imaging in order to rule out tethered cord, myelodysplasia, or other associated cord anomalies. Finally, it is important to rule out other anomalies associated with the

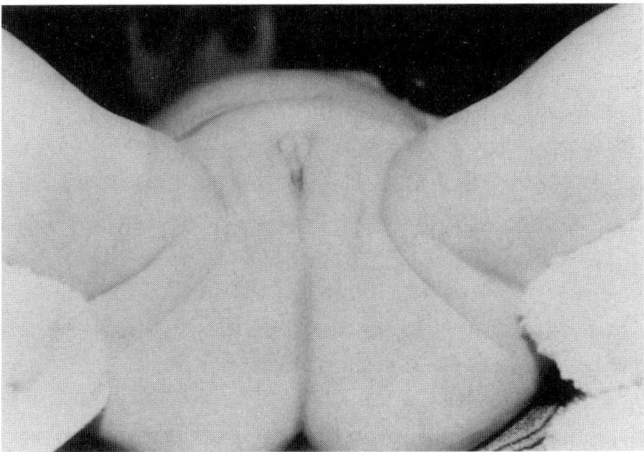

FIG. 1. Typical appearance of a cloacal anomaly.

VACTERL syndrome, e.g., by intubating the stomach or by obtaining an electrocardiogram depending on the clinical circumstance.

TREATMENT

Definitive surgical repair is not feasible in the newborn, although this may be possible in the future. Currently, it is recommended that a divided colostomy be performed proximal to the middle colic artery in order to preserve collateral blood supply to the rectosigmoid via the marginal artery. Since hydrocolpos is a common cause of urinary stasis and sepsis, this should be treated with drainage utilizing one of several techniques. The least invasive technique is clean intermittent catheterization; however, this requires training and strict adherence to a formal catheterization program (5). Furthermore, this may require additional procedures such as cutback and dilatation of the urogenital sinus and/or endoscopic incision of a vaginal septum. Finally, catheterization is not always successful due to the thick, mucous vaginal secretions. A tube vaginoscopy may be utilized, but this too may not provide adequate drainage thereby perpetuating urinary sepsis. Various explanations for this include the tube as a foreign body, hymenal remnants entrapping urine within the vagina, and vaginal septations occurring in approximately 65% of cases. Another solution is to perform a temporary suprapubic vesicostomy (6–12). Vesicostomy is a tubeless form of diversion that may provide temporary urinary drainage, eliminating urinary stasis and allowing regression of the hydrocolpos. In any event, children should always be closely monitored for urinary sepsis and growth failure prior to definitive repair.

The technique of cloacal reconstruction should be guided by the preoperative evaluation and is best performed in patients 9 to 12 months of age. It is advantageous to utilize a posterior sagittal approach because this allows preservation of normal neuromuscular innervation of the sphincter complex and precise reconstruction of the complex around the bladder neck and anorectal canal in the correct anatomic configuration (13). In many cases, the entire reconstructive procedure may be performed through this approach. A critical step in this procedure is the disconnection of the vagina from the urogenital sinus (14). The latter structure is then tubularized to create a neourethra (Fig. 2). The decision to open the entire sinus is based on its length and width. When the urogenital sinus is short and wide, it may be longitudinally opened and tapered in order to enhance urinary continence. However, when it is longer than 2 to 3 cm and/or less than 10 French in diameter, this technique is not necessary and increases the risk of urethral stenosis or urethral vaginal fistula. If the urethra and vagina join distal to the external urinary sphincter, then flap vaginoplasty may be performed via a perineal approach. However, in most cases the vagina enters the urogenital sinus at a higher level, necessitating a more complex pull-through vaginoplasty. In these cases, urine often follows the path of least resistance into the vagina where it becomes entrapped leading to hydrocolpos. Mobilization of the vagina to the perineal skin may be accomplished from below by circumferential dissection and is facilitated by the use of a rectangular vaginal flap or perineal skin flaps (Fig. 3) (15,16).

When insufficient length or vascular compromise of the vaginal pedicle prevents vaginal-perineal anastomosis, transabdominal mobilization of the vagina might be required, thus preserving the ovarian pedicle (Fig. 4) (17). Circumferential dissec-

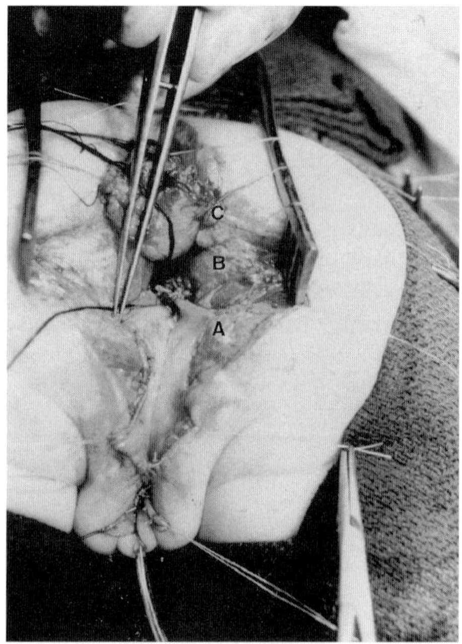

FIG. 2. Posterior sagittal repair of a cloacal anomaly showing urogenital sinus **(A)**, confluence of vagina and bladder neck **(B)**, and rectum disconnected from cloaca **(C)**.

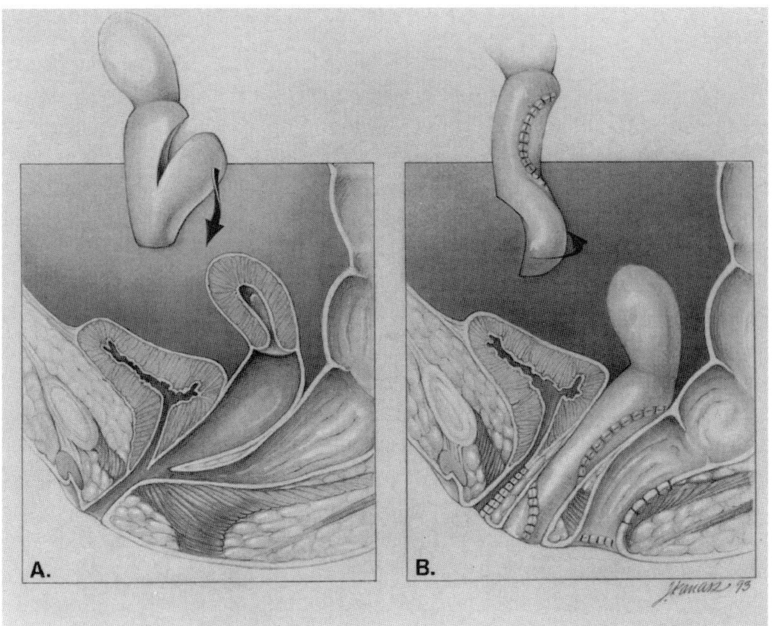

FIG. 3. A and B: Schematic of a rectangular flap vaginoplasty in a posterior sagittal repair.

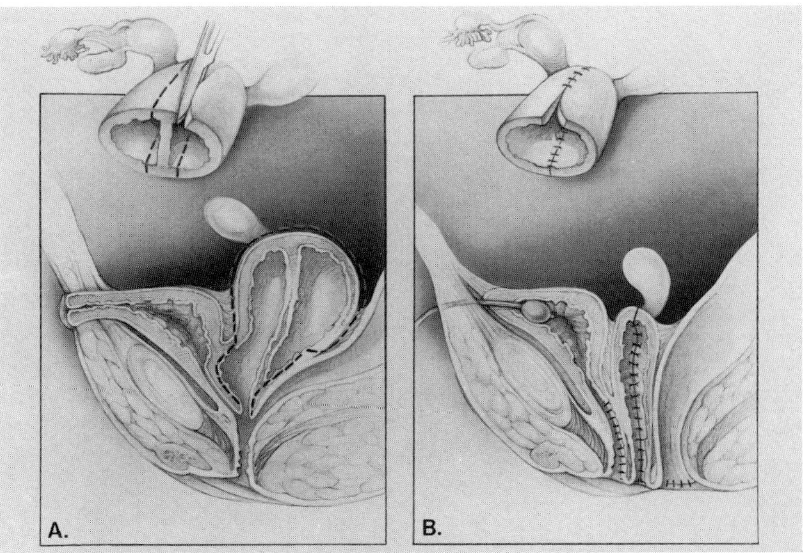

FIG. 4. A and B: Schematic of total vaginal mobilization with excision of vaginal septum in a combined abdominal-posterior sagittal repair. A distal endovaginal dissection is performed with preservation of the vaginal wall down to the level of the cloaca.

tion of the vaginal wall is performed to the vicinity of the bladder neck whereupon the vagina is opened and circumferential endovaginal dissection is continued to the level of the urogenital sinus. The vagina is then disconnected from the proximal edge of the endovaginal plane and pulled through to the perineum on its ovarian pedicle. This transabdominal approach also facilities complete excision of vaginal septations.

Another consideration in the decision to perform a combined abdominal-posterior sagittal procedure is the occurrence of associated congenital urinary malformations (18). Certain malformations such as ureterovesicle junction obstruction, ectopic ureter, or ureteral duplication are more effectively managed by a transabdominal approach. In addition, a new cystotomy or takedown of old vesicostomy with ureteral stents may facilitate dissection of the vaginal cuff.

Vaginal reconstruction in patients with cloacal anomalies and vaginal agenesis usually requires a combined abdominal-posterior sagittal procedure (Fig. 5). The diagnosis is confirmed by the finding of normal ovaries and salpinx along with an absent or dysplastic vagina and uterus. Construction of an artificial vagina in this instance may be accomplished utilizing a tapered segment of sigmoid colon based on a vascular pedicle or creation of a split-thickness skin tube (19). The sigmoid vagina offers several advantages in that it is self-lubricated and does not appear to require

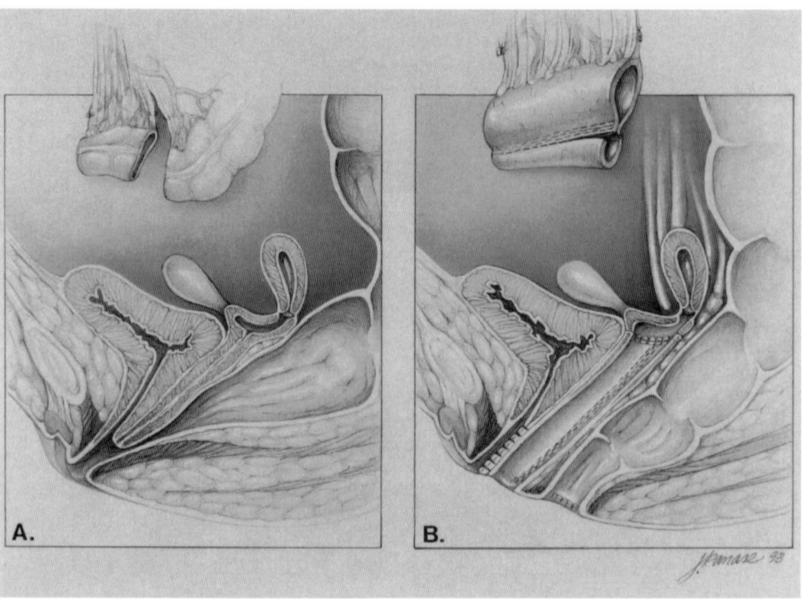

FIG. 5. A and B: Schematic of a sigmoid vagina constructed for vaginal agenesis in conjunction with a cloacal anomaly.

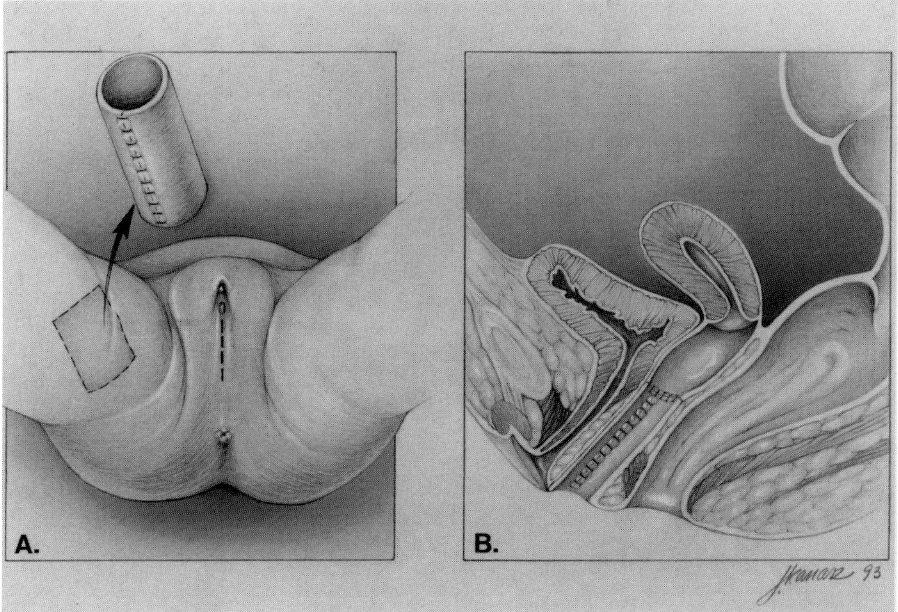

FIG. 6. Schematic of second-stage tubular skin graft for distal vaginal stricture or occlusion.

repeat dilatation. Like the skin tube, the sigmoid vagina may be tapered to any width, but it does not require a postoperative stent or dilatation.

Complications of the cloacal repair are usually related to the vaginal cuff. The most difficult complication is vesical-vaginal or urethrovaginal fistula, which has been reported in 11% of patients (3). This complication may present with urinary sepsis and/or incontinence and is best repaired by colostomy and subsequent redo posterior sagittal exploration in which the anterior wall of the rectum, perineal body, and posterior wall of the vagina are incised in order to expose the neourethra and/or bladder neck.

More commonly, distal vaginal stricture or occlusion may occur due to ischemia of the vaginal flap. This complication may be prevented by gentle handling and adequate mobilization of the vagina. Repair of distal vaginal occlusion depends on the type of reconstruction previously used. For example, after occlusion of a rectangular vaginal flap, transabdominal vaginal reconstruction may be performed by mobilizing the vagina on its ovarian pedicle. Vaginal occlusion after transabdominal vaginoplasty may be salvaged by use of a tubular split-thickness skin graft or perineal skin flaps (Fig. 6). In the event of complete or near-complete loss of the vaginal cuff, reconstruction of an artificial vagina using a vascularized segment of sigmoid colon is advised.

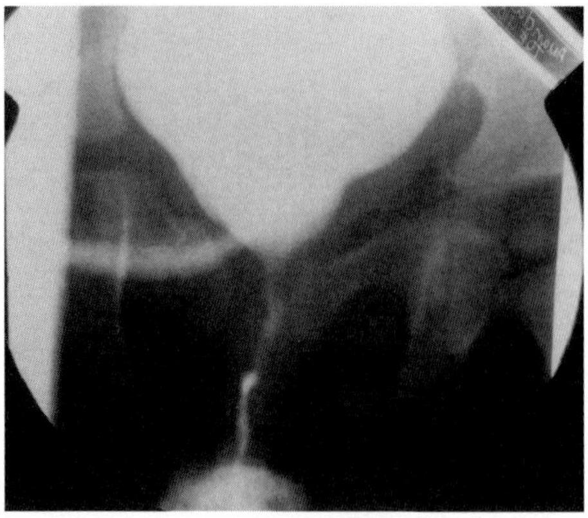

FIG. 7. Voiding cystourethrogram of patient following repair of cloaca. Note the elongated neourethra.

RESULTS

The results of total pelvic reconstruction for cloacal anomalies are generally good, but clean intermittent catheterization and bowel programs are frequently required to ensure that all patients remain clean and dry (Fig. 7). It has been shown in large series that urinary and bowel continence depends at least partially on the integrity of the lumbosacral spine. Fecal incontinence approaches 74% in patients with an abnormal sacrum versus only 30% in patients with a normal sacrum (3). Most patients are potentially fertile; however, revision of the vaginal canal and repeated vaginal dilatation may be required following puberty. Finally, although transvaginal delivery of a fetus is theoretically possible, in most patients delivery by cesarean section is advisable.

REFERENCES

1. Hendren WH. Repair of cloacal anomalies: current techniques. *J Pediatr Surg* 1986;21:1159.
2. Peña A, de Vries PA. Posterior sagittal anorectoplasty: important technical considerations and new applications. *J Pediatr Surg* 1982;17:796.
3. Peña A. The surgical management of persistent cloaca: results in 54 patients treated with a posterior sagittal approach. *J Pediatr Surg* 1989;24:590.
4. Griffin JE, Edwards C, Madden JD. Congenital absence of the vagina. The Mayer-Rokitansky-Küster-Hauser syndrome. *Ann Intern Med* 1976;85:224.
5. Nakayma D, Snyder HM, Schnaufer L, et al. Posterior sagittal exposure for reconstructive surgery for cloacal anomalies. *J Pediatr Surg* 1987;22:588.
6. Alexander F, Kay R. Cloacal anomalies: role of vesicostomy. *J Pediatr Surg* 1974;29:74.
7. Bloksom B. Bladder pouch for prolonged tublis cystostomy. *J Urol* 1957;78:398.
8. Michi AJ, Borns P, Ames MD. Improvement following tubeless superpubic cystostomy of myelomeningocele with hydronephrosis and recurrent acute pyelonephritis. *J Pediatr Surg* 1966;1:347.
9. Noe HN, Jerkins JR. Cutaneous vesicosotomy experience in infants and children. *J Urol* 1985;134:301.
10. Duckett JW. Cutaneous vesicostomy in childhood. *Urol Clin North Am* 1974;1:485–495.

11. Bruce R. Gonzalez ET Jr. Cutaneous vesicostomy: a useful form of temporary diversion in children. *J Urol* 1980;123:927.
12. Snyder HM, Kalichman MA, Charney E, et al. Vesicostomy for neurogenic bladder with spina bifida. *J Urol* 1983;130:724.
13. de Vries PA, Peña A. Posterior sagittal anorectoplasty. *J Pediatr Surg* 1982;17:638.
14. Raffensperger JG, Ramenofsky ML. The management of a cloaca. *J Pediatr Surg* 1973;8:647.
15. Hendren WH. Cloacal malformations: experience with 106 cases. *J Pediatr Surg* 1992;27:890.
16. Hendren WH, Donahoe PK. Correction of longitudinal abnormalities of the vagina and perineum. *J Pediatr Surg* 1980;15:751.
17. Alexander F, Kay R. Technical considerations in the repair of cloacal vaginal deformities. *J Urol* 1995;153:788.
18. Hendren WH. Urological aspects of cloacal malformations. *J Urol* 1988;140:1207.
19. Wesley JR, Coran AG. Intestinal vaginoplasty for congenital absence of the vagina. *J Pediatr Surg* 1992;27:885.

Congenital Malformations of the Female Genital Tract: Diagnosis and Management, edited by G. Gidwani and T. Falcone.
Lippincott Williams & Wilkins, Philadelphia © 1999.

8

Management of Vaginal Agenesis and Nonobstructing Vaginal Septa

Marjan Attaran and Gita Gidwani

Department of Gynecology and Obstetrics, The Cleveland Clinic Foundation, Cleveland, Ohio 44195

Hauser and Schreiner first described the Mayer-Rokitansky-Küster-Hauser (MRKH) syndrome in 1961 after reviewing the autopsy reports described by Mayer in 1829, Rokitansky in 1838, and Küster in 1910 (1,2). Women with this disorder were characterized as having normal secondary sexual characteristics, uterine hypoplasia or aplasia, congenital absence of the vagina, and a spectrum of associated abnormalities. The embryology of the Müllerian-derived organs has been reviewed in Chapter 1. In the ensuing chapter, the evaluation and management of MRKH patients will be discussed via a series of case presentations. In addition, the various nonobstructive vaginal septa will be reviewed.

CLASSIFICATION

Numerous endeavors have been made to classify the Müllerian anomalies. They tend to be either overly simplistic, excluding several anomalies, or too encompassing, which is confusing and unwieldy. However, the necessity of a classification becomes obvious when attempting to compare the various modes of management and their outcomes. The most widely accepted categorization of Müllerian anomalies is from the American Society of Reproductive Medicine (ASRM) (3), which categorizes MRKH as class IA (Table 1). It is based on the degree of failure of normal development. Anomalies are separated into groups with similar anatomic derangement, treatment, and prognosis for fetal wastage. This classification is very similar to the one proposed by Buttram and Gibbons (4) in 1979. One limitation to this categorization is that it primarily focuses on the uterus and does not consider the various associated vaginal anomalies. Although there is no evidence to suggest an etiologic relationship between vaginal septa and fetal wastage, the frequency of this association mandates a classification of vaginal anomalies. Thus, in conjunction with the ASRM classification, we propose including a classification of the vaginal anomalies when

TABLE 1. *ASRM classification of Müllerian anomalies*

Classification	Anomaly
Class I (Agenesis/hypoplasia)	a. Vaginal
	b. Cervical
	c. Fundal
	d. Tubal
	e. Combined anomalies
Class II (Unicornuate)	a. Communicating
	b. Noncommunicating
	c. No cavity
	d. No horn
Class III (Didelphys)	Didelphys
Class IV (Bicornuate)	a. Complete
	b. Partial
Class V (Septate)	a. Complete
	b. Partial
Class VI (Arcuate)	Arcuate
Class VII (DES-related)	DES-related

ASRM, American Society of Reproductive Medicine; DES, diethylstilbestrol.

necessary (Table 2). We believe this modified classification is more clinically oriented and inclusive.

Toaff and colleagues in 1984 classified the various communicating uteri. All types of bicornuate and septate uteri were classified according to accompanying defects in the cervix and vaginal septum. Thus while very complete in categorizing a subclass of the ASRM classification (classes III to V), it is not a complete classification (5).

Rock has suggested an excellent modification of the ASRM classification, which is quite comprehensive. He broadly categorizes uterovaginal anomalies into dysgenesis of the Müllerian ducts, disorders of lateral fusion, disorders of vertical fusion, and unusual configurations of vertical/lateral fusion defects (6). This classification is based on embryologic development and thus provides a natural means of categorization. Although this modification of the ASRM classification is very complete, it is somewhat confusing because the categories do not exactly match the ASRM classes of uterine malformations.

TABLE 2. *Vaginal septa classification*

Classification	Features
Class I	Transverse
	a. Obstructing
	b. Nonobstructing
Class II	Longitudinal
	a. Obstructing
	b. Nonobstructing
Class III	Stenosis/iatrogenic

CLINICAL FEATURES AND DIAGNOSIS

Most investigators cite the incidence of vaginal agenesis to be about 1 in 5,000 phenotypic females (7). It is the second most common cause of primary amenorrhea after gonadal dysgenesis and must be differentiated from vaginal atresia in which the uterus and cervix are typically intact but the lower vagina consists of fibrous tissue. Reindollar et al. demonstrated that 16% of girls presenting to a reproductive endocrinology clinic with primary amenorrhea had Müllerian duct aplasia (8). In our series of 30 patients presenting with primary amenorrhea to an adolescent gynecology clinic, 18 had vaginal agenesis (unpublished data).

Patients with MRKH typically present between the ages of 15 and 18 with primary amenorrhea. They progress through the normal stages of puberty but fail to menstruate. Since their ovaries and adrenal glands are functioning normally, their breast development, pubic hair, and growth spurt are normal. Several studies have documented normal ovarian function, not only by the development of secondary sexual characteristics but by measurement of estradiol, luteinizing hormone (LH), and follicle-stimulating hormone (FSH). The patterns of hormone secretion were within normal limits with the average cycle length varying from 30 to 34 days (9).

The etiology of MRKH is not known. While the majority of MRKH cases have been presumed to be sporadic, a multifactorial mode of inheritance has been postulated (10). Cramer and colleagues demonstrated decreased galactose-1-phosphate uridyl transferase activity in 6 of 13 patients with MRKH syndrome (11). They speculate that increased intrauterine exposure to galactose may lead to delayed vaginal opening. Finally, there is one report of an association between MRKH syndrome and the major histocompatibility complex (12).

Although chromosomal studies are not absolutely necessary for the diagnosis, it may be beneficial when differentiating among the intersex states. Patients in whom the diagnosis of vaginal agenesis is made prior to puberty have not developed any secondary sexual characteristics and their hormonal levels are in the prepubertal range. It may be difficult to differentiate MRKH, androgen insensitivity syndrome (AIS), and other intersex states at this stage of development. Since the presence of a Y chromosome may lead to signs of androgenization at the time of puberty, early documentation of its existence is advantageous to the patient. Finally, artificial reproductive techniques may provide a means of achieving conception; thus a karyotype may help counsel the patient more appropriately regarding her reproductive options.

The association between Müllerian tract anomalies and the renal system is well known. Forty percent of patients diagnosed with MRKH syndrome will have concomitant renal abnormalities that may range from complete absence of the ipsilateral kidney to malposition of the kidney to subtle changes in renal structure (13). Thus a full evaluation of the renal system is warranted in a patient who is diagnosed with MRKH syndrome. The original descriptions of this disease also recognized associated skeletal abnormalities (14,15). The majority of these anomalies involve the spine followed by limb and rib defects. In one series of 574 MRKH cases, a 12% incidence of skeletal malformations was reported (16). An association has also been noted be-

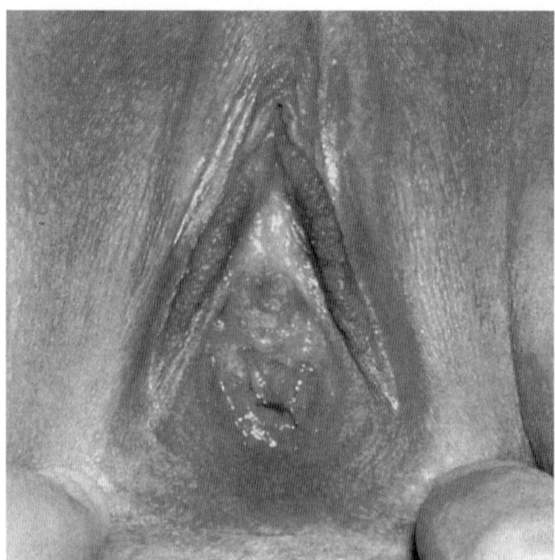

FIG. 1. External genitalia of patient with MRKH.

tween congenital deafness and vaginal agenesis (17). There are also isolated reports of concomitant genital, middle ear, and renal anomalies (18–20). Letterie and Vauss demonstrated a significantly higher rate of auditory defects in patients with genitourinary defects than those with normal Müllerian structures (21). Some of these defects were not clinically evident and could only be detected via sensitive audiometric testing. Finally, an association between MRKH and Klippel-Feil syndrome, which consists of fusion of the cervical spine and a short neck, has been demonstrated.

Physical examination reveals normal secondary sexual characteristics. The lower third of the vagina, which is derived from the urogenital sinus, appears normal (Fig. 1). In many cases a hymenal fringe and a small vaginal pouch is present. In some cases through repeated attempts at intercourse, the patient has increased the length of her blind-ending vaginal pouch. A rectoabdominal examination verifies the absence of a uterus (Table 3).

To confirm the diagnosis of MRKH, the pelvis must be imaged for the existence of ovaries and lack of uterus. Various methods of radiologic evaluation of Müllerian anomalies are presented in Chapter 4. Ultrasound not only delineates the location of the ovary but also determines the extent of uterine development and the existence of a functioning endometrial cavity. In rare instances where ultrasound has been inconclusive or the ovaries have not been located, magnetic resonance imaging (MRI) is indicated. The most common finding consists of normal ovaries and fallopian tubes

TABLE 3. *Criteria for diagnosis*

Primary amenorrhea with absence of vagina
Absent uterus, rudimentary bicornuate cords, or anatomically complete uterus
Normal ovarian function
Normal female breast, body proportions, and hair distribution
Frequent association of renal, skeletal, and other congenital anomalies
46,XX

with only solid nubbins for uterine horns and no vagina. In most cases a surgical procedure is not necessary for the diagnosis of MRKH syndrome. However, if the radiologic findings are inconsistent with the presentation or the patient presents with complaints of cyclic or chronic pelvic pain, then laparoscopy might be necessary to rule out a possible obstructed uterine horn. Therefore, history, physical examination, ultrasound, and cognizance of this entity will lead to the correct diagnosis in the majority of cases. Both communication with the radiologist and his or her degree of experience in identifying Müllerian abnormalities are key factors in arriving at the correct diagnosis. Unfortunately, incorrect interpretation of the pelvic ultrasound and a low index of suspicion have lead to serial attempts at useless hymenectomies in many patients, ultimately leading to suboptimal surgical results.

Case 1

KH is an 18-year-old white woman who presented to the gynecologist a year ago with the complaint of primary amenorrhea. Thelarche initiated at age 10 and she is currently at Tanner stage 5 of breast development. Her mother underwent menarche at age 14. The patient is at the 50th percentile for height and weight. Physical examination revealed normal-appearing external genitalia but the vagina could not be visualized. The patient had an ultrasound, which seemed to reveal a very small uterus. Subsequently, she had two hymenectomies on two separate occasions without restoration of menstruation. In addition, she was unsuccessfully supplemented with estrogen and progesterone to induce menstruation.

The above case illustrates several important points. First, a prepubertal uterus in a patient with normal breast development is inconsistent and thus direct communication with the radiologist should occur concerning the differential diagnosis. Second, the ultrasound has failed to reveal a collection of blood, which would be essential if indeed the patient was suffering from an imperforate hymen or transverse septum. Third, if the patient's presentation cannot be adequately explained, then MRI or laparoscopy is indicated.

MRKH syndrome must be differentiated from AIS and other combinations of male pseudohermaphroditism. The physical examination may be very similar depending on the time of presentation. Patients with AIS have an elevated serum testosterone level. A karyotype must be performed to verify this diagnosis and confirm the existence of a Y chromosome. Since intraabdominal testes must be removed, due to their malignant potential, an imaging procedure such as an ultrasound must be performed to assist in localization of the gonad.

Informing the patient and her parents of this diagnosis demands much tact and sensitivity. The primary issues are the impact of this anomaly on sexuality and subsequent fertility. The former issue will be explored in Chapter 12, while the latter will be reviewed at the end of this chapter.

MANAGEMENT

As with most vaginal surgery, adequate estrogenization of the perineum and lower vagina is necessary for a successful outcome. Since the diagnosis of MRKH syndrome is typically made after puberty, the perineal tissue has been exposed to sufficient estrogen levels. Both physical and emotional maturity are essential for a successful creation of a vagina. At our institution the average age of vaginal construction has been between 16 and 22 years.

With heightened awareness of this syndrome and the increased accuracy of our diagnostic methods, the diagnosis may be made in the prepubertal period. When the external genitalia appear normal, construction of the vagina should not be attempted until the perineum is exposed to estrogen at the time of puberty. A failure rate of 66% was documented in congenital adrenal hyperplasia patients undergoing prepubertal correction of their vagina and external genitalia. However, 70% of patients with congenital absence of the vagina had a successful outcome when they underwent surgical repair in the postpubertal phase (22). Prepubertal patients were typically noncompliant with use of dilators.

Both surgical and nonsurgical routes can be used to create a vagina in MRKH patients (Table 4). Our primary experience is with vaginal dilatation and McIndoe procedures. However the other methods will be discussed for the sake of completeness.

Vaginal Dilatation

The ease with which the vagina can be formed via vaginal dilatation suggests a possible embryologic defect at the level of the pelvic floor. Some patients present with the vaginal pouch already dilated due to repeated attempts at intercourse. These patients must be examined closely for urethral dilatation because at times they are engaging in urethral intercourse (23). In 1938 Frank described a non-operative method of creating a vagina (24) whereby active pressure is applied to the vaginal dimple on a daily basis with a series of vaginal dilators (Fig. 2). Because of awkward positioning and tediousness, this method did not gain popularity until Ingram reintroduced this concept in 1981 (25). He proposed passive vaginal dilatation while sitting on a bicycle seat. As opposed to the surgical methods of vaginal formation, which have a

TABLE 4. *Methods of MRKH management*

Nonsurgical	
Vaginal dilatation	Intermittent pressure (Frank, 1938)
	Sexual activity (D'Alberton, 1972)
	Bicycle seat stool (Ingram, 1981)
Surgical	
Dissection of perineal space	
No graft	Insertion of balsa wood form for continuous dilatation (Wharton, 1938)
Split-thickness skin graft	No mold use (Abbe, 1898)
	Use of mold (McIndoe, 1938)
Peritoneum as graft	With mold use (Davydov, 1969)
Amnion	Brindeau, 1934
Bowel	Ileum (Baldwin, 1907)
	Sigmoid (Pratt, 1961)
Muscle and skin flap	Modified Singapor (Woods, 1992)
Vulvovaginal pouch	Williams, 1964
Traction on retrohymenal fovea	Vecchietti, 1972

MRKH, Mayer-Rokitansky-Küster-Hauser syndrome.

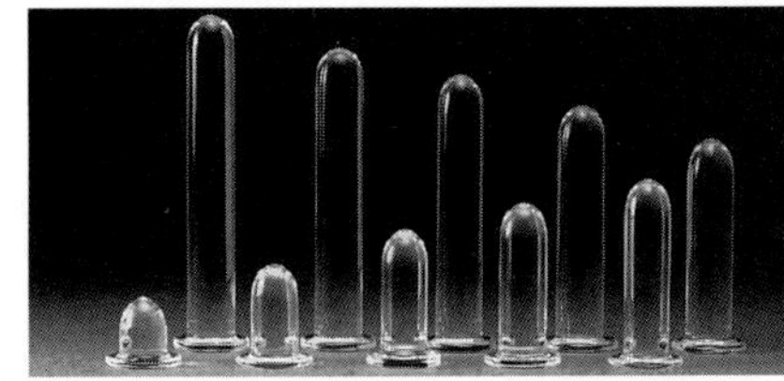
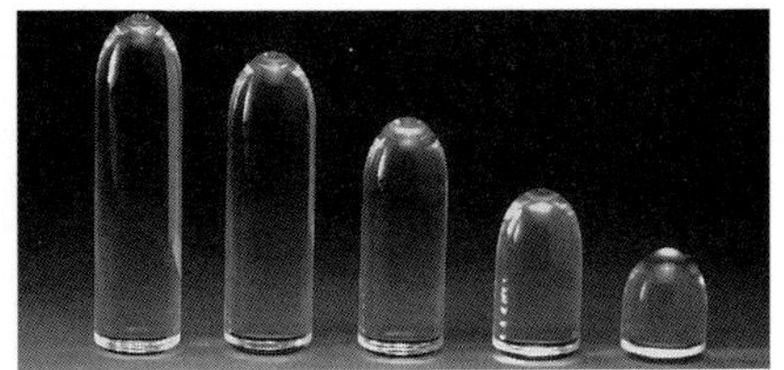

FIG. 2. Lucite dilators.

5% to 10% rate of complications, vaginal dilatation is essentially risk-free (26). Although the possibility of vaginal prolapse and eversion with the Frank method has been described (27), the ease and simplicity of vaginal dilatation behooves its use as the initial form of therapy in MRKH patients. Recently, Edmond et al. presented data on 139 patients who were treated by vaginal dilatation. Eighty-three percent of these patients reported successful intercourse without the need to revert to any further surgery (unpublished data). Despite multiple studies that confirm these findings (25,28), Rock et al. initially presented a series of 21 patients in whom vaginal dilatation was successful in only 9 (29). They now quote a functional success rate of 80% (6). Increased success rates may be attributed to the amount of support, education, and follow-up patients receive during dilatation attempts. Patients must be shown the exact location of the vaginal dimple and the axis of dilator placement, and encouraged to come back for frequent evaluation of the vaginal canal. Thus the success of this technique is dependent not only on the motivation of the patient but also the amount of guidance and support the patient receives.

When mentally and emotionally prepared, these patients appear to be very successful in developing a vagina within a 12-week period. The process is initiated by placing the smallest and thinnest of the Lucite dilators against the vaginal dimple. A peripad is then placed against the dilator followed by normal outer garments. The patient is instructed to sit against a bicycle seat or chair, which passively assists with the pressure application to the perineum (25). Thus, the vagina undergoes passive dilatation while the patient is performing other functions. It is very likely that the adolescent patient is more compliant with a passive dilatation process than with active dilatation. The dilator must be in position for a minimum of 20 minutes per day, 2 to 3 times a day. Typically the patient can change to the next size dilator within a month. Intercourse may be initiated when the patient is successful in using the largest dilator. If intercourse is infrequent, it is recommended that the patient continue to use the dilator. Unlike the surgical route of vaginoplasty, the patient can stop and reinitiate the vaginal dilatation process at any time without any long-term harm to the outcome. While many patients choose to undergo this procedure prior to going to college, the timing of the formation of the neovagina is dependent only on the patient.

McIndoe

Patients who have used dilators unsuccessfully or prefer surgery for the formation of the vagina have several surgical options available (see Table 4). The most widely

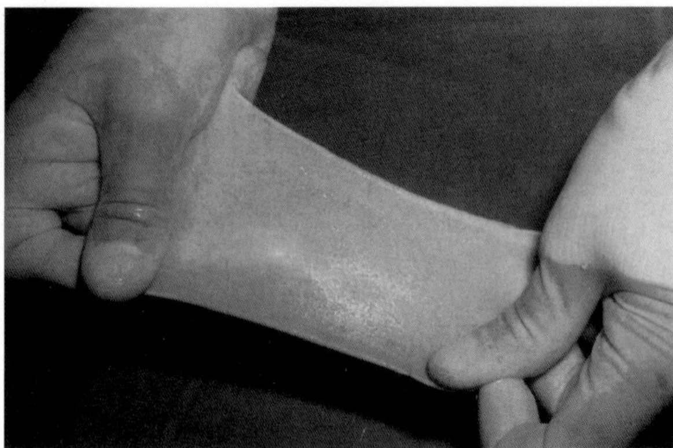

FIG. 3. Skin graft.

used technique is the McIndoe procedure. This method is also indicated in women who have a flat perineum or no vaginal dimple (30). In our institution we work conjointly with the plastic surgery team to obtain a split-thickness skin graft from the buttock area or the inner thigh. The patient is initially placed in the prone position. Great care is taken to ensure that the graft site is at a location that is usually covered by swimwear. The donor site is first soaked with epinephrine saline gauze to allow vasoconstriction of the small punctate bleeding sites. Mineral oil is applied, and an electrodermatome device is utilized to obtain a thick split-thickness skin graft (0.015 to 0.018 in. thick) (Fig. 3). This graft is placed through a 1:1.5 ratio skin mesher. The donor site is then covered with bacitracin followed by Op-site, which is secured in place with a few stitches. Healing occurs within 2 to 3 weeks and there is minimal drainage from the site. Meshing of the skin allows egress of any underlying blood clots or serous fluid. The split-thickness skin graft is sutured with 0000 absorbable suture around the vaginal mold such that it is completely covered (Fig. 4). Great care must be taken to use adequate if not excessive amount of skin graft for this step because areas of the mold not covered by skin graft can lead to formation of granulation tissue in the neovagina.

Next the patient is placed in the lithotomy position and a catheter is placed inside the bladder. A transverse incision is made in the area of the vaginal vestibule between the rectum and urethra (Fig. 5). The surgeon's fingers are used to dissect the areolar tissue in this space. If possible a finger should be placed inside the rectum to ensure

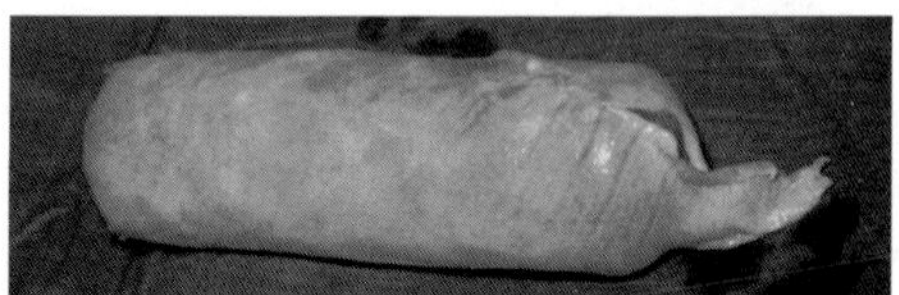

FIG. 4. Skin graft wrapped around mold.

its integrity during the dissection. Hagar dilators can be used to dissect the vaginal cavity, resulting in the formation of two vaginal canals on either side of a median raphe. Dissection of the median raphe connects the two channels. This method may minimize the bleeding that occurs with creation of the neovagina. The dissection continues up till the level of the peritoneum. All bleeding must be controlled meticulously since it may lead to eventual separation of the graft from the vaginal cavity. Prior surgery or irradiation in the perineal area leads to a more difficult dissection, with greater likelihood of damage to bowel and bladder secondary to scarring.

The mold, surrounded by graft, is placed inside the dissected cavity such that the dermal side of the split-thickness skin graft is in contact with the vaginal wall (Fig. 6). A few sites of the skin graft are stitched with 000 absorbable suture to the edges of the incision site or hymenal flaps. Several interrupted nonreactive sutures, such as 00 silk, are placed loosely so the labia cover the site of dissection and provide a barrier to the expulsion of the mold. The urethral catheter is kept in place until the patient returns to the operating room 5 to 7 days later for removal of the mold and evaluation of the graft site. During this time frame, the patient is kept on bed rest, low-residue diet, and an agent to slow bowel motility.

In our institution the primary surgery is performed on a Monday and the patient returns on Friday for removal of the labial stitches and mold, and trimming of the graft. The neovagina is cleansed with warm normal saline and closely evaluated for areas of hematoma or graft separation. Prior to discharge on that day, she is taught to take out and insert the mold atraumatically at the time of urination, defecation, and bathing, since it must be used continuously for a minimum of 3 months. In the ensuing 6 months, the patient must insert the mold every night if she is not sexually active. During periods of prolonged sexual inactivity the patient should revert to use of the mold to avoid progressive contracture of the vagina.

A variety of molds have been used and described by various surgeons. We use a glass mold, which has a diameter of 3 cm and depth of 12 cm. Upon discharge the patient has in place a plastic mold of the same dimensions that allows drainage (Fig. 7). Although some surgeons believe that a hard mold can lead to tissue necrosis and attribute their success to use of a soft mold such as foam, there is no comparative study available. Counseller and Flor advocated the use of a foam rubber mold in which a form is cut from a foam rubber block, covered with a condom, and placed inside the neovagina (31). The foam adapts to the contour of the vagina, thus applying equal pressure to the vaginal wall.

COMPLICATIONS

MRKH patients who have not undergone prior perineal surgical therapy achieve the greatest success rates. Hence the patient must be fully prepared to accept the responsibility of maintaining a neovagina, since postoperative care is very prolonged. The success rate of this procedure is about 80% (32), and although the complication rates have decreased significantly, serious complications still do occur. These include postoperative infection and hemorrhage, fistula formation, and failure of the graft take leading to granulation tissue. We maintain patients on prophylactic antibiotics

 VAGINAL AGENESIS AND VAGINAL SEPTA

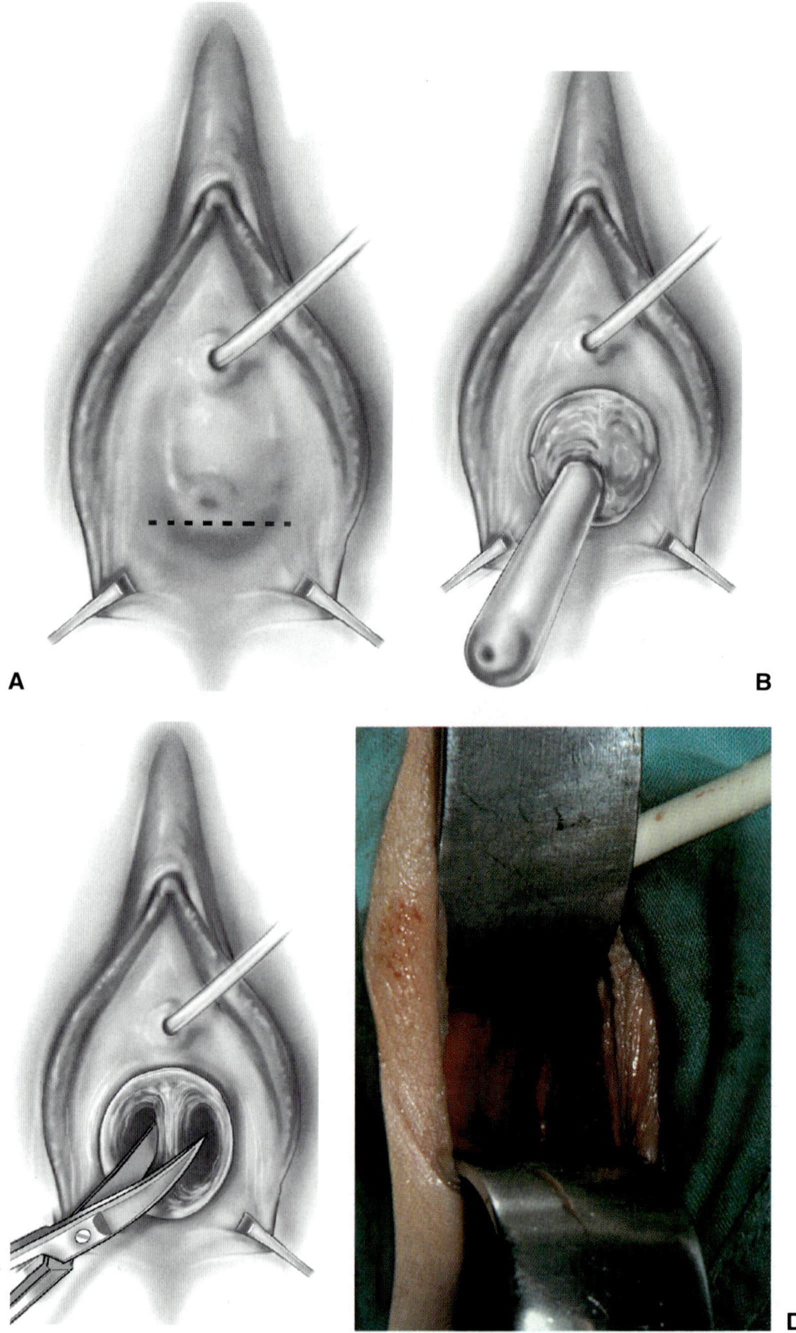

FIG. 5. A: Transverse incision. **B:** Use of dilator for creation of neovagina. **C:** Cutting of median raphe. **D:** Photograph of vaginal space.

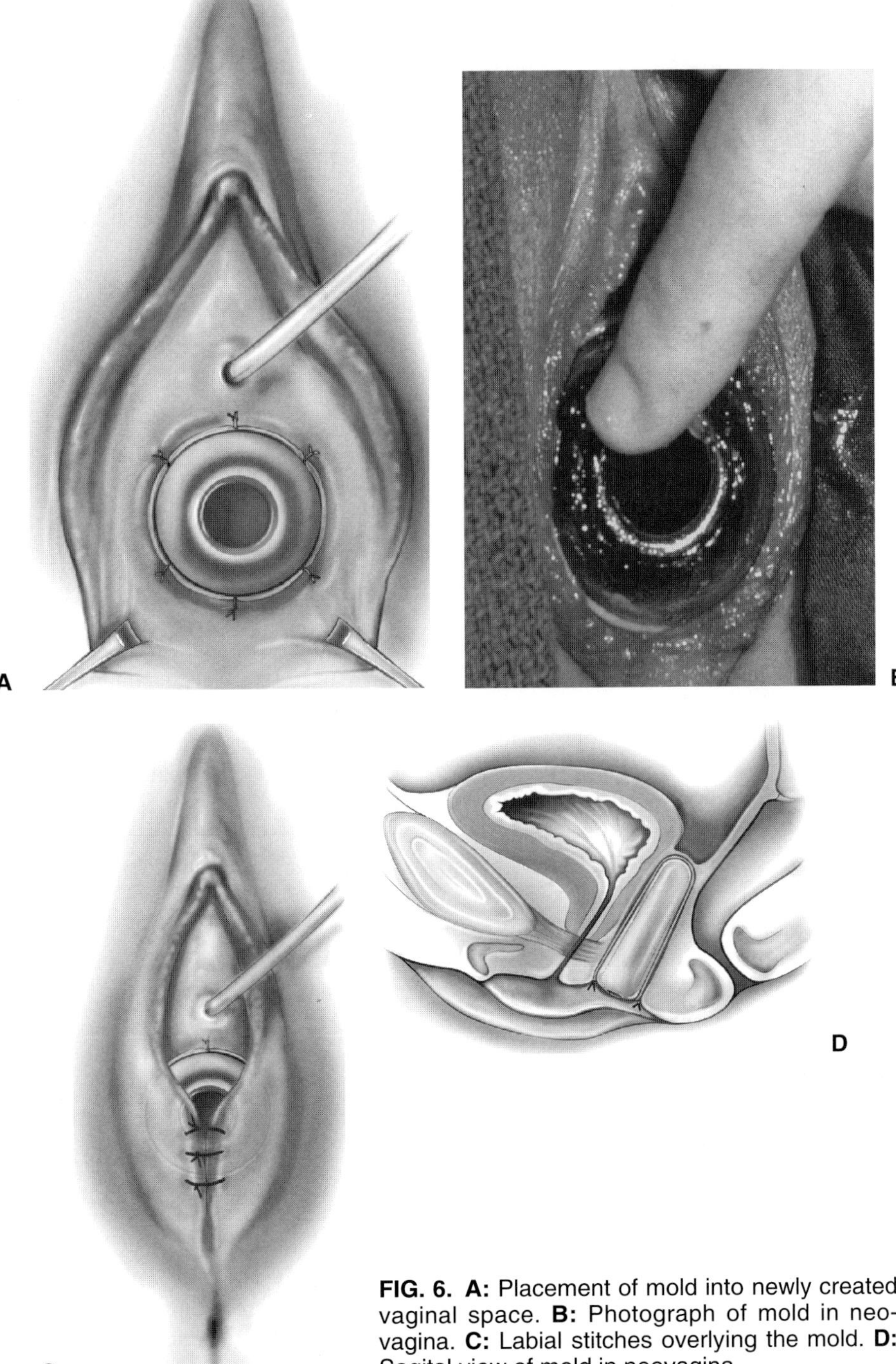

FIG. 6. A: Placement of mold into newly created vaginal space. **B:** Photograph of mold in neo-vagina. **C:** Labial stitches overlying the mold. **D:** Sagital view of mold in neovagina.

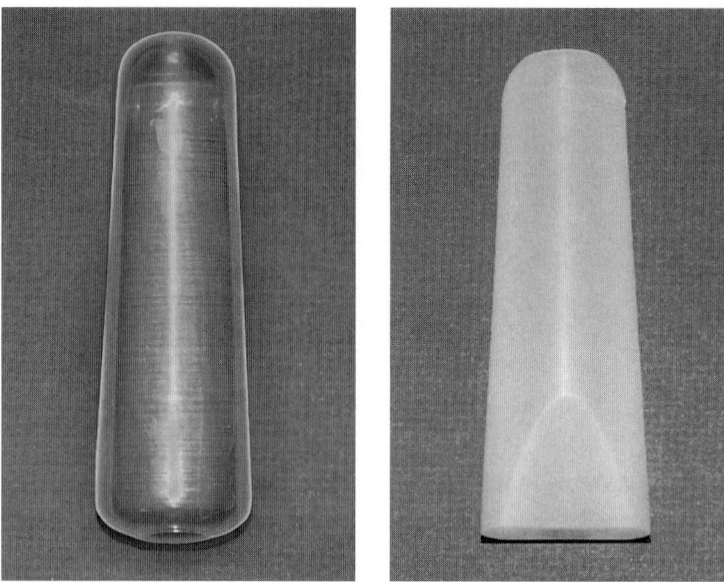

FIG. 7. A: Glass mold. **B:** Plastic mold.

throughout their hospital stay to diminish the chance of graft failure secondary to infection.

In our series of patients, one complication consisted of vaginal bleeding on the fourteenth day postoperatively which led to evaluation under anesthesia and evacuation of clots. No long-term complications were encountered in this patient. Another patient, subsequent to a urinary tract infection during the fifth postoperative week, did not reinsert the mold and required anesthesia for its replacement. She developed some adhesions of the vagina.

In a larger series at the Mayo Clinic, Buss and Lee reviewed data on 50 patients who had a McIndoe procedure performed during a 10-year interval (27). Forty-six of these patients had MRKH. They reported 2 rectovaginal fistulas, 1 graft failure, and 5 of the 50 patients required additional reconstructive procedures. In a questionnaire follow-up, 85% of patients considered their operation to be successful, but only 90% remained sexually active. Alessandrescu et al. from Romania have also presented a series of 202 patients in whom the rate of rectal perforation was 1%, graft infection 4%, and graft site infection 5.5% (33). Other reports confirm the low rate of complication associated with this procedure (1,34).

More operative difficulties are encountered in certain patients. The rectovaginal space is difficult to dissect in those who have had previous operations. These patients are at increased risk of bleeding and fistula formation. Problems are also encountered in patients with narrow subpubic arch, strong levators, shorter perineum, more rigid male-type perineum, prior hymenectomy, pelvic kidney, and congenitally deep pelvic cul de sac (27).

Amnion

The original McIndoe procedure required the use of a split-thickness skin graft, which potentially resulted in scarring and pain at the graft site. Amnion has been used successfully to line the neovagina, thereby avoiding the external reminder of the procedure (35,36) (Fig. 8). Epithelialization of the neovagina occurs in a very short time. Indeed, Dhall in 1984 demonstrated that by 8 to 10 weeks the resulting epithelium was histologically identical to normal vaginal epithelium (37). Amnion does not express histocompatibility antigens, thus it is not rejected by the body (38). In addition, it is believed to have an antibacterial effect by covering the wound (39). Because of the possibility of transmitting a viral infection with the use of amnion, this method, despite good results and lack of graft site, has not become popular.

Our experience is limited to two patients. Although the results were satisfactory, one patient had cicatration of the vagina and postoperative fever of 105°F. She was diagnosed with pseudomembranous colitis secondary to prophylactic antibiotic therapy. The other patient was diagnosed with human papilloma virus (HPV) infection at the cuff of the vagina. Because two strips of amnion were applied on separate occasions, both patients were hospitalized for a longer duration than those in whom a split-thickness skin graft was utilized.

Bowel

Another structure used to line the new vaginal cavity is the bowel. Pediatric surgeons are the primary advocates of this type of surgery. The patient must undergo a laparotomy to obtain a portion of small or large bowel with a preserved vascular pedicle, which is then sutured into the neovagina. The resulting abdominal scar requires a longer healing time than the site of a split-thickness skin graft. These patients do

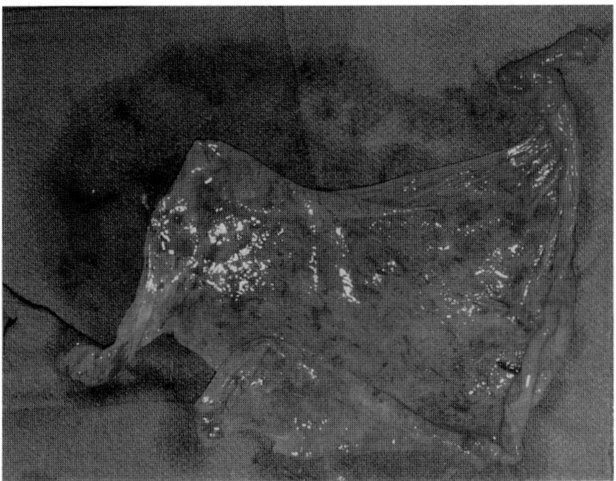

FIG. 8. Amnion.

not require the use of dilators, although they may have complaints of vaginal constriction especially with the use of ileum. In addition many patients complain of profuse foul vaginal discharge which does not necessarily dissipate with daily douching. Finally, there are case reports of adenocarcinoma formation in these grafts (40).

We have not used this method for patients with MRKH syndrome. Its use may be primarily indicated for correction of complex cloacal abnormalities. In the two instances when we utilized bowel to line the neovagina, the patients had complex vaginal anomalies. Both patients had complications, which included prolapse of the sigmoid neovagina and introital constriction. Vulvovaginoplasty and resection of the prolapsed bowel in two separate procedures corrected these complications. Freundt, who reported three such cases, echoed this experience (41). Although in the long term these patients are described as having anatomically satisfactory vaginas, it appears that more reoperative procedures may have been necessary (42).

Nongrafting Method of Vaginal Construction

Interceed Absorbable Adhesion Barrier (Johnson & Johnson Patient Care Inc, New Brunswick, NJ) is another agent that may be used to line the new vaginal canal. Unlike other neovagina linings, which must be harvested during a separate operative procedure, Interceed is a synthetic agent made of oxidized regenerated cellulose. By forming a gelatinous layer on raw surfaces, Interceed prevents adherence and scar formation. These properties have led to its use in the neovagina. Jackson and colleagues report the successful use of Interceed in 18 MRKH patients (unpublished data). Only one of these patients required a repeat surgery. Epithelialization occurred within 3 to 6 months in these women (43).

Wharton first proposed the use of a mold in the dissected perineal space in MRKH patients. Theoretically, if the space is dilated for long periods of time then epithelialization should occur. The success rate with this method was variable since some patients after years of using the mold failed to epithelialize adequately and thus had prolonged vaginal discharge and spotting from granulation tissue. In many cases the upper portion of such a vagina became constricted. Thus use of a perineal mold without graft fell out of favor. Makinoda et al. report the successful formation of a new vagina in 18 patients using a combination of initial vaginal dilatation, followed by dissection of the vaginal space, and suturing of the uterine remnants and uterosacral ligaments to the vaginal wall (44). Patients were required to use a vaginal mold for a minimum of 6 months and a graft was not utilized in this procedure. Complete epithelialization was not seen until 6 months after the operation. Indeed, only fibrin deposition is seen at the site of the new vagina at 7 to 10 days.

Williams Vulvovaginoplasty

The premise of this procedure is the formation of a perineal bridge (Fig. 9). A U-shaped incision is made leading from one labia down across the perineum and up to the other labia. The inner skin margins are undermined and sewn together. The next

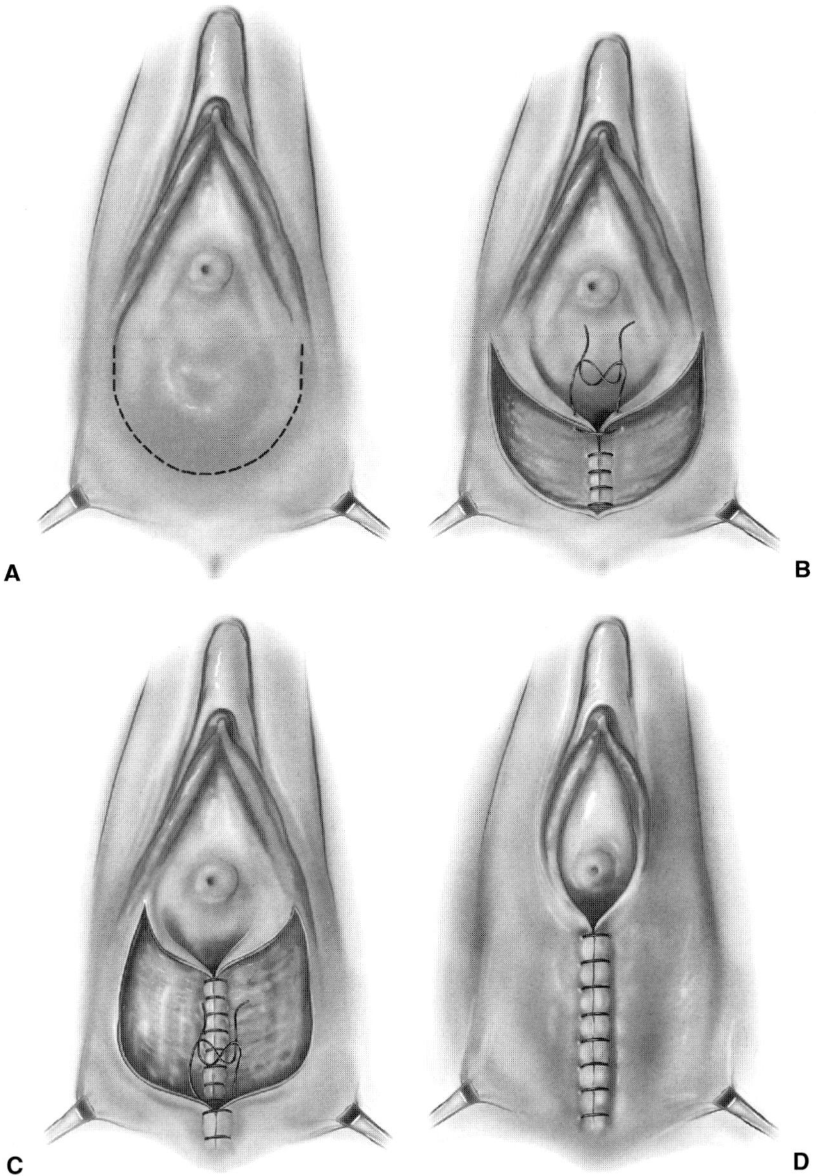

FIG. 9. A: U-shaped incision in a Williams vulvovaginoplasty. **B:** Reapproximation of inner incision margins. **C:** Reapproximation of outer incision margins. **D:** Completed perineal pouch.

layer of subcutaneous tissue is then sewn in the same manner and finally the outer skin margins are reapproximated with interrupted sutures. Since the pouch is formed parallel to the perineum, the axis of the vagina is abnormal. A dilator may be used for a short duration after the area has healed to rectify the abnormal direction of the vagina (45). This method should be considered the procedure of choice in cases where the patient has failed a prior vaginoplasty, or situations in which the vaginal introitus is extremely small due to prior irradiation. Since access is not gained into the pelvic cavity, the complication rate is very low.

Modified Sheares

The Sheares operation is less commonly known and used than the McIndoe. The objective of this method is placement of perineal skin into the space between the bladder and rectum. The presence of embryonic elements in this area may exert a growth-activating influence, leading to more rapid epithelialization of the newly created tunnel. Indeed, circumferential epithelialization from the edge of the isograft is noted to be rapid and complete (46). Initially a racquet-shaped incision is made in the perineal area between the urethra and rectum. The handle of the racquet extends over the fourchette toward the rectum. The skin is undermined and reflected posteriorly where it retains its attachment. In the manner described for the McIndoe, the tissue between the rectum and bladder is dissected carefully to a depth of 12 cm. The racquet-shaped tissue is then placed inside the newly formed cavity such that it covers the posterior aspect of the cavity. Several 00 absorbable sutures are utilized to hold the isograft in place. A vaginal mold must be inserted and kept in place by several interrupted non-absorbable sutures on the labia majora. After 14 days the mold is removed and the area is irrigated with warm saline. The patient must then accept the responsibility of using the mold on a twice-daily basis for a minimum of 15 minutes. According to Fliegner et al., after 3 months the epithelial layer in the neovagina is thick and strong enough to permit intercourse (46). We do not have any personal experience with this method of vaginoplasty for MRKH. However a modification of this technique has been used on occasion for some patients presenting with ambiguous genitalia. Ratnam has performed this operation on 44 patients with long-term follow-up of 4 months to 10 years. Good anatomical results were obtained in 39 of the patients (47). One vesicovaginal fistula was reported by this group. The Royal Women's Hospital in Melbourne reports satisfactory coitus in 10 of 11 patients who underwent this procedure (46). Cicatration and apical stenosis were rare complications of this surgery.

Muscle and Skin Flaps

Patients who have been exposed to heavy irradiation or multiple surgical procedures commonly have a major defect in the vulvar area. Muscle and skin flaps are indicated for the reconstruction of this defect. This is not the procedure of choice in a patient with MRKH syndrome (48). While gracilis myocutaneous flaps have been used successfully by some, others report an unacceptably high failure rate of 33%, which is attributed to tenuous vascularity of the flaps (49). In addition, the thigh scars can be quite prominent and conspicuous.

To overcome the vascular problem inherent in gracilis myocutaneous flaps, Wee and Joseph in Singapore designed flaps that maintained good blood supply and innervation (50). This technique was applied to their MRKH patients with success. Woods et al. further modified this technique and refer to it as the modified Singapore method (51). While they had no flap failure, they had problems with dehiscence, infection, and drainage in their patients. However, their cases involved high-risk patients who had multiple prior surgical procedures and irradiation to the area.

Labial Flaps

Song et al. (52) describe the use of labia majora and labia minora to create a new vagina. The resulting vagina is described as being soft, pliable, durable, and sensate. However, because of the scarring of the labia majora and minora, the vulva is distorted. Labiovaginal flaps created by tissue expansion have also been successfully employed in the creation of a neovagina (53).

Laparoscopy

Vecchietti's method (54) of upward traction on the retrohymenal fovea has been modified by Fedele et al. to be performed laparoscopically (55). After the pelvis is explored with the laparoscope, Vecchietti's needle is passed under direct vision through the subperitoneal tissue via the ancillary ports downward and medially until it reaches the pseudohymen. Upon perforation of the pseudohymen the thread of the olive device is hooked into the eye of the needle and brought back onto the abdominal wall where it is attached to a traction device. The same procedure is repeated through the other ancillary port. Thus graduated pressure on the olive by traction on the sutures via a spring appliance positioned on the patient's abdomen leads to formation of the neovagina. The Food and Drug Administration has not approved the use of this device in the United States. Care must be taken not to kink the ureters with placement of the stitches, so a cystoscopy must be performed at the time of stitch placement to ensure ureteral function.

LONG-TERM FOLLOW-UP

Long-term data on these patients is sparse and because of the individual variations used in vaginal construction, comparisons are rather difficult. Mobus and colleagues presented long-term data on 44 patients on whom they had used peritoneum for the construction of the vagina (1). Eighty-two percent of these patients had excellent results. The length of the measured vagina ranged from 3.5 to 15 cm. A minimum of a 6-cm vagina was necessary for unimpaired sexual intercourse. This finding concurs with our experience that the length of the vagina does not seem to have any correlation with the final result as perceived by the patient and her partner. Masters and

Johnson investigated the functional response of five MRKH women with neovaginas. Similar to an endogenous vagina, they noted a functional expansion of 2 to 3 cm in the vaginal depth during the excitement phase of sexual intercourse in MRKH patients. This extension may explain the self- and partner-reported satisfaction with sexual intercourse. Within 30 to 40 seconds of sexual stimulation, lubrication of the vaginal wall by mucoid material is noted. All had normal excitement, plateau, orgasmic, and resolution phases of sexual function with the neovagina (56).

The skin that has been grafted into the neovagina can transform and develop many of the characteristics of the normal vaginal mucosa (57). Vaginal swab reveals superficial squamous and large intermediary epithelial cells. In addition, the glycogen content of these cells approaches that seen in endogenous vaginal mucosa. It appears that the degree of epithelial differentiation is comparable to that of other women. However, even 13 years after the operation, keratinization could still be seen on the Pap smears. Complete loss of hair and sweat glands has been reported in a patient 20 years after her vaginal construction (58). Since both gonococcal infection and human papillomavirus have been reported in these patients (59,60), regular Pap smears are indicated.

Some suggest that an embryologic deficit in the pelvic floor fascia may account for the ease of vaginal dilatation and subsequent formation of the vagina. However, this deficit may also explain enterocele formation in some of these patients (6,61). While there are several case reports of such a complication, they are quite rare and it is unclear as to whether they are incidental or truly related to MRKH pathology. In our combined long-term follow-up of 30 years we have not experienced such a complication.

Endometriosis has also been reported in MRKH patients. In most instances a uterine remnant with a functioning endometrial lining is present and the patient has cyclic pelvic pain. Removal of the remnant results in resolution of the symptoms. In our series we have had only two patients with endometriosis.

Prior to in vitro fertilization (IVF), MRKH patients had no options in achieving pregnancy. While under stimulation with gonadotropins these patients have similar ovarian responses as non-MRKH patients undergoing IVF. High placement of the ovaries can make access to the follicles more difficult. Thus a laparoscopic approach to the ovaries may be necessary. Petrozza et al. report 34 live births from MRKH patients in whom only one congenital defect was noted (62). Thus it is unlikely that this anomaly is transmitted in a dominant fashion. Once the legal issues of surrogacy are further clarified, this avenue may become a more common course for MRKH patients.

RUDIMENTARY UTERINE BULBS (CLASS IE)

Congenital absence of the vagina is often associated with a rudimentary upper duct system. These rudimentary uterine bulbs usually do not cause symptoms but may occasionally be appreciated on rectal examination as a thickened central band. If there is a functional endometrium, then symptoms such as cyclical pelvic pain may occur.

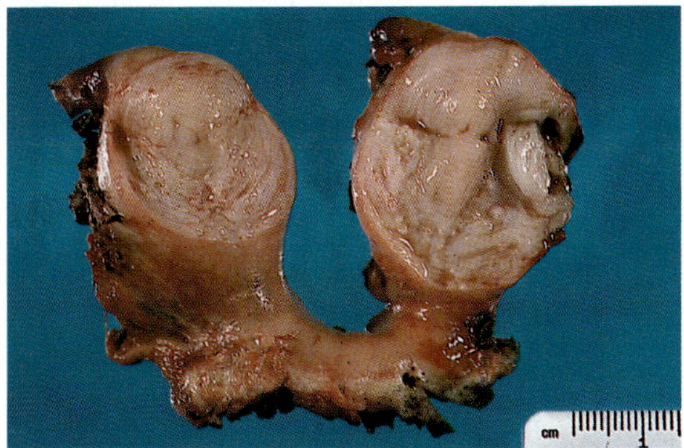

FIG. 10. Obstructing rudimentary horns.

The rudimentary uterine bulbs may be associated with fallopian tubes that are patent. In this case endometriosis may develop. If the fallopian tubes are occluded then a hematometra or hematosalpinx may occur. A thickened band of tissue (Fig. 10) often connects the uterine bulbs to each other. At times it may be many years before the patient is symptomatic; thus the initial laparoscopy may not be diagnostic.

Laparoscopy or laparotomy can accomplish excision of these rudimentary bulbs. We usually perform this procedure by laparoscopy as an outpatient. The following is a description of the laparoscopic approach, but the procedure is performed similarly by laparotomy. An umbilical port and two lower quadrant accessory ports are utilized for this procedure. Placing contralateral traction on the uterine bulbs can identify rudimentary round ligaments. Once the round ligaments are electrocoagulated and cut, the retroperitoneal space is opened and the ureter is identified. The incision is carried anteriorly to create a bladder flap. This dissection is carried down caudad until the fibrous band that connects the two uterine bulbs is identified. Excision of the fallopian tubes must occur without compromising the blood supply to the ovaries. The uteroovarian ligament is then cauterized and cut. The uterine artery is identified near the uterine horns and is dissected. The only remaining tissue is the fibrous band between the uterine horns.

Attempts have been made to reconstruct the rudimentary bulbs into a functioning uterus. Its usefulness is questionable since there are associated problems of stenosis and obstruction (63).

NONOBSTRUCTING VAGINAL SEPTA

Longitudinal

Incomplete resorption of the Müllerian ducts and urogenital sinus may cause the formation of a longitudinal vaginal septum. These septa account for only 12% of the malformations of the vagina. Nonobstructed longitudinal septa are typically asymp-

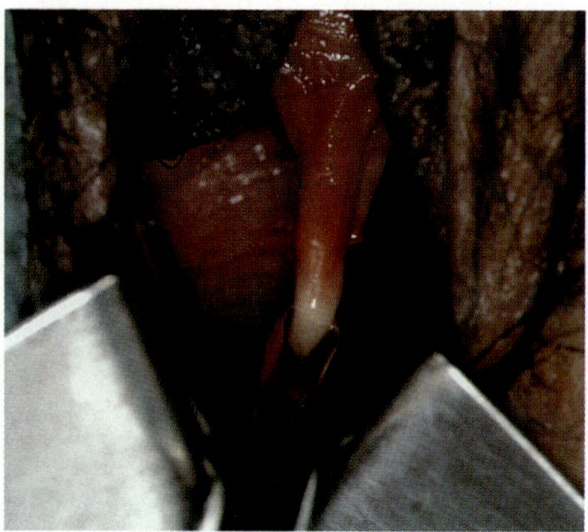

FIG. 11. Nonobstructing longitudinal septum.

tomatic (Fig. 11) (64,65). Thus the initial physical exam is very important in identifying these septa. Occasionally, the patient will complain of bleeding despite the placement of a tampon. The two vaginal cavities may be unequal in diameter, explaining why the diagnosis may be missed. In cases where the septum is incomplete, the patient may complain of a hooked tampon or pain with intercourse, which may be secondary to bruising of the septum.

Once a longitudinal vaginal septum is diagnosed, the Müllerian and renal collecting systems must be evaluated to rule out any associated abnormalities. In a review of 202 patients with longitudinal vaginal septa, 60% of the patients had a septate uterus (64). Heinonen, however, reports a predominance of didelphic uteri in these patients (65). Since uterine anomalies are associated with a poorer obstetric outcome, the uterine anatomy must be evaluated once a longitudinal vaginal septum is discovered.

Resection of the septum is indicated when the patient wishes to use a tampon effectively or when intercourse is painful. If the two cavities are equal in size and the septum is thick it may be necessary to remove the septum prior to delivery in order to avoid problems such as dystocia and tearing of septum during delivery.

Prior to initiating the surgery, a Foley catheter is placed in the bladder. Since these septums are typically well vascularized, Kelly clamps are systematically applied to the anterior portion of the septum and then cut with a knife or electrocautery device. Sutures are applied to each pedicle for hemostasis. The same procedure is applied to the posterior aspect of the septum. Great care must be used when approaching the most superior portion of the septum to avoid injury to the cervix. In this repair, use of a mold is not necessary. Although complications are very rare, a bladder wound has been reported.

Transverse

Since these patients do not have complete obstruction (Fig. 12), they present with complaint of inability to insert a tampon, and difficulty or injury during intercourse.

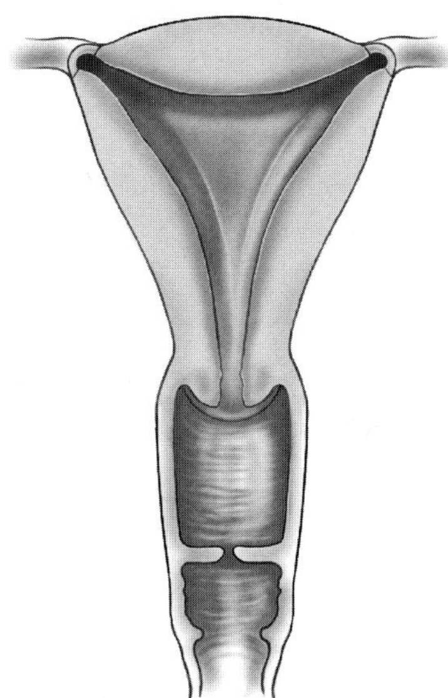

FIG. 12. Incomplete transverse septum.

On rare occasions they may present with fever and symptoms of an ascending pelvic infection. Physical examination reveals a short vagina and close inspection usually fails to demonstrate the pinpoint orifice, which must be present. Rectal exam will reassure the physician of lack of a hematocolpos, but the uterus should be palpable. In these patients it is important to perform an imaging procedure such as ultrasound during the luteal phase to delineate the anatomy.

Resection of the septum is an elective, nonemergent surgery. Thus the patient must be mentally mature enough to assume the responsibility of postoperative care. It is best to schedule the patient for surgery during her menstrual period at which time it is easier to identify the pinhole opening through the septum. The opening may be gradually dilated with dilators at which time an Allis clamp may be utilized to grasp the septum. The full diameter of the septum is excised, and the proximal and distal portions of the vagina are reapproximated with 00 absorbable suture. A mold must be kept in place for a minimum of 3 months to avoid cicatration.

Iatrogenic/Stenosis

Vaginal stenosis and septa may also occur as a result of prior surgery or irradiation in the area. Occasionally, it is necessary to tailor the repair by using a variety of surgical techniques. Case 2 illustrates this example.

Case 2

DB is a 22-year-white woman who was diagnosed with rhabdomyosarcoma of the vagina and bladder at age 3. At that time she underwent resection of the bladder and

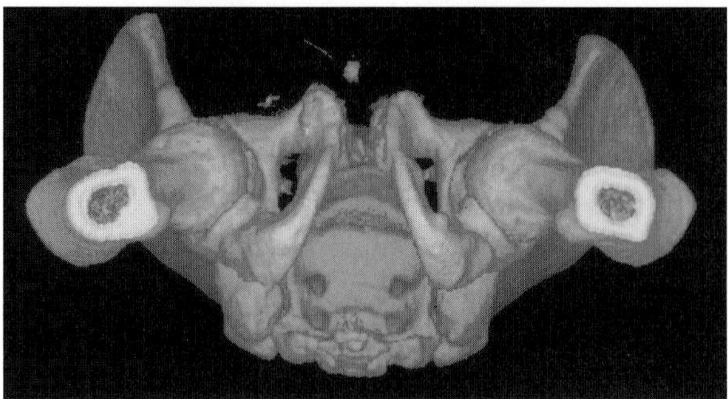

FIG. 13. CT scan of pelvis of patient exposed to radiation for rhabdomyosarcoma.

irradiation to the area. No recurrences were noted in the ensuing years. However, she failed to undergo puberty and was diagnosed with premature ovarian failure. Hormonal replacement therapy resulted in cyclic menstruation. She eventually presented at age 22 with inability to have intercourse. Examination revealed a small introital opening, narrow subpubic arch (Fig. 13), and a partial transverse septum originating at the 9 o'clock position, 2.5 cm into the vaginal cavity.

After undergoing cystoscopy and vaginoscopy to confirm the anatomy, she was scheduled for resection of the septum. The septum was excised and radial incisions were developed to enlarge the diameter of the vagina. Since the tissue had been irradiated, a split-thickness skin graft was applied to the area of dissection and a mold was placed inside. Due to a narrow subpubic arch, only a small-diameter mold could be inserted within the vaginal canal.

SUMMARY

Patients presenting with MRKH syndrome and vaginal septa should be evaluated thoroughly for concomitant Müllerian and renal anomalies. Both surgical and non-surgical routes of therapy have high rates of success if the patient is mentally and emotionally prepared. Thus she and her family must be counseled extensively and issues of sexuality, fertility, and pregnancy must be addressed with sensitivity and tact.

REFERENCES

1. Mobus VJ, Kortenhorn K, Kreienberg R, Friedberg V. Long term results after operative correction of vaginal aplasia. *Am J Obstet Gynecol* 1996;175:617–624.
2. Hauser GA, Schreiner WE. Das Mayer-Rokitansky-Küster syndrom. *Schweiz Med Wochenschr* 1961;91:381–384.
3. American Fertility Society classification of Müllerian anomalies. *Fertil Steril* 1988;49:952.
4. Buttram VC, Gibbons WE. Mullerian anomalies: a proposed classification (an analysis of 144 cases). *Fertil Steril* 1979;32:40–46.
5. Toaff ME, Lev-Toaff AS, Toaff R. Communicating uteri: review and classification with introduction of two previously unreported types. *Fertil Steril* 1984;41:661–679.
6. Rock JA. Surgery for anomalies of the Müllerian ducts. In: Rock JA, Thompson JD, eds. *Te Linde's operative gynecology,* 8th ed. Philadelphia: Lippincott-Raven Publishers, 1997:687–729.

7. Evans TN, Poland ML, Boving RL. Vaginal malformations. *Am J Obstet Gynecol* 1981;141:910–920.
8. Reindollar RH, Tho SPT, McDonough PG. Pubertal amenorrhea: a subset of 290 patients. *Adolesc Pediatr Gynecol* 1993.
9. Fraser IS, Baird DT, Hobson BM, et al. Cyclical ovarian function in women with congenital absence of the uterus and vagina. *J Clin Endocrinol Metab* 1973;36:634–637.
10. Carson SA, Simpson JL, Malinak LR. Heritable aspects of uterine anomalies. II. Genetic analysis of mullerian aplasia. *Fertil Steril* 1983;40:86–90.
11. Cramer DW, Goldstein DP, Fraer C, Reichardt JKV. Vaginal agenesis (Mayer-Rokitansky-Kuster-Hause syndrome) associated with the N314D mutation of galactose-1-phosphate uridyl transferase (GALT). *Mol Hum Reprod* 1996;2:145–148.
12. Dabirashrafi H, Mohammad K, Nikbin B, Moghadami N, Azari A. Histocompatibility leukocyte antigens in Rokitansky-Kuster-Hauser syndrome. *Am J Obstet Gynecol* 1995;172:1504–1505.
13. Buttram VC. Mullerian anomalies and their management. *Fertil Steril* 1983;40:159.
14. Rokitansky C. Uber die sogenannten Verdoppelungen des Uterus. *Med Jb Ost Staat* 1838;26:39–77.
15. Kuster H. Uterus bipartitus solidus rudimentarius cum vagina solida. *Z Geb Gyn* 1910;67:692–718.
16. Griffen JE, Creighton E, Madden JD, Harrod MJ, Wilson JD. Congenital absence of the vagina: the Mayer-Rokitansky-Kuster-Hauser syndrome. *Ann Intern Med* 1976;85:224–236.
17. Willemsen WNP. Renal skeletal ear and facial anomalies in combination with Mayer-Rokitansky-Kuster (MRK) syndrome. *Eur J Obstet Gynecol Reprod Biol* 1982;14:121.
18. King LA, Sanchez-Ramos L, Talledo OE, et al. Syndrome of genital, renal, and middle ear anomalies. A third family and report of a pregnancy. *Obstet Gynecol* 1987;69:491.
19. Turner G. A second family with renal, genital, and middle ear anomalies. *J Pediatr* 1970;76:641.
20. Winter JSD, Roaan G, Mellmaan WJ, et al. A familial syndrome of renal, genital and middle ear anomalies. *J Pediatr* 1968;72:88.
21. Letterie MGS, Vauss MN. Müllerian tract abnormalities and associated auditory defects. *J Reprod Med* 1991;36:765–768.
22. Goerzen JL, Gidwani GP, Bailez MM, Merritt DF, Caughey S, Yang M. Outcome of surgical reconstructive procedures for the treatment of vaginal anomalies. *Adolesc Pediatr Gynecol* 1994;7:76–80.
23. Taneja PP, Heera D, Gulati SM, et al. Urethral coitus in a case of vaginal agenesis. *Br J Urol* 1973;45:451.
24. Frank RT. The formation of an artificial vagina without operation. *Am J Obstet Gynecol* 1938;35:1053–1055.
25. Ingram JM. The bicycle seat stool in the treatment of vaginal agenesis and stenosis: a preliminary report. *Am J Obstet Gynecol* 1981;140:867–873.
26. Wabrek AJ, Millard PR, Wilson WB, et al. Creation of a new vagina by the Frank non-operative method. *Obstet Gynecol* 1971;37:408–413.
27. Buss JG, Lee RA. McIndoe procedure for vaginal agenesis: results and complications. *Mayo Clin Proc* 1989;64:758–761.
28. Wabreck AJ, Millard PR, Wilson WB Jr. Creation of the neovagina by the Frank nonoperative method. *Obstet Gynecol* 1971;37:408–413.
29. Rock JA, Reeves LA, Retto H, et al. Success following vaginal creation following mullerian agenesis. *Fertil Steril* 1983;39:809.
30. Rock JA, Jones HW Jr. Construction of a neovagina for patients with a flat perineum. *Am J Obstet Gynecol* 1989;160(4):845–851.
31. Counseller VS, Flor FS. Congenital absence of the vagina. *Surg Clin North Am* 1957;37:1107.
32. Hojsgaard A, Villadsen I. McIndoe procedure for congenital vaginal agenesis: complications and results. *Br J Plast Surg* 1995;48:97–102.
33. Alessandrescu D, Peltecu GC, Buhimschi CS, Buhimschi IA. Neocolpopoiesis with split-thickness skin graft as a surgical treatment of vaginal agenesis: retrospective review of 201 cases. *Am J Obstet Gynecol* 1996;175:131–138.
34. Wiser WL, Bates W. Management of agenesis of the vagina. *Surg Gynecol Obstet* 1984;159:108–112.
35. Morton KE. Human amnion in the treatment of vaginal malformations. *Br J Obstet Gynaecol* 1986;93:50–54.
36. Ashworth MF, Morton KE, Dewhurst J, Lilford RJ, Bates RG. Vaginoplasty using amnion. *Obstet Gynecol* 1986;67:443–446.
37. Dhall K. Amnion graft for treatment of congenital absence of the vagina. *Br J Obstet Gynaecol* 1984;91:279–282.
38. Akle CA, Adinolfi M, Welsh KI. Immunogenicity of human amniotic epithelial cells after transplantation into volunteers. *Lancet* 1981;2:1003.

39. Robson MC, Krizek TJ. The effect of human amniotic membranes on the bacterial population of infected rat burns. *Ann Surg* 1973;136:904.
40. Andryjowicz E, Qizilbash MB. Adenocarcinoma in a cecal neovagina—complication of irradiation: report of a case and review of the literature. *Gynecol Oncol* 1985;21:235.
41. Freundt I, Toolenaar TA, Jeekel H, Drogendijk AC, Huikeshoven FJ. Prolapse of the sigmoid vagina: report of three cases. *Obstet Gynecol* 1994;83(5pt2):876–879.
42. Freundt I, Toolenaar TAM, Huikeshoven FJM, Jeekel HJ, Drogendijk AC. Long term psychosexual and psychosocial performance of patients with a sigmoid neovagina. *Am J Obstet Gynecol* 1993;169:1210–1214.
43. Jackson ND, Rosenblatt PL. Use of interceed absorbable adhesion barrier for vaginoplasty. *Obstet Gynecol* 1994;84:1048–1050.
44. Makinoda S, Nishiya M, Sogame M, et al. Non-grafting method of vaginal construction for patients of vaginal agenesis without functioning uterus (Mayer-Rokitansky-Kuster-Hauser syndrome). *Int Surg* 1996;81:385–389.
45. Williams EA. Congenital absence of the vagina: a simple operation for its relief. *J Obstet Gynecol Br Commonw* 1964;71:511.
46. Fliegner JR. Congenital atresia of the vagina. *Surg Gynecol Obstet* 1987;165(5):387–391.
47. Ratnam SS. Vaginal atresia. In: Ratnamm SS, Soon-Chye N, Sen DK, eds. *Contributions to obstetrics and gynecology,* Vol. 2. Singapore: Longman Singapore, 1991.
48. Tobin GR, Day TG. Vaginal and pelvic reconstruction with distally based rectus abdominus myocutaneous flaps. *Plast Reconstr Surg* 1988;81:62.
49. McCraw JB, Massey FM, Shanklin KD, Horton CE. Vaginal reconstruction with gracilis myocutaneous flaps. *Plast Reconstr Surg* 1976;58:176.
50. Wee JTK, Joseph VT. A new technique of vaginal reconstruction using neurovascular pudendal-thigh flaps: a preliminary report. *Plast Reconstr Surg* 1989;83:701–709.
51. Woods JE, Alter G, Meland B, Podratz K. Experience with vaginal reconstruction utilizing the modified Singapore flap. *Plast Reconstr Surg* 1991;90:270–274.
52. Song R, Wang X, Zhou G. Reconstruction of the vagina with sensory function. *Clin Plast Surg* 1982;9:105.
53. Chudaff RM, Alexander J, Alvero R, Segars J. Tissue expansion vaginoplasty for treatment of congenital vaginal agenesis. *Obstet Gynecol* 1996;87:865–868.
54. Vecchietti G. Le neovagin dans le syndrome de Rokitansky-Kuster-Hauser. *Rev Med Suisse Romande* 1979;99:593–601.
55. Fedele L, Bianchi S, Tozzi L, Borruto F, Vignali M. A new laparoscopic procedure for creation of a neovagina in Mayer-Rokitansky-Kuster-Hauser syndrome. *Fertil Steril* 1996;66:854–857.
56. Masters WH, Johnson VE. The artificial vagina; anatomy and physiology. In: Masters WH, Johnson VE, eds. *Human sexual response.* Boston: Little, Brown & Co, 1966:101–110.
57. Lele RJ, Heidenreich W, Schneider J. Cytological findings after construction of a neovagina using two surgical procedures. *Surg Gynecol Obstet* 1990;170:21–24.
58. Pierce GW, Klabunde EH, O'Conner GB, Long AH. Changes in skin flap of a constructed vagina due to environment. *Am J Surg* 1956;92:4–8.
59. Bodsworth NJ, Price R, Davies SC. Gonococcal infection of the neovagina in the male-to-female transsexual. *Sexually Transm Dis* 1994;21(4):211–212.
60. Haney AF. Vaginal condylomata acuminata after McIndoe neovagina creation. *Sexually Transm Dis* 1990;17(2):102–105.
61. Peters WA III, Uhlir JK. Prolapse of a neovagina created by self dilatation. *Obstet Gynecol* 1990;76(5 Pt 2):904–906.
62. Petrozza JC, Gray MR, Davis AJ, Reindollar RH. Congenital absence of the uterus and vagina is not commonly transmitted as a dominant genetic trait: outcomes of surrogate pregnancies. *Fertil Steril* 1997;67:387–389.
63. Singh KJ, Devi L. Hysteroplasty and vaginoplasty for reconstruction of the uterus. *Int J Gynecol Obstet* 1980;17:457.
64. Haddad B, Louis-Sylvestre C, Poitout P, Paniel BJ. Longitudinal vaginal septum: a retrospective study of 202 cases. *Eur J Obstet Gynecol Reprod Biol* 1997;74:197–199.
65. Heinonen PK. Longitudinal vaginal septum. *Eur J Obstet Gynecol Reprod Biol* 1982;13:253–258.

Congenital Malformations of the Female Genital Tract: Diagnosis and Management, edited by G. Gidwani and T. Falcone. Lippincott Williams & Wilkins, Philadelphia © 1999.

9

Obstructive Müllerian Anomalies

Marjan Attaran, Tommaso Falcone, and Gita Gidwani

Department of Gynecology and Obstetrics, The Cleveland Clinic Foundation, Cleveland, Ohio 44195

Although Müllerian anomalies are believed to occur in 0.1% to 3.8% of the population, the true incidence of obstructive Müllerian anomalies is not known. In this chapter the various Müllerian anomalies that present with an obstruction to the outflow tract and their management will be reviewed. Cervical agenesis will be discussed in much greater detail in Chapter 10. Patients with obstructive anomalies may not necessarily present with pelvic pain at menarche or even close to the time of menarche. Since their presentation is quite variable, physicians must be attuned to the existence of these anomalies and actively consider them in their differential diagnosis.

CLASSIFICATION

The obstructive anomalies can be classified according to the American Society of Reproductive Medicine (ASRM) (1) classification as described in Chapter 8 (Table 1). This classification does not describe most vaginal anomalies. A proposed classification of vaginal anomalies is described in Table 2. Thus a patient presenting with uterine didelphys and a longitudinal obstructive vaginal septum has a class III uterine anomaly and class IIA vaginal anomaly.

IMPERFORATE HYMEN

Incomplete canalization of the urogenital sinus with the Müllerian system can lead to this anomaly. These patients may present at different stages of life. While in utero the infant is exposed to high levels of maternal estrogen; the vaginal tract and cervix respond by producing secretions. Obstruction leads to accumulation of these secretions and formation of a hydrocolpos (mucocolpos). This anomaly has been diagnosed while in utero (2,3). The incidence of congenital imperforate hymen is estimated to be 0.1%. It is typically considered to be an isolated finding. But rare associated anomalies may include polydactyly and duplication of the ureter (4), urethral membrane (5), imperforate anus (6), hypoplastic kidney with ectopic ureter and vascular anomalies (7), multicystic dysplastic kidney, and bifid clitoris (8). Although

TABLE 1. *ASRM classification of Müllerian anomalies*

Classification	Anomaly
Class I (Agenesis/hypoplasia)	a. Vaginal
	b. Cervical
	c. Fundal
	d. Tubal
	e. Combined anomalies
Class II (Unicornuate)	a. Communicating
	b. Noncommunicating
	c. No cavity
	d. No horn
Class III (Didelphys)	Didelphys
Class IV (Bicornuate)	a. Complete
	b. Partial
Class V (Septate)	a. Complete
	b. Partial
Class VI (Arcuate)	Arcuate
Class VII (DES-related)	DES-related

ASRM, American Society of Reproductive Medicine; DES, diethylstilbestrol.

in most cases imperforate hymen is a sporadic phenomenon, there have been reports of familial imperforate hymens suggesting genetic causes (9). Thus a family history should be sought.

The majority of infants will be asymptomatic and can be followed carefully without any surgical intervention. On occasion the hydrocolpos leads to urinary tract infections or is large enough to obstruct the bladder and cause urinary retention. In this situation surgical management is mandated immediately. When all other causes of a hymenal bulge have been ruled out, the imperforate hymen may be opened in the hospital or office setting after application of a topical anesthetic composed of 2.5% prilocaine and 2.5% lidocaine.

In some cases, due to increased awareness of this diagnosis, an asymptomatic prepubertal child is referred for evaluation of absent vagina. Since the prepubertal child is not estrogenized, the evaluation of the vagina can be quite difficult. The differential diagnoses at this point are labial adhesion, imperforate hymen, or absent vagina.

TABLE 2. *Vaginal classification*

Classification	Features
Class I	Transverse
	a. Obstructing
	b. Nonobstructing
Class II	Longitudinal
	a. Obstructing
	b. Nonobstructing
Class III	Stenosis/iatrogenic

Close inspection can typically differentiate labial adhesions (Fig. 1). Labial agglutination occurs in girls between the ages of 18 months and 6 years. The exact cause is unknown, but persistent irritation and poor hygiene might be contributing factors. If posterior in location, small, and not associated with any concomitant urinary tract problems, these adhesions may be left untreated. At the time of puberty with estrogenization, spontaneous separation of these adhesions will occur. In cases where the degree of adhesion is quite extensive, application of estrogen containing cream (e.g., Premarin) to the area twice a day for 2 weeks has been helpful. Once the adhesion has opened the patient may be switched to the use of a bland ointment to the area in addition to maintaining good hygiene. In cases where local application of estrogenic hormone cream has not been successful, a topical anesthetic may be applied to the area an hour before an attempt is made in the office to gently pull apart and loosen the adhesions. On occasion, in extreme cases, labial separation under anesthesia may be necessary.

Since the perineum is not estrogenized, an external genitalia inspection is unlikely to elucidate the difference between imperforate hymen and absent vagina. A rectal exam may be helpful in determining the existence of a uterus. An ultrasound of the pelvis, performed by a radiologist conversant with pediatric anatomy, should be obtained if there is any doubt concerning the existence of the uterus. If a uterus is present, the patient and her guardian are instructed to return at the time of initial breast development when a more thorough genital examination may be performed, but prior to the presumed time of menarche.

The final group of patients will present at the perimenarchal stage with complaint of cyclic abdominal pain and amenorrhea. Physical examination of the external gen-

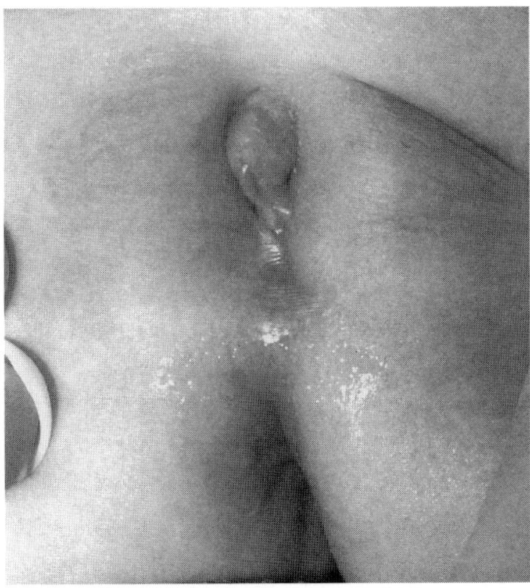

FIG. 1. Labial adhesion.

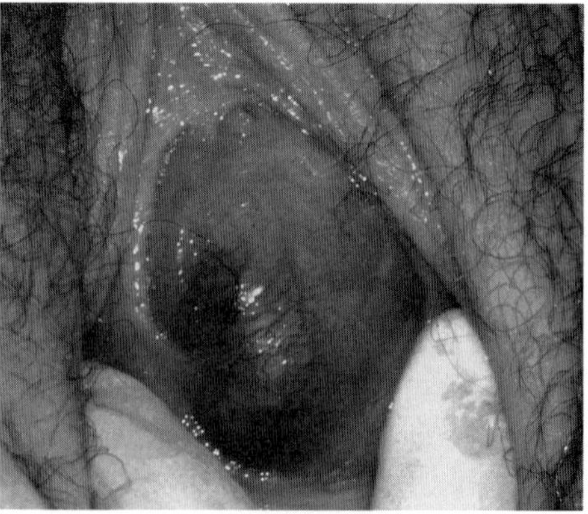

FIG. 2. Imperforate hymen.

italia is quite revealing. The imperforate hymen is noted to be bulging with a bluish hue (Fig. 2). Occasionally, the hematocolpos leads to distention of the abdominal cavity. This is one of the few emergency situations associated with congenital anomalies. These patients must be taken to the operating room where a cruciate incision is made through the hymen resulting in release of the hematocolpos (Fig. 3). Since the anatomy is distorted, examination of the cervix and vagina at this time is unrevealing and should be reserved for follow-up visit when the uterus and vagina have diminished in size. Under no condition should this hematocolpos be pierced in a nonsterile condition in the emergency room. Nonadherence with the proper technique may result in adhesion formation and recurrence of the obstruction.

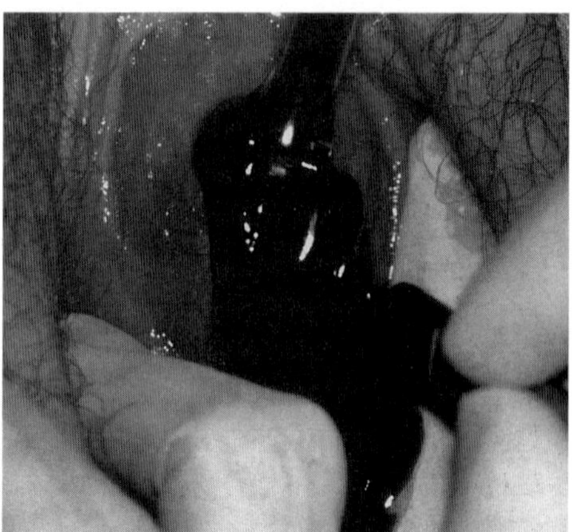

FIG. 3. Cruciate incision with release of hematocolpos.

Case 1

A 14-year-old girl presented to her physician with the complaint of cyclic abdominal/pelvic pain. Puberty had progressed normally. Patient had Tanner 3 breast development at the time of presentation. External genitalia examination revealed a bulging, bluish hue hymen. The patient underwent a hymenotomy but the edges of the hymen were not sutured. She re-presented at age 17 with difficulty using a tampon. Examination at that time revealed a cribriform-type hymen.

Case 2

A 14-year-old girl presented with abdominal pain and palpable pelvic mass. She was diagnosed with an imperforate hymen and had a hymenectomy performed with subsequent drainage of hematocolpos. One month later the patient again presented with pelvic pain. Examination failed to reveal a vaginal opening. But a rectal exam was consistent with hematocolpos.

She had a second surgery in which the low transverse septum was resected with appropriate reapproximation of the vaginal mucosa. One year later the patient presented with cyclic periods but an inability to place tampons inside the vagina. On physical examination a vaginal opening could not be detected. Surgery was timed to coincide with her period. At that time a pinpoint opening was noted and dilated grad-

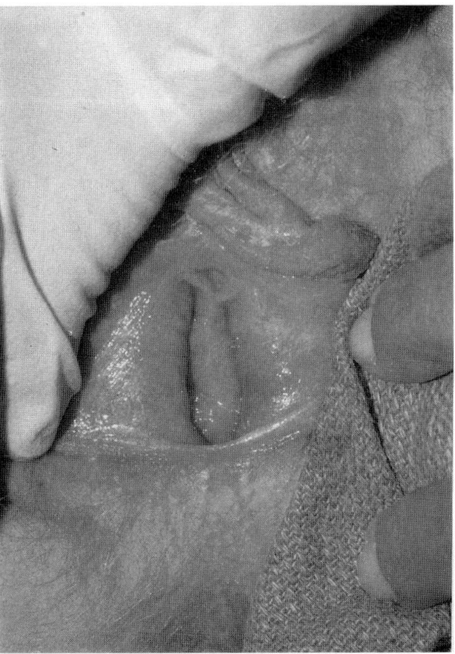

FIG. 4. Low transverse vaginal septum.

ually with Hagar dilators. After the cervix was visualized the septum was transected and excised. An obturator was placed in the vagina.

An imperforate hymen in the perimenarchal stage must be differentiated form a low transverse septum (Fig. 4). The Valsalva maneuver is advocated to differentiate these two entities. The imperforate hymen should bulge with the Valsalva maneuver, whereas the transverse septum should not. This differentiation is quite important because it will determine whether or not a mold is utilized in the postoperative period.

TRANSVERSE VAGINAL SEPTUM

Clinical Presentation

The incidence of transverse vaginal septum is reported to range from 1 in 2,100 to 1 in 72,000 (10). Transverse septa may result from incomplete canalization of the Müllerian system and the urogenital sinus. The exact cause of this incomplete canalization is unknown; however, there has been a report of familial transmission of this entity within the Amish community (11). Lodi et al. determined that 46% of transverse vaginal septa occur in the upper vagina, 40% in the midvagina, and 14% in the lower vagina (12). Rock and his colleagues have confirmed these results (4) (Fig. 5).

A transverse vaginal septum may be complete or incomplete. Patients with complete transverse vaginal septa usually present after puberty with a complaint of primary amenorrhea or pelvic pain. In our series of patients the mean age of presentation was 14 and the principle complaint was primary amenorrhea. Patients with a high complete transverse septum are likely to present earlier since there is less vaginal space for distention. Endometriosis is also more likely to be observed in these patients (13). When the obstruction is not complete the primary symptoms may be profuse vaginal discharge, inability to insert a tampon or have intercourse, or coital injury. On examination a perineal bulge may not be evident since the hematocolpos might be high in the vagina. Rectal examination may reveal a pelvic mass. Since associated anomalies include coarctation of the aorta, atrial septal defect, and malformations of the lumbar spine and urinary tract (4), a thorough history and physical examination is warranted and the renal system must be evaluated.

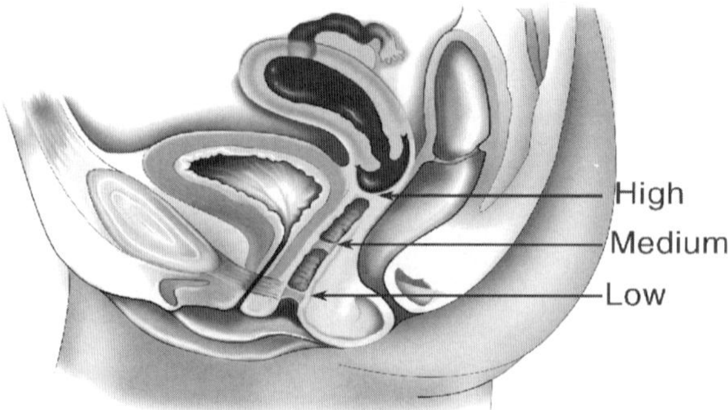

FIG. 5. Various levels of transverse septa.

In some instances a transverse septum may be diagnosed in young children and infants. They present with a hydrocolpos, which is composed of vaginal and cervical secretions. Occasionally, a large hydrocolpos causes obstruction at the level of the ureters leading to hydronephrosis. In severe cases the mass may be large enough to compress the vena cava and lead to cardiopulmonary failure (10). These circumstances would dictate the removal of the septum at the time of diagnosis. But the tendency for subsequent vaginal stenosis is quite high since the area is not estrogenized. Many of these patients will require vaginal reconstruction in the postpubertal years.

The obstructed portion of the vagina may have a different appearance than the nonobstructed vagina. Histologic evaluation of the transverse septum has revealed a diversity of epithelia (14). In most instances histopathologic evaluation of the septum reveals the obstructed side to be composed of glandular epithelium and the nonobstructed side of squamous epithelium.

These patients must undergo radiologic evaluation prior to surgery to help discriminate among the various Müllerian anomalies. Magnetic resonance imaging (MRI) has been particularly helpful in delineating the thickness of the vaginal septum. This information assists in better planning and execution of the appropriate surgery. Thus in instances where the septum is very thick and mucosal reapproximation may be difficult, the patient and her parents are prepared for prolonged use of a mold and possible skin grafting.

Surgical Repair

The goal of surgical repair is to excise the septum and re-anastomose the adjoining vaginal mucosa. A urethral catheter is positioned in the bladder to assist with confirmation of the location of the bladder. If the vaginal septum is not very thick, the perineal bulging of the hematocolpos may be clearly seen. Placement of a needle into the protruding part of the septum results in extrusion of old blood from the needle and assists with confirming the axis of dissection (Fig. 6A, B). The septum is then excised with cautery or knife until access is gained into the cavity behind the septum. After the full thickness of the septum is grasped with Allis clamps, it must be excised in its entirety up to the border of the vaginal mucosa. This mucosa is then undermined enough to be able to adjoin the upper portion of the vagina to the lower portion with delayed absorbable suture (Fig. 6C, D). A mold must then be kept in the vagina for a minimum of 6 weeks until complete epithelialization has occurred. At this time the patient can become sexually active. If she is not considering sexual activity at that time, then she must continue to use the mold on a daily basis. The commonest problem with resection of transverse septa is formation of stenosis and cicatration at the site of the excised septum. Thus prolonged use of the mold is recommended.

If the septum is high and thick it may be impossible to undermine enough vaginal mucosa for reanastamosis. In these cases a bulge is not necessarily noted; thus the dissection is somewhat blind. The axis of dissection is maintained between the bladder and the rectum. A finger in the rectum is helpful in guiding this dissection. The tissue that is being cut may be areolar in nature. Eventually the cervix may be palpated through

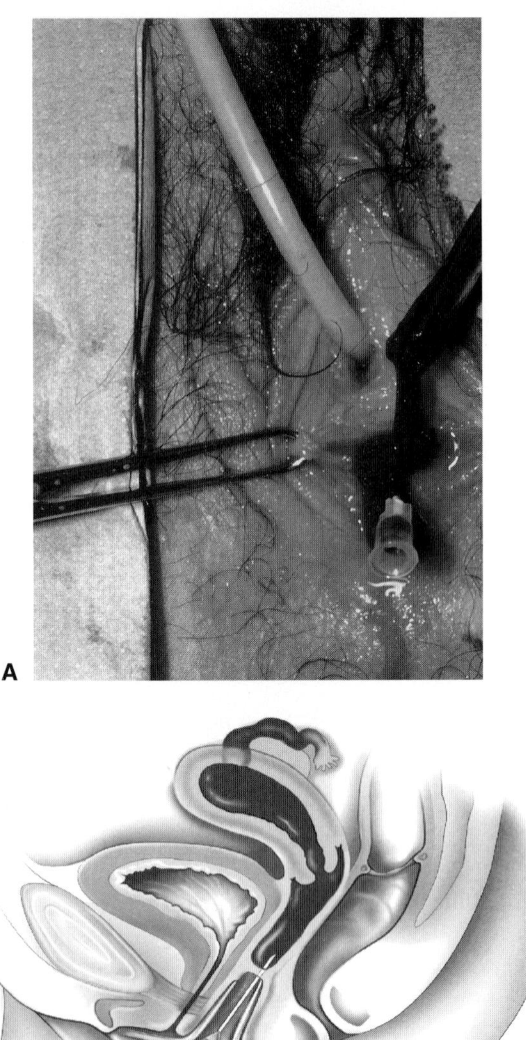

FIG. 6. A: Placement of needle into transverse septum. **B:** Sagittal schematic of above.

the areolar tissue and the two cavities can be joined. Since a significant portion of the vaginal mucosa is missing in these patients, a spilt-thickness skin graft may be sutured into place. A mold must be kept in place for a minimum of 3 months. In cases where a skin graft is not utilized the mold must be sutured into place for a longer duration of time. If anatomy is distorted and the location of dissection is unclear, one must be

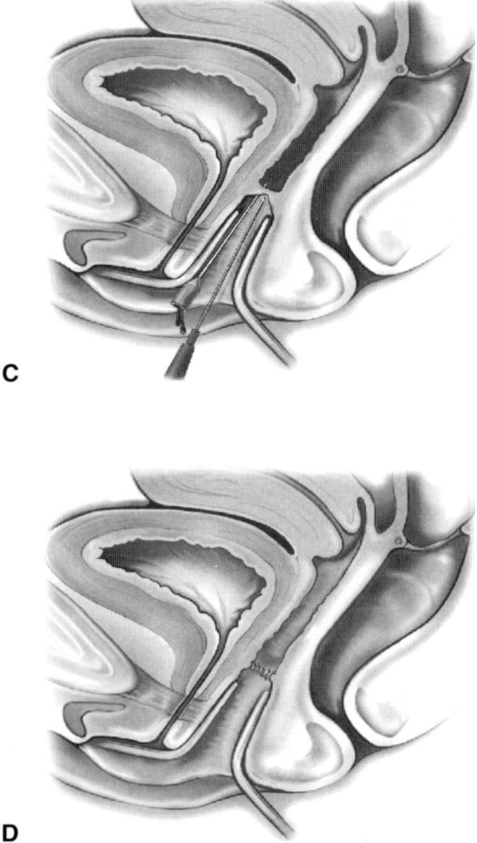

FIG. 6. *Continued.* **C:** Cutting through septum. **D:** Re-approximation of upper and lower vaginal mucosa with absorbable suture.

prepared to proceed with laparoscopic evaluation at the time. We have also intra-operatively utilized ultrasound to determine the correct axis of dissection. It is not uncommon to confirm correct anatomic landmarks by seeking another opinion intrasurgically.

Case 3

MC presented at age 22 with a complaint of chronic vaginal discharge and pelvic pain. She had been diagnosed with a bicornuate uterus at the time of her laparoscopy many years earlier for pelvic pain. In addition, she had had a hypoplastic right kidney and ureter removed. She specifically complained of a brownish discharge for many years that occurred postmenstrually till midcycle.

On physical exam, the right vaginal apex felt slightly thickened but no pelvic masses were palpable. A MRI revealed a uterine didelphys, two cervices, and two vaginas. A hematocolpos was seen in the right obstructed vagina. At the time of surgery, the hematocolpos could not be appreciated by exam. An ultrasound in the operating room assisted in locating the site of obstruction. A pinpoint opening was then noted adjacent to the normal left cervix. The opening was extended and access gained into the obstructed vagina.

In extreme cases where the direction of the dissection is unclear, it may be necessary to proceed with a laparotomy and place a probe through the fundus of the uterus past the cervix and into the obstructing septum. The septum may then protrude and provide evidence for the direction of the dissection (10). These patients must be counseled about the possible problems associated with surgery. They must have a bowel prep, and the colorectal team may be consulted if access is inadvertently gained into the rectum. In our experience it is best to terminate the definitive surgery at this point and proceed at another time. However the hematocolpos should be evacuated prior to terminating the procedure.

Whereas with vaginal agenesis surgery may be postponed until the patient is ready to assume the responsibility of a new vagina, patients with transverse vaginal septa have pelvic pain and must undergo surgery at the time of diagnosis regardless of whether they are mentally prepared. Thus compliance may be poorer in these pubertal patients. Hurst and Rock have reported delaying this procedure in three patients with a high septum (15). They were able to successfully decompress the hematocolpos via transvaginal needle aspiration. The patients were then placed on continuous oral contraceptive pills (OCPs) to prevent reoccurrence of the hematocolpos. They all underwent vaginal dilatation for several months followed by successful resection of the septum and reanastamosis of the upper and lower vagina.

Long-Term Outcome

There is a paucity of information on the outcome of these patients. In a series of 19 patients attempting pregnancy following resection of a transverse septum, 47% of attempts were successful (4). In this same study, 13 of 15 patients with imperforate hymen conceived and the spontaneous miscarriage rate was 5% versus 50% in the transverse septum group. Six of 7 patients with transverse vaginal septa who underwent laparotomy had endometriosis. In our series, 2 of 6 patients with complete transverse septa were noted to have endometriosis (Table 3). It may be that the lower pregnancy rates are due to higher rates of endometriosis in the transverse vaginal septa group.

TABLE 3. *Series of patients presenting with obstructive Müllerian anomalies from 1983 to 1998*

Class	Age at presentation	Symptoms	Prior surgery	Renal agenesis	Surgical procedure	Diagnosis	Outcome
Vaginal Ia	13	Dysmenorrhea	1	IVP-R	Excision of septum, laparoscopy	High transverse septum, hydrosalpinx	Repeat surgery for repair of transverse septum stenosis, split-thickness skin graft utilized, normal sexual activity
Vaginal Ib	14	Vaginal discharge, could not complete Pap test	0	Not known	Resection of septum	Low transverse incomplete septum	Normal sexual activity
Uterine IIb Vaginal Ia	16	Primary amenorrhea and 6-month history of worsening abdominal pain	1	US-N	Excision of septum, excision of uterine horn, laparoscopy	Complete transverse septum, left unicornuate, right rudimentary horn	Resolution
Vaginal Ia	14	Pelvic pain and abdominal mass, primary amenorrhea	2	IVP-bilateral hydro-nephrosis	Laparotomy with introduction of stent to drain hematocolpos, resection of transverse septum and placement of mold for 6 months	High transverse septum, extensive endometriosis, hemtosalpinges hydronephrosis	Regular periods, normal intercourse
Vaginal Ia	16	Primary amenorrhea, pelvic mass	0	N	Laparoscopy, resection of transverse septum, mold for 6 months	Transverse septum upper 2/3 of vagina	Resolution

Continued

TABLE 3. *Continued*

Class	Age at presentation	Symptoms	Prior surgery	Renal agenesis	Surgical procedure	Diagnosis	Outcome
Vaginal 1a	14	Pelvic pain, primary amenorrhea	1	N	Resection of transverse vaginal septum, laparoscopy	Transverse septum bilateral hydrosalpinges, pelvic adhesions, endometriosis	No follow-up
Vaginal Ia	14	Pelvic pain	2	N	Resection of transverse septum, laparoscopy	Transverse vaginal septum in the lower one third of the vagina	No follow-up
Uterine III Vaginal IIb	13	Dysmenorrhea, pelvic mass, malodorous discharge	2	IVP-R	Excision of longitudinal septum, excision of uterovaginal fistula, laparoscopy	Right incomplete longitudinal vaginal septum with pinpoint opening, uterine didelphys	Resolution of symptoms
Uterine III Vaginal IIb	16	Malodorous vaginal discharge, admission for salpingitis	0	U/S-L	Excision of longitudinal vaginal septum, laparoscopy	Left incomplete longitudinal vaginal septum	Resolution
Uterine III Vaginal IIa	14	Dysmenorrhea	0	U/S-L	Excision of left longitudinal vaginal septum, L hemihysterectomy	Longitudinal vaginal septum, uterine didelphys, endometriosis	Established full-term pregnancy
Uterine III Vaginal IIa	14	Lower abdominal pain, pelvic mass	2	IVP-N	Excision of R longitudinal septum, diagnostic laparoscopy	Complete R longitudinal vaginal septum, didelphic uterus, R hydrosalpinx, endometriosis	Established full-term pregnancy

Uterine III Vaginal IIa	13	Pelvic pain	1	R	R fimbrioplasty, laparoscopy, resection of longitudinal septum	Longitudinal vaginal septum, R hematosalpinx, with hematocolpos, uterine didelphys, adhesions	Resolution of symptoms
Uterine III Vaginal IIa	15	Severe dysmenorrhea	1	R	Resection of R obstructing longitudinal septum, R salpingectomy, lysis of adhesions, laparoscopy	Longitudinal vaginal septum, right hematosalpinx, endometriosis, uterine didelphys	Resolution of pain, cicatration of septum leading to resurgery
Uterine III Vaginal IIb	16	Irregular bleeding	1	L	Resection of longitudinal septum	Uterine didelphys, with longitudinal vaginal septum with small opening	Resolution of symptoms
Uterine III Vaginal IIa	26	Vaginal mass and pain	2	R	Laparoscopy, hysteroscopy, resection of R vaginal septum	Longitudinal vaginal septum communication in lower uterine segment, uterine didelphys	Pregnant
Uterine III Vaginal IIb	19	Pelvic pain, irregular bleeding	1	L	Laparoscopy, resection of septum	L longitudinal vaginal septum, uterine didelphys	Continued pain
Uterine III Vaginal IIa	12	Severe dysmenorrhea, pelvic mass	0	L	Laparoscopy, resection of L obstructing vaginal septum	Longitudinal vaginal septum uterine didelphys	Resolution of symptoms
Uterine III Vaginal IIb	18	Profuse vaginal discharge, neurofibromatosis, bulging vaginal mass	0	L	Laparoscopic resection of vagina septum, hysteroscopy	Longitudinal vaginal septum, with pinpoint opening, uterine didelphys	Resolution

Continued

TABLE 3. *Continued*

Class	Age at presentation	Symptoms	Prior surgery	Renal agenesis	Surgical procedure	Diagnosis	Outcome
Uterine III Vaginal IIa	15	Incidental finding on MRI	0	R	Laparoscopy, resection of vaginal septum	Obstructing longitudinal vaginal septum, uterine didelphys	No symptoms
Uterine III Vaginal IIb	26	Periodic profuse vaginal discharge	2	R hypo-plastic	Laparoscopy, resection of obstructing R vaginal septum	Obstructing longitudinal vaginal septum with pinpoint opening, uterine didelphys	Resolution
Uterine IIb	32	Failed induction of intrauterine fetal demise at 20 weeks	1	IVP-N	Laparoscopy, hysteroscopy, resection of rudimentary horn	Unicornuate uterus with L rudimentary horn non-communicating, hemato-salpinx, endometrioma	Attempting pregnancy
Uterine Ie	28	Pelvic pain, fever, primary amenorrhea	1	N	Laparoscopic resection of rudimentary bulbs	MRKH, obstructing rudimentary bulbs, R ovarian endometrioma	Resolution
Uterine IIb	17	Dysmenorrhea	1	IVP-N	Laparoscopy, continuous OCPs, resection of blind horn	Unicornuate uterus on the L with noncom-municating rudimentary horn on the R	No follow-up
Uterine III	18	Severe dysmenorrhea	0	IVP-N	Laparoscopy, Strassman operation	Uterine didelphys with stenosis of R cervix, obstruction of R uterus scoliosis, moderate endometriosis	Resolution of pain and endometriosis

MRI, magnetic resonance imaging; IVP, intravenous pyelogram; R, right; L, left; N, normal; US, ul-trasound; OCP, oral contraceptive pill; MRKH, Mayer-Rokitansky-Küster-Hauser syndrome

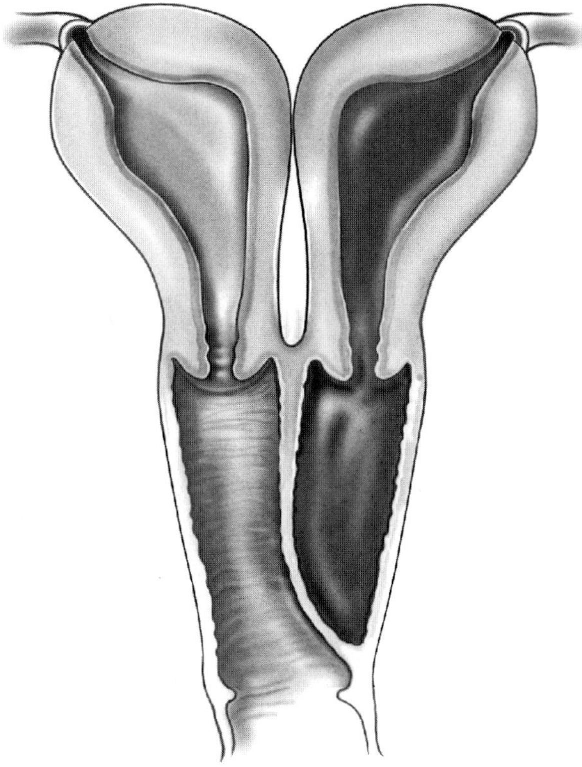

FIG. 7. Complete obstructing longitudinal vaginal septum.

OBSTRUCTING LONGITUDINAL SEPTUM

Patients with obstructing longitudinal septum can have either complete or incomplete obstructing vaginal septa (Figs. 7 and 8). Those with complete obstructing longitudinal septa present with cyclic menstruation but increasingly severe dysmenorrhea, and on physical examination the majority of patients have a paravaginal mass (16) (Fig. 9). Patients with incomplete longitudinal obstructing septa have a pinpoint vaginal communication and thus may complain of profuse or intermittent vaginal discharge. They may also present with irregular or prolonged vaginal bleeding because the incompletely obstructed vagina may drain more slowly than the unobstructed vagina. On rare occasions the pinpoint opening in the vaginal septum may allow access of organisms leading to symptoms of pelvic inflammatory disease and pyocolpos. Pelvic examination may not necessarily reveal an anatomic problem in cases of incomplete obstructing longitudinal septum. Thus a high index of suspicion is necessary to make this diagnosis.

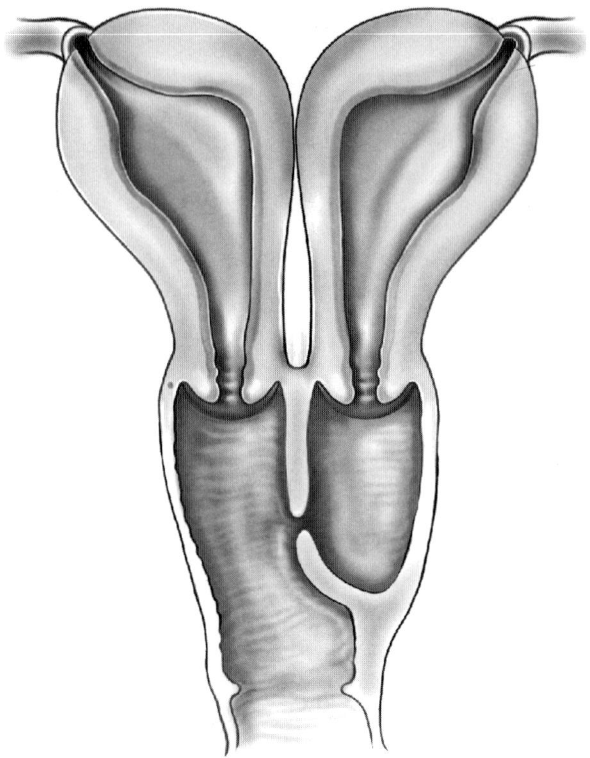

FIG. 8. Incomplete obstructing longitudinal vaginal septum.

Case 4

MD is a 16-year-old girl who presented with a complaint of profuse foul vaginal discharge. Her periods were described as regular and her past history was significant for neurofibromatosis with café-au-lait spots. An ultrasound revealed a uterine didelphys. Since the vaginal exam failed to reveal both cervices, she underwent an exam under anesthesia with subsequent finding of incomplete obstructed longitudinal vaginal septum. Resection of the septum revealed the second cervix and after several months the discharge diminished significantly.

Associated anomalies include a uterine didelphys and an absent or hypoplastic kidney typically on the same side as the obstructing septum. In our series of patients (see Table 3), 13 patients presented with longitudinal septa, 7 of which were completely obstructing. This group had cyclic pelvic pain, pelvic mass, notable bulge in the vagina, and both regular and irregular cycles. Six patients had an absent kidney, one had a hypoplastic kidney, and the other had normal kidneys. They all had uterine didelphys.

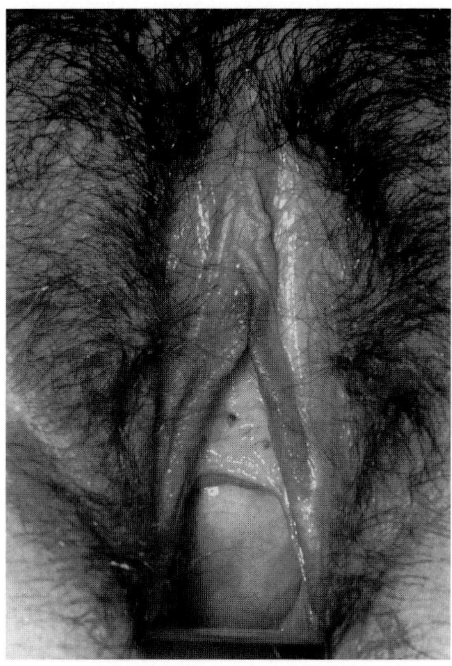

FIG. 9. Bulging vaginal mass in patient with complete obstructing longitudinal vaginal septum.

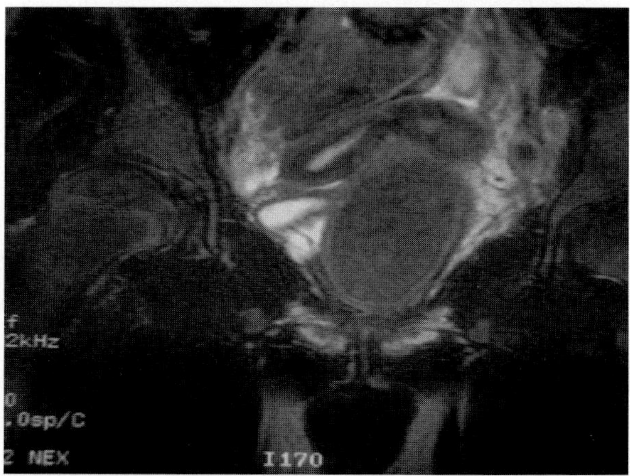

FIG. 10. Magnetic resonance image of hematocolpos due to obstructing longitudinal vaginal septum. Note the uterine didelphus.

Patients are primarily evaluated by means of an ultrasound to document uterine didelphus and the existence of the kidneys. In cases where the anatomy is unclear an MRI may be obtained, which provides good visualization of the hematocolpos and concomitant information on the renal system (Fig. 10). An absent kidney in the adolescent and pediatric population warrants an evaluation of the Müllerian system.

Surgical Repair

Initially a Foley catheter is inserted into the bladder and the patient is started on broad-spectrum prophylactic antibiotics. If she has a complete obstruction, examination of the vagina will reveal a bulge. A needle is positioned into this mass and the contents of the hematocolpos are noted to extrude through the needle. Next an electrocautery device is utilized to gain access into the obstructed cavity following the same axis as the needle. The septum, which is typically thick, is excised in its entirety and the upper and lower portion of the vaginal mucosa are reapproximated in a similar fashion to the transverse septum repair. Care must be taken when cutting the medial portion of the septum since it is in very close proximity to the unobstructed cervix. Failure to reapproximate the vaginal mucosa of the excised septum can lead to reformation of an incomplete septum and difficulty with future visualization of the cervix.

Both visually and tactilely, the cervix on the obstructed side appears abnormal (Fig. 11). It is typically flush with the vaginal fornix and appears erythematous and glandular. Both cervices should be sounded and a diagnostic hysteroscopy should be performed to confirm the existence of two separate cavities because on very rare oc-

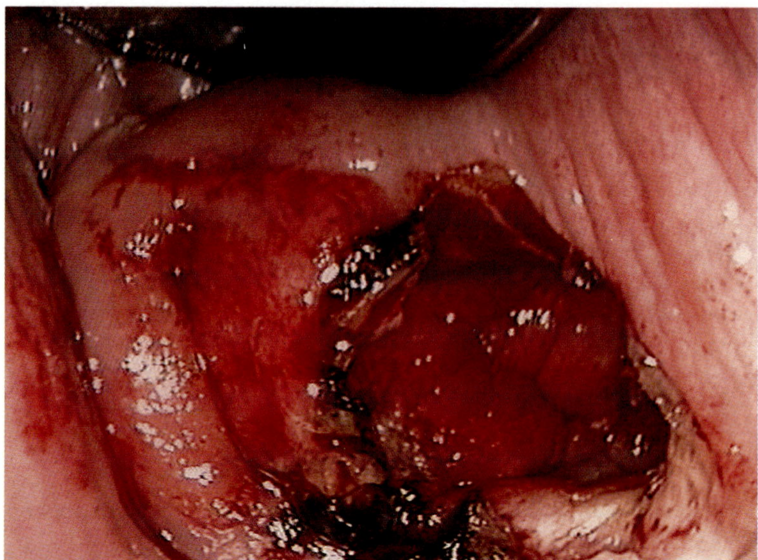

FIG. 11. Excised vaginal septum showing underlying cervix *(to viewer's right)* adjacent to normal left cervix.

casions the cavities are connected (Patient 15, Table 3). Histologic evaluation of the septum reveals columnar epithelium with glandular crypts on the obstructed side of the septum and vagina. Metaplastic transformation of the obstructed vagina to mature squamous epithelium may take many years (16).

The existence of endometriotic implants in patients with obstructive anomalies has been well documented (13). In the majority of cases relief of the obstruction leads to regression of the endometriotic lesion (13). Thus the decision to proceed with laparoscopy in these patients may be difficult. Stassart and colleagues noted endometriosis in all of their patients who had incomplete longitudinal vaginal septa (17). We advocate the liberal use of laparoscopy in the management of patients presenting with obstructing longitudinal septum. On occasion, the obstruction may have led to the formation of endometriomas and hematosalpinges, which rarely may need to be excised.

Case 5

KM is a 15-year-old girl who presented with chronic pelvic pain. Menarche began at age 13. Within several months of menarche she began experiencing dysmenorrhea. Referral to a surgeon for pelvic pain resulted in the finding and subsequent repair of a right inguinal hernia. Her pain did not resolve and at the time of her presentation she described the pain as continuous throughout the cycle.

She appeared emaciated and in significant pain. Rectal examination revealed a bulging tense pelvic mass. An adequate vaginal examination could not be performed due to the size of the mass. An MRI was performed which revealed an absent right ureter, a uterine didelphys, obstructed hematocolpos, and a right hematosalpinx. Laparoscopy at the time of vaginal septum resection confirmed the hematosalpinx and stage III endometriosis. Although the peritoneal endometriotic implants were not excised, the hematosalpinx was considered to be irreparable and was removed.

Due to the extent of the endometriosis and inadequate excision of the septum, permission was obtained to repeat a diagnostic laparoscopy at the time of the septum excision. Complete regression of the endometriotic implants was noted.

Long-Term Outcome

There are very few long-term studies on these patients. In the largest series presented thus far, when serial vaginal biopsies were obtained from the obstructed side, foci of hyperplasia of the basal reserve cells were seen and on occasion characteristics of mild dysplasia were noted (16). Indeed, these investigators report two cases of dysplasia of the vagina and three cases of vaginal adenosis. This vaginal histopathology may explain the occasional patient who complains of profuse vaginal discharge. Since the vaginal mucosa undergoes a slow transformation after the obstruction is relieved, caution should be used in interpreting the cytology and histopathology of these septa and vaginas. This dynamic environment warrants performing Pap smears on both cervices.

In our series as with others, chronic pelvic pain and dysmenorrhea resolved in almost all cases after surgical correction (see Table 3). Candiani and colleagues report a pregnancy rate of 87% and a live birth rate of 77% following surgical correction. Pregnancy outcome appears to be comparable with that reported for uterine didelphys associated with a longitudinal nonobstructing vaginal septum (16).

CERVICAL AGENESIS (CLASS IB)

The true incidence of congenital cervical agenesis is not known. These patients will present with primary amenorrhea and recurring cyclic pelvic pain in their early teens. Cervical agenesis may occur with or without the presence of a normal vagina. Rock attempts to differentiate between cervical agenesis and cervical dysgenesis in which a portion of the cervix is developed (10). On one end of the spectrum are patients with complete cervical agenesis, whereas on the other end are patients in which the cervix is hypoplastic. The problem lies in identifying the specific abnormality of the patient. At the time of surgery the anatomy can be distorted due to the hematocolpos, pelvic adhesions, and endometriosis.

Management of these patients is controversial, consisting of a hysterectomy versus a canalization procedure. In a recent review of the literature, Fugimoto et al. (18) reported on 58 cervical agenesis patients, in whom 40 initially underwent a canalization procedure. Seventy percent of these patients experienced normal vaginal bleeding although some required repeat canalizations. Women with both cervical agenesis and vaginal agenesis had poorer patency rates (40%) and greater likelihood of infection. The higher failure rate associated with vaginal atresia may dictate a more aggressive therapy such as hysterectomy. Cervical canalization has been reported to result in fulminant sepsis leading to death (19,20).

In short, patients who are diagnosed with cervical dysgenesis with an intact vagina may benefit from cervical canalization, whereas those with complete cervical agenesis may be better candidates for a hysterectomy. Other factors such as degree of pelvic adhesions, presence of endometriosis, number of attempts at surgery, success of medical therapy, and ability to correctly define anatomy will contribute to the final decision regarding hysterectomy.

Emotionally, the patient and her parents may not be able to accept the concept of a hysterectomy at the time of initial presentation. In such cases, after evacuation of the hematocolpos and relief of pain, some time may be gained by stopping menstruation via medroxyprogesterone (e.g., Depo-Provera) or continuous OCPs. During this quiescence period, not only may anatomic information be obtained by measures such as MRI, but also the patient has time to mature and understand the consequences of therapy. Spontaneous pregnancy has been reported in three patients who underwent canalization for cervical dysgenesis (21–23).

OBSTRUCTED UTERINE ANOMALIES (CLASS II)

Vertical fusion defects can result in a didelphic, bicornuate, or septate uterus. If there are no associated vaginal abnormalities, these defects are not associated with obstructive symptoms but usually are found in patients who are being investigated for

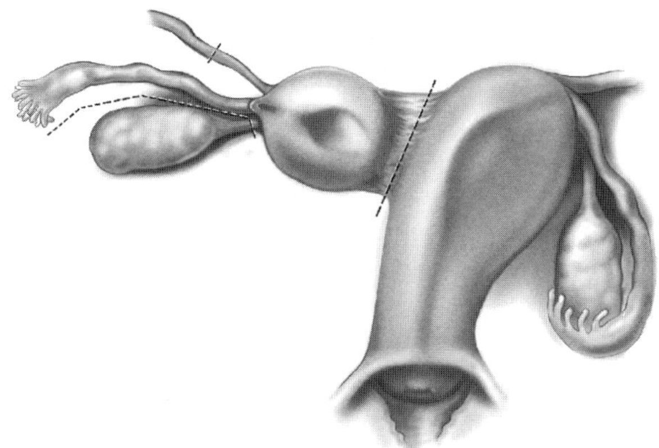

FIG. 12. Rudimentary horn attached to the unicornuate uterus with a band of tissue. Dotted lines represent the dissection planes.

infertility, recurrent pregnancy loss, or obstetric problems. These will be addressed in a subsequent chapter. A didelphic uterus can be associated with obstructive symptoms if there is agenesis of the cervix or, more commonly, if there is an associated obstructing vaginal septum.

Vertical fusion defects can also result in a unicornuate uterus (class II). Obstructive symptoms can occur if there is an associated rudimentary horn. Most patients with a unicornuate uterus will have an associated rudimentary horn, which can vary in three basic ways. First, there may or may not be a functional endometrium. Second, if an endometrial cavity is present, it may or may not communicate with the uterine cavity of the unicornuate uterus. Finally, the uterine horn might be part of the unicornuate uterus or it might be attached by a fibrous band (24) (Figs. 12 and 13).

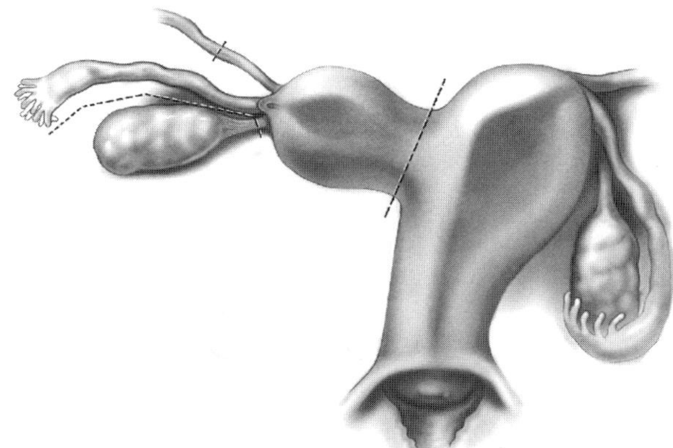

FIG. 13. Rudimentary horn attached to the unicornuate uterus without intervening tissue. Dotted lines represent the dissection planes.

Noncommunicating cavitated rudimentary horns are the most clinically significant as they are most likely to be associated with pelvic pain from hematometra or from endometriosis due to retrograde menstruation. Pregnancy in a rudimentary horn is a life-threatening condition because it is usually diagnosed late when rupture occurs in the second trimester (25). These patients usually present with severe dysmenorrhea since menarche, which is not alleviated by nonsteroidal antiinflammatory analgesics or oral contraceptives. Physical examination may reveal an adnexal mass or signs of endometriosis. The uterus may feel deviated to one side even if the adnexal mass is difficult to appreciate. The external genitalia, vagina, and cervix are normal. Preoperative ultrasound may reveal an adnexal mass that could be interpreted as an endometrioma. An obstructing Müllerian anomaly should always be in the differential diagnosis of this symptom complex in an adolescent or young adult. Preoperative MRI should be considered in this group of patients. Accurate diagnosis of the type of anomaly is critical to properly assess the appropriate surgical approach. A search for associated renal anomalies should be performed routinely. Anomalies of the urinary tract are often associated with a unicornuate uterus. A pelvic mass appreciated on examination may be a pelvic kidney.

Müllerian anomalies have increasingly been managed by surgical approaches that avoid laparotomy with excellent reproductive outcome. The rudimentary horns of a unicornuate uterus can also be managed by surgical techniques that avoid laparotomy. Many have described the techniques utilized for laparoscopic removal of a rudimentary horn (26–29). The surgical approach is the same whether it is performed by laparotomy or laparoscopy.

Access to the pelvic cavity can be obtained through a lower abdominal transverse incision or laparoscopically. The access is different but the procedure is the same. With the laparoscopic approach, a 10-mm trocar is placed intraumbilically and two additional trocars are introduced under direct vision into the peritoneal cavity (one 10-mm port in the left lower quadrant and one 5-mm port in the right lower quadrant). The tube associated with the rudimentary horn should be removed to prevent the possible risk of ectopic pregnancy from transmigration of sperm. Initially the round ligament is ligated and cut. The retroperitoneal space is opened and the ureter identified. The bladder peritoneum over the rudimentary horn is sharply dissected downward. A salpingectomy is then carried out starting at the fimbriated end. The tube is left attached to the rudimentary horn. The ovary may be malpositioned and the tube may lie above the pelvic brim. Therefore removal of the tube may require that surgery be initiated with a search for the tube and ovary above the pelvic brim. Finally, the uteroovarian ligament, which is the only remaining attachment, is ligated and cut.

The blood supply to the rudimentary horn is from the uterine artery. It courses up the side of the lower part of the unicornuate uterus. If the rudimentary horn is attached to the unicornuate uterus with a band of tissue (see Fig. 12), then tension on the horn away from the uterus will identify a plane that can be clamped and divided (a stapling device can be used laparoscopically). The blood supply to the rudimentary horn will be in this pedicle. Occasionally, there may be aberrant vessels to the rudimentary horn directly from the internal iliac artery.

If the rudimentary horn is firmly attached to the uterus, the blood supply to the rudimentary horn is not easily seen or dissected and is contiguous with the underlying myometrium. In this case, the uterine artery should be ligated as it ascends under the horn (see Fig. 13). The most difficult part of the procedure is dissecting the rudimentary horn that is firmly attached to the uterus. It is quite vascular and caution must be used not to dissect deeply into the myometrium of the unicornuate uterus. If the correct plane is identified, only a few sutures are required to reapproximate the myometrium. Reperitonealization is not required. The hemiuterus can then be removed by extending the 10-mm port or by morcellating and then removing the specimen.

Although it is clear that a noncommunicating rudimentary horn with a functional endometrium should be removed, removal of a communicating or nonfunctional rudimentary horn is controversial. There is no apparent risk to leaving a nonfunctional uterine horn. Patients with a communicating uterine horn with a functional endometrium should probably have the horn removed (30).

An unusual appearance of a class II Müllerian anomaly is a unicornuate endometrial cavity but a symmetric normal external surface. It is usually diagnosed when a unicornuate uterus is identified during a hysteroscopy or hysterosalpingogram and a normal uterus is seen at laparoscopy. These patients do not have obstructive symptoms but only those associated with the unicornuate uterus.

SUMMARY

Obstructive Müllerian anomalies are very unusual and can result in reproductive morbidity. Their diagnosis necessitates a high index of suspicion and their management is very challenging. Since anatomy can be very difficult to elucidate, we strongly advocate concomitant vaginal and laparoscopic evaluation of the patient. Multiple disciplines may be necessary to confirm anatomy. Thus treatment should be performed at centers that are familiar with these abnormalities.

REFERENCES

1. American Fertility Society classification of Müllerian anomalies. *Fertil Steril* 1988;49:952.
2. Winderl LM, Silverman RK. Prenatal diagnosis of congenital imperforate hymen. *Obstet Gynecol* 1995;85(5Pt2):857–860.
3. Kahn R, Duncan B, Bowes W. Spontaneous opening of congenital imperforate hymen. *J Pediatr* 1975;87:768–770.
4. Rock JA, Zacur HA, Dlugi AM, Jones HW, Te Linde RW. Pregnancy success following surgical correction of imperforate hymen and complete vaginal septum. *Obstet Gynecol* 1982;59:448–451.
5. Doyle JC. Imperforate hymen: with and without hematocolpos. *Calif Western Med* 1942;56:242–247.
6. Sen NC. Hydrocolpos. *Lancet* 1949;ii:991–993.
7. Iuchtman M, Assa J, Blatnoi I. Urometrocolpos associated with retroiliac ureter. *J Urol* 1980;124:283–285.
8. Fevre M. L'hydrocolpos et ses accidents. *Bull Acad Natl Med* 1957;141:619.
9. Usta IM, Anwad JT, Usta JA, Makarem MM, Karam KS. Imperforate hymen: report of an unusual familial occurrence. *Obstet Gynecol* 1993;82:655–656.
10. Rock JA. Surgery for anomalies of the Müllerian ducts. In: Rock JA, Thompson JD, eds. *Te Linde's operative gynecology,* 8th ed. Philadelphia: Lippincott-Raven Publishers, 1997:687–729.
11. McKusich VA, Koop CE, Bauer RL, Scott RB. Hydrometrocolpos as a simply inherited malformation. *JAMA* 1964;189:119–122.

12. Lodi A. Contributo clinico statistico sulle malformazioni della vagina osservate nella clinica ostetrica e ginecologica di Milano dal 1906 al 1950. *Ann Obstet Ginecol* 1951;73:1246.
13. Sanfilippo JS, Wakim NG, Schikler KN, Yussman MA. Endometriosis in association with uterine anomaly. *Am J Obstet Gynecol* 1986;154(1):39–43.
14. Suidan FG, Azoury RS. The transverse vaginal septum: a clinicopathologic evaluation. *Obstet Gynecol* 1979;54:278.
15. Hurst BS, Rock JA. Preoperative dilatation to facilitate repair of the high transverse vaginal septum. *Fertil Steril* 1992;57:1351–1353.
16. Candiani GB, Fedele L, Candiani M. Double uterus, blind hemivagina, and ipsilateral renal agenesis: 36 cases and long term follow-up. *Obstet Gynecol* 1997;90:26–32.
17. Stassart JP, Nagel TC, Prem KA, Phipps WR. Uterus didelphys, obstructed hemivagina, and ipsilateral renal agenesis: the University of Minnesota experience. *Fertil Steril* 1992;57:756–761.
18. Fugimoto VY, Miller JH, Klein NA, Soules MR. Congenital cervical atresia: report of seven cases and review of the literature. *Am J Obstet Gynecol* 1997;177:1419–1425.
19. Geary W, Weed J. Congenital atresia of the uterine cervix. *Obstet Gynecol* 1973;42:213–217.
20. Niver D, Barrett G, Jewelewicz R. Congenital atresia of the uterine cervix and vagina: three cases. *Fertil Steril* 1980;33:25–29.
21. Hampton H, Meeks G, Bates W, Wiser W. Pregnancy after successful vaginoplasty and cervical stenting for partial atresia of the cervix. *Obstet Gynecol* 1990;76:900–901.
22. Fraser I. Successful pregnancy in a patient with congenital partial cervical atresia. *Obstet Gynecol* 1989;74:443–445.
23. Zarou G, Esposito J, Zarou D. Pregnancy following surgical correction of congenital atresia of the cervix. *Int J Gynaecol Obstet* 1973;11:143–146.
24. Pinsonneault O, Goldstein DP. Obstructing malformations of the uterus and vagina. *Fertil Steril* 1985;44:241–270.
25. O'Leary JL, O'Leary JA. Rudimentary horn pregnancies. *Obstet Gynecol* 1963;22:371.
26. Falcone T, Hemmings R, Kalife R. Laparoscopic management of a unicornuate uterus with a rudimentary horn. *J Gynecol Surg* 1995;11:105–107.
27. Falcone T, Gidwani G, Paraiso M, Beverly C, Goldberg J. Anatomical variation in the rudimentary horns of a unicornuate uterus: implications for laparoscopic surgery. *Hum Reprod* 1997;12:263–265.
28. Canis M, Wattiez A, Pouly JL, Mage G, Manhes H, Bruhat MA. Laparoscopic management of a unicornuate uterus with a rudimentary horn and unilateral extensive endometriosis: case report. *Hum Reprod* 1990;7:819.
29. Nezhat F, Nezhat C, Bess O, Nezhat CH. Laparoscopic amputation of a noncommunicating rudimentary horn after a hysteroscopic diagnosis. *Surg Laparosc Endosc* 1994;2:155–156.
30. Andrews MC, Jones HW. Impaired reproductive performance of the unicornuate uterus: intrauterine growth retardation, infertility, and recurrent abortion in five cases. *Am J Obstet Gynecol* 1982;144:173.

Congenital Malformations of the Female Genital Tract: Diagnosis and Management, edited by G. Gidwani and T. Falcone.
Lippincott Williams & Wilkins, Philadelphia © 1999.

10

Diagnosis, Clinical Presentation, and Management of Cervical Agenesis

D. Keith Edmonds

Queen Charlotte's and Chelsea Hospital, London, W6 OXG, United Kingdom

Congenital absence of the cervix, or cervial agenesis, is a rare anatomic developmental abnormality. The literature has a limited number of described cases (1–35), but obviously not all cases of cervical agenesis are reported in the literature. Therefore its incidence remains completely unknown. In terms of the description in the literature, it is almost impossible to differentiate between cases of cervical agenesis and those in which the cervix is atretic, and while reference to the literature gives some descriptive evidence, it is far from clear.

The situation of classification is also made more complex because of the relationship between the development of the cervix, the uterus, and the vagina. In the Mayer-Rokitansky-Küster-Hauser syndrome circumstances exist whereby the hemiuteri may be functional; this is known as functional anlage. Whether these circumstances are due to the same etiologic process as that involved in cervical agenesis is very likely; therefore this syndrome of cervical agenesis is probably a midpoint in a developmental abnormality spectrum from normality to complete absence of the uterus and vagina (Fig. 1A, B). Because it is difficult to classify these abnormalities, management is controversial; certainly there is no consensus of opinion as to whether or not attempts should be made to salvage these uteri or whether they are best removed to prevent further problems. In addressing the anatomic problems, none of the published reports look at the psychological impact of this situation and authors report solely on the anatomic and surgical experiences.

This psychological aspect is extremely important as the age of presentation of these cases is usually very early in puberty. Generally at this stage, the pubertal child is unable to express an opinion as to her wishes other than those imprinted on her by her parents, and while it is most likely that she would choose to salvage her uterus, the true magnitude of the problem is difficult to impart to both parents and patient.

CLINICAL PRESENTATION

These girls usually present between the ages of 12 and 17 with primary amenorrhea and cyclical abdominal pain in the presence of normal secondary sexual charac-

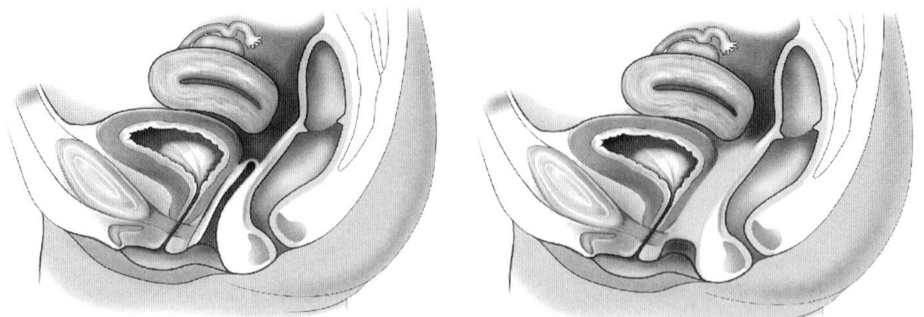

FIG. 1. A: Cervical atresia with normal vagina. **B:** Cervical atresia with vaginal atresia.

teristics. The cyclical abdominal pain is probably due to severe dysmenorrhea, following distention of the uterus by retained menstrual blood, pressure buildup during the shedding process, and the failure of uterine contraction to expel blood swiftly through any outlet. The pressure required to expel the blood through the fallopian tube and into the peritoneal cavity is considerably greater than that required to expel blood through a normal cervix, and it is this uterine spasm that causes the dysmenorrhea-type pain. It is, in my opinion, a fallacy to believe that retrograde menstruation is the etiology of the pain, as retrograde menstruation is a normal phenomenon in women, and while there may be an increased amount of menstrual blood appearing in the peritoneal cavity, it is unlikely that this is the cause of the pain. What is apparent is the increased incidence of endometriosis if these situations are not resolved reasonably quickly, and these circumstances are well described in congenital abnormalities that are associated with retrograde menstruation (36,37).

The presence of endometriosis might give a clinical picture of secondary dysmenorrhea but this is difficult to define in the amenorrheic girl.

Recurrent retrograde menstruation may lead to a hematosalpinx as the fimbrial end of the tube becomes occluded due to distal adhesion formation. These hematosalpinges can become very large indeed, and might present as a pelvic mass that itself can exert pressure on the bladder or rectum. This may lead to urinary frequency and occasional tenesmus.

These girls usually present as an acute surgical emergency due to abdominal pain. Examination of the patient will disclose that secondary sexual characteristics are normal, that the external genitalia are normal, and that the vagina is short and blind; occasionally, abdominal palpation will reveal a mass. However, in these circumstances rectal examination should be avoided because it is an unpleasant examination for an adolescent girl to undergo and it reveals no information that cannot be discovered with ultrasound or magnetic resonance imaging (MRI). As these two imaging techniques are mandatory in these patients, this is where efforts for diagnosis should be directed.

DIAGNOSIS

The diagnosis of cervical atresia will be made in one of four ways. First, ultrasound imaging of the pelvis may reveal the whole anatomic situation, and an experienced ultrasonographer, in conjunction with the gynecologist who is experienced with dealing with congenital abnormalities, will mean that it is rarely necessary to carry out any more sophisticated imaging techniques (Fig. 2).

All too often the problem of diagnosis on ultrasound concerns the clinician not taking the trouble to be present at the time of the ultrasound and the ultrasonographer not having sufficient experience in congenital abnormalities to be able to give a diagnosis. I would urge, therefore, that clinicians make it their duty to be with the patient at the time of imaging.

Rarely, the ultrasound image may be very complicated. For example, the presence of hemosalpinges and endometriomata can make interpretation of the ultrasound image difficult. Here MRI may be useful, and careful analysis of the films with the radiologist may help to define the anatomy and the diagnosis.

Occasionally, sadly, surgical intervention occurs as a result of the ignorance of clinicians to recognize in the adolescent the possibility of a congenital abnormality as a cause of abdominal pain. These girls are often laparoscoped on the misunderstanding that they might have a torted ovarian cyst or an appendicitis, and at this stage the congenital abnormality might become apparent. This situation requires the presence of an experienced clinician, if a final opinion is to be given, and occasionally general surgeons or gynecologists may perform a laparotomy because of the presence of a pelvic mass, only to find that the mass is in fact the result of a congenital abnormality, not some other form of pathology. Again, one can only emphasize the importance of clinical examination and adequate imaging in order to assess these girls very carefully before embarking on surgery.

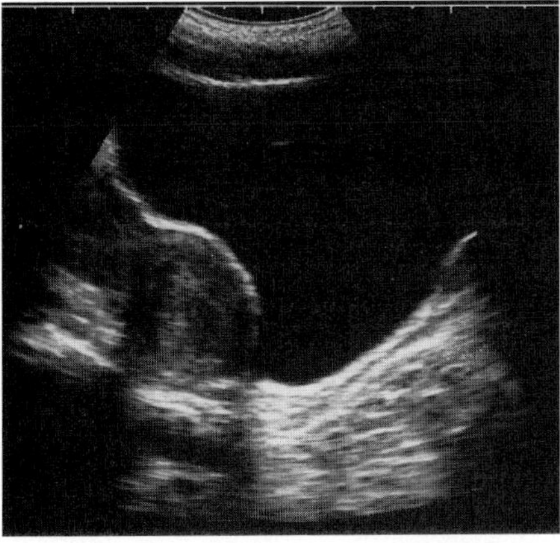

FIG. 2. Ultrasound indicating a hematometra in the presence of an absent cervix.

MANAGEMENT

The management of congenital cervical atresia is controversial. Such cases are extremely rare, and therefore there can be little doubt that each country should have centralized services to ensure that girls with this condition receive the best care possible. At present this does not occur and therefore the girls are managed by individuals with very limited experience. This cannot be in the best interest of the girls or their parents, and organizational avenues need to be opened in order to achieve the best results.

These services are not solely about the surgeon. In fact, they are about experienced ultrasonographers and radiologists, and about the availability of an experienced psychologist and experienced nurses with specialist knowledge. Finally, the clinician with more experience in these circumstances will be better able to counsel the parents and the patient as to the best outcome for them all.

The immediate management of these circumstances involves pain relief. This may require particularly potent analgesia, but as the pain will subside over 2 to 4 days in virtually all cases, there is no urgency to embark on surgery. Once the pain has receded, the appropriate imaging can be performed to make the diagnosis.

The medium-term management is then to take control of the pain until such time as surgery needs to be embarked upon. So long as these teenagers do not menstruate, they are pain-free.

Menstruation can be controlled either by the continuous oral contraceptive pill, depo-progestogens, or gonadotropin-releasing hormone analogs. All of these will ensure that time is available for a patient and her parents first to come to terms with the abnormality, and second to come to terms with the strategic options that face them, as well as the longer term sequela of sterility which often is the end result. It is therefore important to consider both the patient and her parents' request in terms of the choice of surgical options. There are two options that the surgeon faces: (a) hysterectomy or (b) an attempt at vaginoplasty and a uteroneovaginal reconstruction. The clinical features of the patient will determine which of these options is most appropriate. When the vagina is very short and the uterus very small, particularly if it is a hemiuterus, then it is very unlikely that any attempt at surgical reconstruction will be successful, and the literature supports this (20,22).

Conversely, when the vagina is reasonably long and the uterus is well formed, then attempts at reconstruction might be successful. Here, through a joint vaginal and abdominal approach, the upper vagina is opened from below. The uterus is exposed through a Pfannenstiel incision and a midline incision is made through the anterior wall of the uterus to enter the uterine cavity. The atretic part of the lower uterus is exposed, and a passage through which menstrual blood will subsequently flow is created where the cervix should have been. The open part of the vagina is then apposed to the posterior part of the uterus, and a Foley catheter is sutured into the uterine cavity and laid through the neocervix into the vagina. The uterine body is then reconstructed and the anterior vagina attached to the lower part of the uterus (Figs 3 to 5).

The stent that has been inserted then remains present for 6 to 12 weeks, in an attempt to create a permanent sinus for drainage. The author's own experience now includes 15 patients and 8 of these are currently menstruating regularly.

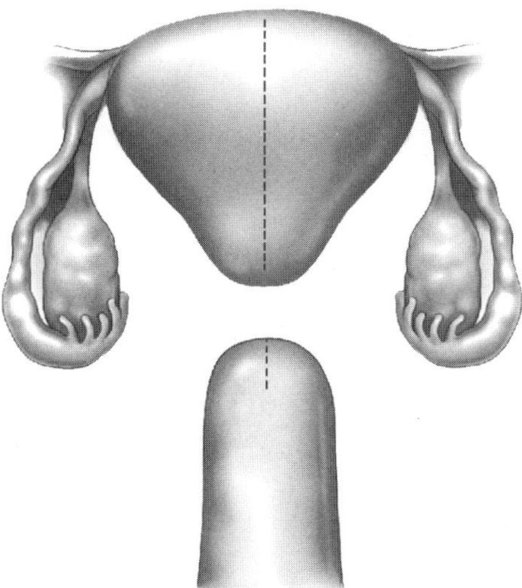

FIG. 3. Incisions on the vagina and anterior uterine wall.

However, seven have failed to menstruate and have subsequently required a hysterectomy. It is a very limited experience, and the rest of the world literature is limited to some 70 to 80 cases (1–35). However, in those cases in which reconstruction has been attempted, a 50% success rate seems to be realistic. However, this figure must be given very cautiously as no randomized trials have ever been carried out or are ever likely to be. The complications of this reconstructive-type procedure may be considerable and serious sepsis has occurred in two cases, resulting in death of the

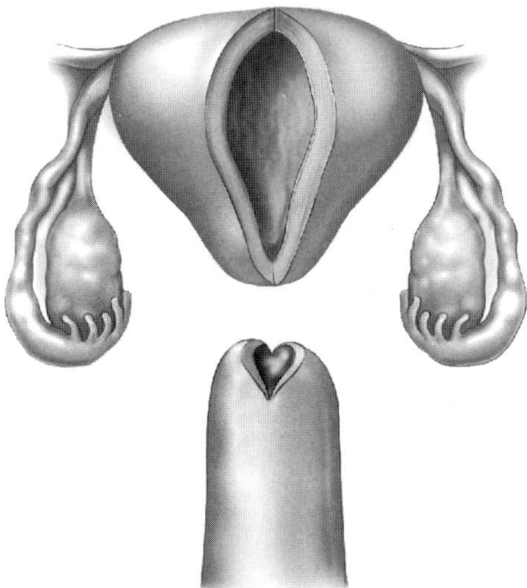

FIG. 4. Opened uterus and vaginal vault.

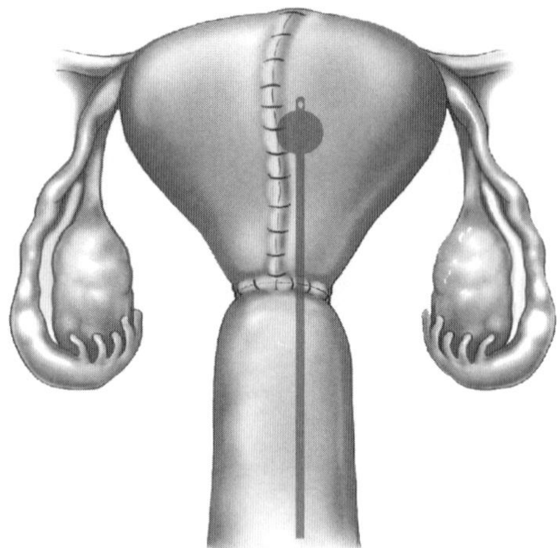

FIG. 5. Vagina sutured to lower uterine pole.

patient (10,17). As a result of this, embarking on this type of surgery is fraught with danger. As we are only talking about some 70 described cases, this surgery should only be carried out by extremely experienced surgeons with knowledge about reconstruction of congenital abnormalities.

An advantage of this type of reconstruction is that the uterus is conserved for fertility; in fact, there have been four pregnancies in patients with this type of disorder, in which the uterus has been conserved. Three of them are allegedly spontaneous pregnancies, and one occurred through assisted reproductive technologies (11,25,28,29). It is therefore important to understand that the salvation of the uterus is for reproductive purposes only and that because there is a surgical risk in the procedure careful assessment is required.

The surgery is arduous and for young teenage girls may not be desirable immediately after the diagnosis is made. The medical strategy of buying time while the family come to terms with the difficulty is one that should be carefully considered. Acceptance of the difficulties can take many months or even years before surgery is requested, but we have an obligation to try to help these patients through difficult times and not to rush them through their surgery, whatever the decision of outcome.

CONCLUSION

This very rare condition of cervical atresia is complex, primarily because of the management options. There are no clear guidelines as to whether or not reconstruction of the genital tract should be attempted, or whether or not hysterectomy should be the operation of choice. The psychological difficulties that are faced by these young girls and their parents require attention in just the same way as the anatomic abnormality does. These psychological problems need to be addressed over the long term, whereas the surgical decision is a short-term one. Care must be taken to centralize these services so that a holistic approach to the management of the patient can be available, as is in her best interests. Currently, this cannot be said to be the case and one must hope that the future will hold a more optimistic outlook for girls with this rare congenital abnormality.

REFERENCES

1. Ludwig A. Cervical absence. *Contralbl Gynak* 1900;25:652–655.
2. Berard J. Absent cervix. *Lyon Med J* 1911;117:493.
3. Sherwood M, Speed T. Congenital atresia of the cervix. *Tex J Med* 1941;37:215–219.
4. Puterman A. Congenital absence of the cervix. *NY State J Med* 1951;51:1748.
5. Rotter C. Surgical correction of congenital atresia of the cervix. *Am J Obstet Gynecol* 1958;76:643–646.
6. Zarou G, Acken H, Brevett R. Surgical management of congenital atresia of the cervix. *Am J Obstet Gynecol* 1961;82:923–928.
7. Williams B. Congenital cervical and vaginal atresia. *J Obstet Gynaecol Br Commonw* 1963;70:301–304.
8. Inverson S. Congenital atresia of the cervix uteri. *Nordisk Medicin* 1966;75:41–44.
9. Scott JR, Galask R, Yannone M. Congenital atresia of the uterine cervix. *Int J Gynaecol Obstet* 1971;9:249–251.
10. Geary W, Weed J. Congenital atresia of uterine cervix. *Obstet Gynecol* 1973;42:213–217.
11. Zarou GS, Gsposito JM, Zarou DM. Pregnancy following the surgical correction of congenital atresia of the cervix. *Int J Gynaecol Obstet* 1973;11:143–146.
12. Farber M, Marchant DJ. Congenital absence of the uterine cervix. *Am J Obstet Gynecol* 1975;121:414–418.
13. Farber M, Marchant DH. Reconstructive surgery for congenital atresia of the uterine cervix. *Fertil Steril* 1976;27:1277–1282.
14. Maciulla G, Heine M, Christian C. Functional endometrial tissue and vaginal agenesis. *J Reprod Med* 1978;21:373–376.
15. Dillon W, Mudaliar N, Wingate M. Congenital atresia of the cervix. *Obstet Gynecol* 1979;54:126–129.
16. Monks P. Uterus didelphys associated with unilateral cervical atresia and renal agenesis. *Aust NZ J Obstet Gynaecol* 1979;19:245–246.
17. Niver D, Barrett G, Jewelewicz R. Congenital atresia of the cervix and vagina: three cases. *Fertil Steril* 1980;33:25–29.
18. Nunley WC, Kitchen JD. Congenital atresia of the cervix with pelvic endometriosis. *Arch Surg* 1980;115:757–762.
19. Valdes C, Malini S, Malinak L. Sonography in the surgical management of vaginal and cervical atresia. *Fertil Steril* 1983;40:263–265.
20. Rock JA, Schlaff WD, Zacur HA, Jones HW. The clinical management of congenital absence of the uterine cervix. *Int J Gynaecol Obstet* 1984;22:231–235.
21. Ragni N, Foglia G, Boccardo E, Pinto P. A case of congenital cervical atresia. *Am Obstet Ginecol Med Perinat* 1984;105:14–19.
22. Regan L, Dewhurst CJ. Atresia of the cervix. *Pediatr Adol Gynecol* 1985;3:83–102.
23. Markham SM, Parmley TH, Murphy AA, Huggins GR, Rock JA. Cervical agenesis combined with vaginal agenesis by magnetic resonance imaging. *Fertil Steril* 1987;48:143–145.
24. Jacob J, Griffin W. Surgical reconstruction of the congenitally atretic cervix: two cases. *Obstet Gynecol Surv* 1989;44:556–568.
25. Fraser I. Successful pregnancy in a patient with partial cervical atresia. *Obstet Gynecol* 1989;74:443–445.
26. Satoh T, Igarashi Y, Itoh T, Kotah T, Yamaguchi A. Cervical atresia combined with vaginal agenesis diagnosed by MRI. *Rinsho Hoshason* 1989;34:391–394.
27. Sherer DM, Beyth Y. Ultrasonic diagnosis and assisted surgical management of haematotrachelos and haematometra due to uterine cervical atresia with associated vaginal agenesis. *J Ultrasound Med* 1989;8:321–323.

28. Hampton H, Meeks G, Bates W, Wiser W. Pregnancy after successful vaginoplasty and cervical stenting for partial atresia of the cervix. *Obstet Gynecol* 1990;76:900–901.
29. Thÿssen R, Hollander J, Willemsen W, Van Der Heyden P, Van Dongen P, Rolland R. Successful pregnancy after ZIFT in a patient with congenital cervical atresia. *Obstet Gynecol* 1990;76:902–904.
30. Bakri Y, Al Sugair A, Hugosson C. Bicornuate nonfused uterine horns with functioning endometria and complete cervico-vaginal absence: magnetic resonance diagnosis. *Fertil Steril* 1992;58:620–621.
31. Salas-Cerniceros S, Paulin-Gonzalez D. Cervical agenesis with secondary endometriosis. *Ginecol Obstet Mex* 1996;64:477–481.
32. Chen CD, Wu MY, Ho HN, Huang SC, Cheng CJ, Yong YS. Congenital atresia of the cervix and vagina; a report of a case. *Acta Obstet Gynecol Scand* 1996;75:770–771.
33. Mami A, Ade-Ajayi N, Malone PS. Colovaginoplasty for cervicovaginal atresia. *J Urol* 1997;157:333–340.
34. Fujimoto V, Miller H, Klein N, Soules M. Congenital cervical atresia: report of seven cases and review of the literature. *Am J Obstet Gynecol* 1997;177:1419–1425.
35. Badawy S, Prasad M, Powers C, Wojtowycz A. Congenital cervicovaginal aplasia with septate uterus and functioning endometrium. *J Pediatr Adol Gynecol* 1997;10:213–217.
36. Sanfilippo J, Wakim N, Schikler K, Yussman H. Endometriosis in association with uterine anomaly. *Am J Obstet Gynecol* 1986;154:39–43.
37. Sanfilippo J, Lobe TE. Laparoscopic surgery in girls and adolescents. *Semin Pediatr Surg* 1998;7:62–72.

Congenital Malformations of the Female Genital Tract: Diagnosis and Management, edited by G. Gidwani and T. Falcone.
Lippincott Williams & Wilkins, Philadelphia © 1999.

11

Müllerian Anomalies: Reproduction, Diagnosis, and Treatment

Jeffrey M. Goldberg and Tommaso Falcone

Department of Gynecology and Obstetrics, The Cleveland Clinic Foundation, Cleveland, Ohio 44195

Abnormalities of the Müllerian ducts are associated with a significant risk of pregnancy loss. The incidence of Müllerian abnormalities in the general population, as well as in women with infertility or recurrent pregnancy loss (RPL), is unknown. Most studies have a selection bias in that they include patients who present with a reproductive problem. The diagnostic modalities used to classify the patients into different groups may be less sensitive to subtle defects such as a small septum. Even at surgery there may be a difference of opinion as to the correct diagnosis. This could lead to patients being excluded from study groups because the results were not thought to be clinically significant. The distinction between an arcuate uterus, mildly septate uterus, or mildly bicornuate uterus might be difficult and might affect reporting of these anomalies.

The incidence of Müllerian abnormalities in women undergoing a hysterosalpingogram (HSG) to confirm tubal occlusion after a tubal ligation has been reported to be 3.2% (1). The incidence was 2.3% in patients undergoing transcervical tubal sterilization (2). The diagnosis was made by hysteroscopy or HSG. The patients in these studies had a normal reproductive outcome prior to the tubal ligation.

In patients with RPL the incidence depends on whether they are investigated after two or three pregnancy losses. Furthermore, some centers may have a particular interest in certain problems associated with RPL that could result in overestimation of the incidence of a specific disorder. The overall incidence of Müllerian defects, including minor defects such as arcuate uterus, in 2,311 patients with RPL was 14% (3–9).

In a study by Meis et al. (10), Müllerian abnormalities carried the highest odds ratio for medically indicated preterm induction of labor or cesarean section primarily for intrauterine growth retardation or third-trimester bleeding. Müllerian anomalies were not associated with an increased probability of spontaneous preterm delivery (PTD). However, these patients constituted only 0.4% of the study population. Green and Harris (11), in a 10-year review of 31,836 deliveries who presented with premature labor or abnormal presentation, found only 80 cases (0.25%) of Müllerian duct anomaly. These anomalies are associated with malpresentation, especially breech. The cesarean section rate in patients with Müllerian anomalies is reported to be 30% to 80% (12).

Most reports on Müllerian anomalies have not documented any increase in infertility. Tulandi et al. (13) reviewed over 2,000 HSGs in infertile patients and found that only 1.3% of patients had a Müllerian anomaly. Life table analysis in patients with a unicornuate uterus revealed a cumulative pregnancy rate after 7 years of 77% and with didelphic uterus a pregnancy rate of 81% (12). Maneschi et al. (14) reported 24-month cumulative pregnancy rates and monthly fecundity rates in patients with Müllerian anomalies incidentally detected at hysteroscopy for abnormal uterine bleeding. The pregnancy rates were similar to those of the control group without Müllerian anomalies. Surgery for correction of a Müllerian anomaly should rarely be performed as a treatment for infertility.

The American Fertility Society classification of uterine anomalies is the current standard. Some of these anomalies are illustrated in Fig 1. The anatomy of the uni-

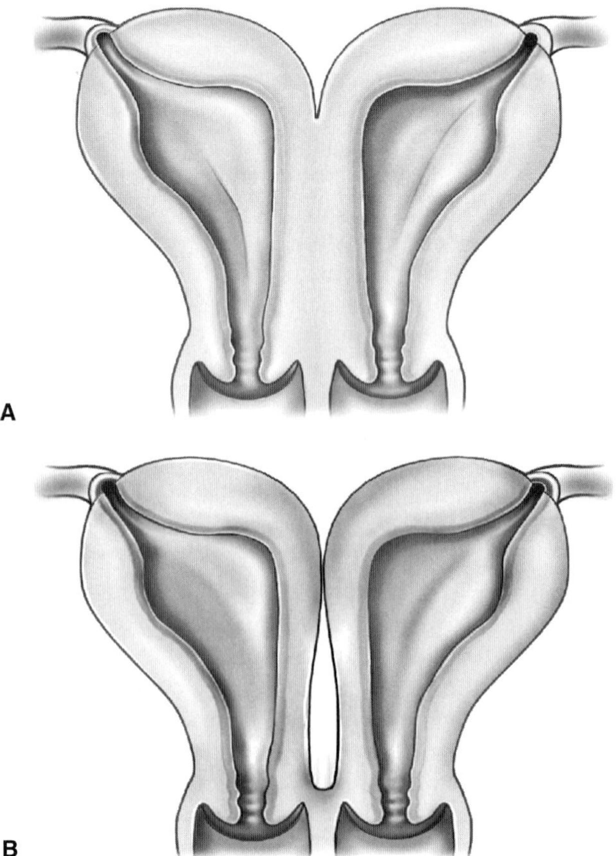

FIG. 1. **A:** Didelphic uterus. **B:** Bicornuate bicollis uterus.

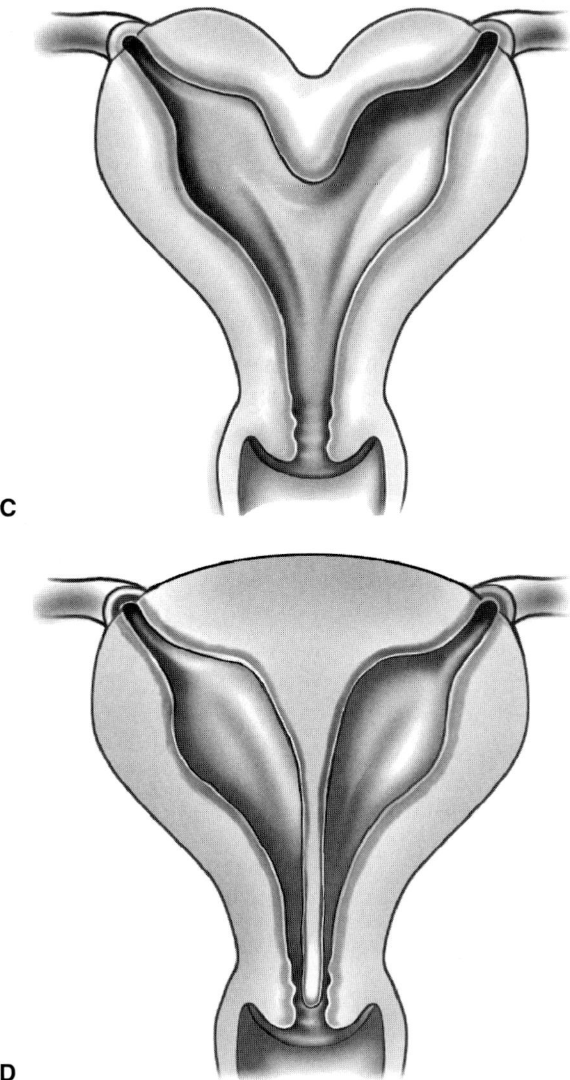

FIG. 1. *Continued.* **C:** Mild bicornute uterus. **D:** Septate uterus, complete.

cornuate uterus (class II) is described in the chapter on obstructive Müllerian anomalies. The didelphic uterus (Class III) is essentially two separate unicornuate uteri with little or no connection above the level of the cervix. It may appear similar to a bicornuate bicollis uterus. The bicornuate uterus (class IV) can be complete (division of the cavity to the internal os) or partial. The complete bicornuate uterus may have one or two cervices. The septate uterus (class V) can be also be partial or complete (septum to the internal os) and some patients may have a double cervix. The external appearance of the uterine fundus is normal. Acien (15) reviewed the published literature on the frequency of each type of defect. In 1,770 cases he noted the following distribution from most common to least common: bicornuate, arcuate, partial septum, didelphys, complete septum, and unicornuate. It is possible that the arcuate uterus is underreported as it is not thought to be clinically relevant.

UNICORNUATE/DIDELPHIC UTERUS

Unicornuate and didelphic uteri have not been commonly reported in the infertility or obstetric literature. They are more often reported in association with obstructive symptoms. This is due to an associated rudimentary horn with the unicornuate uterus and an obstructing longitudinal vaginal septum with the didelphic uterus. Andrews and Jones (16) reported only five cases of unicornuate uterus in their 12-year experience in infertility and obstetric practice at Norfolk General Hospital and Johns Hopkins Hospital. A recent report of all cases diagnosed with unicornuate uterus or didephic uterus over a 40-year period at Johns Hopkins Hospital revealed only 29 cases in the former group and 25 cases in the latter group (12). Most reports in the literature also reflect a low incidence of these anomalies. These anomalies may be associated with renal abnormalities especially renal agenesis on the contralateral side to the unicornuate uterus or the side of an obstructing hemivagina with a didelphic uterus. Other renal anomalies include hypoplastic, pelvic, and horseshoe kidneys.

The diagnosis of these abnormalities is usually made during an investigation for infertility or recurrent pregnancy loss (Table 1). These patients also present with pelvic pain or a pelvic mass if there are associated obstructing abnormalities. They can be found incidentally at laparotomy, laparoscopy (LS) or cesarean section. They may also be diagnosed in patients who become pregnant with an intrauterine device in place.

These anomalies are associated with a poor reproductive outcome. It is difficult to compare different studies as many did not differentiate between first and second trimester losses. In a review of a large number of case series over the last 30 years, it appears that there is an overall increase in spontaneous abortion (SAB) and preterm delivery with these anomalies (Table 2). Both anomalies are associated with an increased incidence of malpresentation and cesarean section rates. Intrauterine growth

TABLE 1. *Presenting symptoms of unicornuate/didelphic uteri*

Recurrent pregnancy loss
Obstetric complications (malpresentation, bleeding, preterm labor, intrauterine growth retardation)
Pelvic pain[a]
Pelvic mass
Abnormal uterine bleeding
Incidental[b]

[a] Usually in association with obstructive anomalies such as a rudimentary horn or a vaginal septum.
[b] Usually at the time of investigation for infertility or recurrent pregnancy loss.

TABLE 2. *Pregnancy outcome with unicornuate/didelphic uteri*

Uterus	Spontaneous abortion, 1st and 2nd trimester	Preterm birth	Term birth
Unicornuate (*N* = 185)	44%	12%	44%
Didelphic (*N* = 213)	36%	19%	45%

N, number of pregnancies.
Data from Moutos (12), Fedele (20,134), Andrews (16), Beernink (135), Stein (39), Ludmir (19), Musich (27), and Capraro (136).

retardation has been reported inconsistently with these anomalies and is thought to be a contributing cause to the prematurity rate (10). The etiology of these obstetric problems with unicornuate and didelphic uteri is not clear. The most popular theory is that the diminished capacity of the uterine cavity cannot adequately accommodate the growing fetus.

Patients with poor reproductive outcomes in association with these anomalies should have thorough history, physical examination, and investigation for other causes of pregnancy loss. The history should include details of specific chronic diseases such as lupus erythematosus, inflammatory bowel disease, diabetes, and thyroid and renal disease. Other possible causes of recurrent fetal wastage include submucous myomas, polycystic ovarian syndrome, and endometrial infections such as mycoplasma. The evaluation should also include karyotypic analysis on both partners, serum thyroid-stimulating hormone (TSH), anticardiolipin antibodies and circulating lupus anticoagulant, and an endometrial biopsy to rule out a luteal phase defect.

Patients with an associated obstructive component should have this corrected. Most patients with a didelphic uterus have an associated longitudinal vaginal septum. The septum should be excised if it is causing obstruction or dyspareunia. It should also be removed in infertility patients because of the possibility that intercourse may occur with the hemivagina contralateral to the ovulating ovary.

A rudimentary horn can be found in most patients with a unicornuate uterus though most do not have a functioning endometrium. Although it is clear that a noncommunicating rudimentary horn with a functional endometrium should be removed, removal of a communicating or nonfunctional rudimentary horn is controversial. There does not appear to be any risk in retaining a nonfunctional uterine horn. Patients with a communicating uterine horn with a functional endometrium should probably have the horn removed (16).

Some authors have recommended prophylactic cervical cerclage in patients with uterine malformations even if there is no documented cervical incompetence (17,18). Since these opinions are not based on any controlled trials, we share the opinion of other authors (12,19,20) that cervical cerclage should be recommended only if cervical incompetence is documented. A Strassmann metroplasty for unification of a didelphic uterus is rarely indicated and is usually limited to fusion of the fundus. Surgery to unify the cervix is difficult and may result in cervical incompetence or stenosis.

BICORNUATE UTERUS

Incidence

The following discussion will be limited to the symmetric bicornuate uterus as the asymmetric bicornuate uterus has been addressed in the chapter on obstructed uterine anomalies. The incidence of bicornuate uterus, and congenital uterine anomalies overall, in the general population and in patients with infertility or fetal wastage is unknown (21,22). This is due to the fact that in many studies the evaluation was incomplete and the diagnosis was not definitively established. Many patients may have escaped detection because reproductive performance is generally acceptable and gynecologic difficulties do not necessarily occur. Comparison of studies is also complicated by different classification systems (23). The incidence in the fertile population has been estimated to be between 0.1% to 0.6% based on three studies that performed tubal ligation followed by HSG on a combined total of 2,135 patients (1,22,24). Five of 1024 (0.5%) infertility patients and 16 of 868 (1.9%) patients with RPL or PTD undergoing evaluation by HSG and laparoscopy (LS) had a bicornuate uterus. Bicornuate uterus accounted for 26/128 (20.3%) of all uterine anomalies (22).

Diagnosis

A symmetric bicornuate uterus may be diagnosed by an abnormal fundal contour during pregnancy or delivery, by the occurrence of pregnancy with an intrauterine device (IUD) in place, or as an incidental finding during surgery. Most are diagnosed by HSG during the evaluation for infertility or RPL (23). Many of the earlier studies used the angle between the uterine cavities to distinguish between septate and bicornuate uteri without surgical confirmation of the external fundal contour. In other studies they were grouped together as a "double uterus." Most authors agree that differentiating these entities by HSG is very unreliable and that LS is required for a definitive diagnosis (17,23,25,26). Buttram and Gibbons (26) noted that 38 of 39 patients reported to have a bicornuate uterus on HSG were found to have a uterine septum at LS. Similarly, Musich and Behrman (27) reported that 8 of 12 septate uteri were diagnosed as bicornuate on preoperative HSG. In the past, both of these conditions were managed by abdominal metroplasty via laparotomy, and making the distinction preoperatively was less critical than it is now, as septoplasty is currently performed by operative hysteroscopy.

Other imaging studies were evaluated in an effort to avoid an invasive LS. The combination of HSG and ultrasound (US) was stated to provide a correct diagnosis in 94% of the 63 patients as validated by LS (28). Wu et al. (29) performed three-dimensional US on 40 infertility or RPL patients with a uterine abnormality noted on HSG or conventional US. They claimed to have correctly identified 11 of 12 (92%) of the septate and all 3 bicornuate uteri. However, the diagnosis was not confirmed by LS in all cases. They felt that three-dimensional US provided more detailed images than standard two-dimensional US.

Magnetic resonance imaging is currently being used as a diagnostic alternative to LS. Carrington et al. (30) state that MRI of the bicornuate uterus reveals a fundal concavity and that the "septum" is composed entirely of myometrium whereas the septate uterus has a normal shape with a low signal intensity from the septum consistent with fibrous tissue. Mintz et al. (31) make the distinction based solely on the medium-intensity signal band from the myometrium of the bicornuate uterus versus the low-intensity signal from the septum. They claim that the evaluation of the fundal contour was not helpful or necessary to distinguish between the two anomalies. Conversely, others (32,33) note that the signal from the septum of the septate uterus may be of low or intermediate intensity, or both, and that the external fundal contour is the key feature in differentiating the septate from the bicornuate uterus. The most comprehensive study examined six patients with bicornuate and six with septate uteri by HSG, transabdominal and transvaginal US, MRI, and diagnostic LS and hysteroscopy. The sensitivity and specificity of US (73% and 33%, respectively) and MRI (73% and 66%, respectively) was not sufficient to make a reliable diagnosis. They conclude that US and MRI do not provide adequate visualization of the fundal contour to differentiate between septate and bicornuate uteri and that LS is still the most accurate modality (34).

Reproductive Performance

The bicornuate uterus does not impair conception (17,21,23). Most patients with symmetric uterine abnormalities have no obstetric difficulty, whereas those who do seem to do so on a repetitive basis. The etiology for this is not clear (21). A bicornuate uterus was diagnosed as an incidental finding during unrelated surgery in 36 patients (35). Of the 56 pregnancies established in these patients, 47 (84%) were successful and all patients carried at least one infant to term (35). The bicornuate uterus is associated with a higher incidence of SAB, PTD, and malpresentation. Postpartum hemorrhage is also stated to be more common due to incomplete expulsion of the placenta (17).

The obstetric outcomes in several series of untreated patients with a bicornuate uterus are presented in Table 3. Two patients did have a metroplasty and five were treated with cervical cerclage in the Acien et al. study (36). In that study, the patients with a bicornuate unicollis had the worst reproductive outcome of all uterine anomalies, with only 40% delivering a viable infant. The study also included a normal

TABLE 3. *Pregnancy outcome of bicornuate uteri before surgery*

	No. patients	No. pregs.	SAB	PTD	Term	Live
Raga (22)	26	56	14 (25%)	14 (25%)	26 (46%)	35 (63%)
Maneschi (40)	21	41	16 (39%)	5 (12%)	16 (39%)	17 (41%)
Ayhan (55)	40	97	81 (84%)	15 (16%)	1 (1%)	3 (3%)
Ludmir (19)	25	45	11 (24%)	10 (22%)	17 (38%)	23 (51%)
Acien (36)	57	160	67 (42%)	31 (19%)	49 (31%)	71 (44%)
Controls	26	47	3 (6%)	2 (4%)	40 (85%)	42 (87%)
Combined[a]	169	399	189 (47%)	75 (19%)	109 (27%)	149 (37%)

SAB, spontaneous abortion; PTD, preterm delivery.
[a] "Combined" excludes the controls from the Acien (36) study.

uterus control group for comparison. Overall, it can be seen that a bicornuate uterus confers a higher risk of early SAB and PTD, and lower term and viable pregnancy rates.

Two factors that likely contribute to the higher fetal wastage are uteroplacental insufficiency and cervical incompetency. Leible et al. (37) noted that 10 of 15 (67%) septate/bicornuate uteri had laterally located placentas compared with 1 of 30 (3%) controls. There was a clear association between a lateral placenta and high systolic-to-diastolic ratios of the nonplacental uterine artery. In patients with these uterine anomalies and poor pregnancy outcome, 11 of 12 (92%) had abnormal systolic-to-diastolic ratios of the uterine arteries versus only 1 of the 4 in the control group. It is believed that lack of anastomosis between the two uterine arteries where Müllerian duct fusion is incomplete prevents the nonplacental uterine artery from reaching the placental circulation. Patients with abnormal resistive indices in both uterine arteries had the worst pregnancy outcomes. The bicornuate uterus has been noted to have the highest incidence of cervical incompetence of all the uterine anomalies (38%) (38). However, in this study the authors relied solely on the HSG appearance to differentiate a septate from bicornuate uterus. It is interesting that they had previously reported that LS is necessary to make the final diagnosis, as these anomalies may appear identical on HSG (17). Also, the appearance of cervical dilatation on HSG and the ability to pass a cervical dilator were included in the diagnosis of cervical incompetency in addition to the more agreed on prior history of painless cervical dilatation during pregnancy.

Furthermore, the rate of fetal malpresentation ranged from 25% to 77% (19,36,39,40). There are no data describing the labor patterns of patients with bicornuate uteri and vertex presentation, though uterine contractility during various phases of the menstrual cycle and in response to oxytocin and methylergobasin was similar between the horns of symmetric bicornuate and normal uteri (41). Obstetric complications such as uterine inversion (42) and torsion (43) have been described with bicornuate uteri but there is no evidence that they are increased in this condition. Fetal deformations, however, may be more common due to the abnormal uterine cavity (44–47).

Treatment

The results of treatment for the bicornuate uterus must be interpreted cautiously. In several studies it is not clear if other causes of reproductive failure were excluded or corrected. Metroplasty was also performed for dysmenorrhea and menorrhagia in some of the earlier series. Most importantly, the chance for a liveborn increases with each pregnancy loss due to improved vascularization, myometrial stretching, or other factor(s) (23). In young patients with one or two SABs the indication for metroplasty is questionable as the viable birth rate is progressively increasing. In patients over 35 years of age and those needing sophisticated infertility treatments, proceed to surgical correction to immediately achieve the highest probability of success (40). The treatment options for the bicornuate uterus are metroplasty and cervical cerclage. Metroplasty may be considered in the face of reproductive failure with no other causative factors even though its benefit has never been tested in a controlled trial (48).

Although abdominal metroplasty with Tompkins and Jones procedures has been applied to the bicornuate uterus, the Strassmann technique is the appropriate procedure (49). If a rectovesical ligament is present, it needs to be excised prior to the procedure. Dilute pitressin is infiltrated into the myometrium, or tourniquets are placed around the uterine and ovarian vessels for hemostasis. A transverse fundal incision is made into the uterine cavities taking care to avoid the cornua. The uterus then assumes its "intended" configuration. The defect is repaired in layers in the anterior/posterior plane (Fig. 2). It is debated as to whether or not a divided cervix should be unified as originally described. There is concern that incising the cervical septum may compromise the competency of the cervix. In the case of a bicornuate bicollis uterus, the cervices should not be joined (23).

Several of the original cases reported by Strassmann in 1907 were performed via a colpotomy incision (50). Recently, Pelosi (51) described performing a Jones metroplasty for a bicornuate uterus through a posterior colpotomy following the creation of the initial uterine incision by LS with hysteroscopic guidance. While the combined endoscopic/vaginal approach has the advantage of avoiding a laparotomy, the Jones procedure excises a wedge of myometrium, which reduces the final intrauterine volume. It does demonstrate that this approach should be feasible for the Strassmann procedure as well.

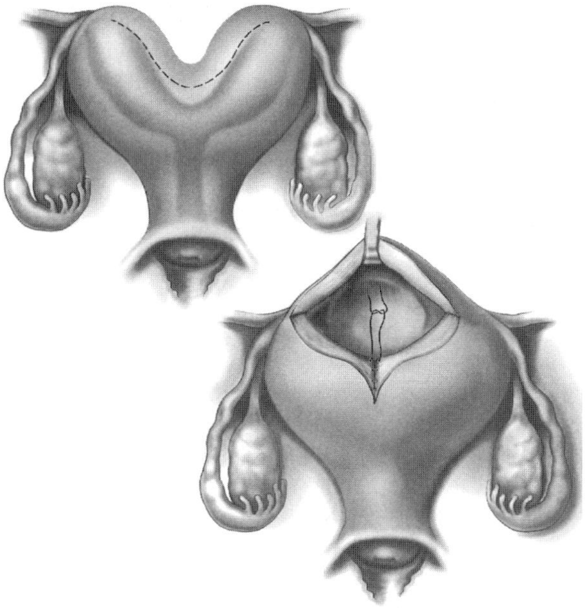

FIG. 2. Strassmann metroplasty.

TABLE 4. *Pregnancy outcome after metroplasty for bicornuate uteri*

Study	No. patients	No. Pregs.	SAB	PTD	Term	Live
Maneschi (40)	8	10	2 (20%)	0	8 (80%)	8 (80%)
Ayhan (55)	40	54	6 (11%)	19 (35%)	29 (54%)	45 (83%)

SAB, spontaneous abortion; PTD, preterm delivery.

Data on the success rates following metroplasty are severely limited (Table 4). Musich and Behrman (27) reported that only 10% of the 31 pregnancies in 12 patients with bicornuate uteri were viable prior to unification. Six of those patients underwent metroplasty and four of the five subsequent pregnancies resulted in a live birth. Maneschi et al. (40) performed metroplasty on 8 of the 21 patients with bicornuate uteri and a history of SABs. Two of the 10 pregnancies (20%) were lost in the first trimester. The remaining 80% delivered a viable infant at term. Contrast these rates with their preoperative rates in Table 3. In addition, there was a 40% malpresentation rate at term prior to surgery while all of the postoperative pregnancies were vertex. The cumulative pregnancy rates at 12 and 24 months were similar before and after surgery. Prior to surgery, the probability of a live birth was 30% for the first pregnancy, 58% for the second, and 79% for the third. After surgery these rates rose to 71% for the first pregnancy and 86% for the second. They conclude that metroplasty is successful in reducing first- and second-trimester fetal losses and the time needed to produce a live birth.

The question of mode of delivery for pregnancy following abdominal metroplasty is unsettled. Despite evidence that the uterine scar after unification is as strong, if not stronger, than after a cesarean section, most still recommend an elective cesarean section. This is especially true if there is a septate or double cervix that may lead to dystocia (23). In Strassmann's (52) extended series, 61 of 71 pregnancies delivered vaginally without rupture. Others have also allowed vaginal delivery and claimed no cases of rupture (53,54). Ayhan et al. (55) advocate elective cesarean section based on the occurrence of uterine rupture in 2 of 48 pregnancies even though there were no intrapartum ruptures among the 12 patients who delivered vaginally.

It is generally agreed that cervical incompetency is increased with the bicornuate uterus; however, there are no reliable estimates of its incidence (38,48). This has led some to recommend prophylactic cervical cerclage for all patients with bicornuate uteri (18,38,56). Heinonen et al. (56) reported an increase in fetal salvage from 53% to 100% and a reduction in prematurity from 53% to 31% after cerclage. Blum (57) performed cervical cerclage on 23 patients with a reduction in SABs from 69% to 5%. Golan et al. (38) also advised routine prophylactic cerclage for the bicornuate uterus based on a decrease in late SAB and PTD from 50% to 22% with a corresponding increase in term deliveries from 50% to 78%. However, they used HSG to distinguish between septate and bicornuate uteri. Although the risk of cervical incompetence appears to be higher, prophylactic cerclage cannot be endorsed based on available studies (48).

In an interesting study, Ludmir et al. (19) managed 61 pregnancies in 25 patients with a high-risk obstetric protocol that included weekly cervical exams, decreased physical activity, home uterine monitoring, tocolysis for preterm labor, and cervical cerclage if effacement or dilatation before 22 weeks or with a history of cervical incompetency. Tocolysis was required in 13 pregnancies and a cerclage was placed in 3. The rates of term and viable pregnancies (39% and 54%, respectively) were essentially the same for the 45 pregnancies in the same patients prior to the treatment (38% and 51%). They conclude that patients with a bicornuate uterus and history of pregnancy wastage may benefit more from metroplasty than cerclage, though no trial comparing these modalities has been reported.

SEPTATE UTERUS

The septate uterus has been classified as complete or partial depending on the extent that the septa descends into the uterine cavity. As with other Müllerian anomalies, the septate uterus is associated with increased fetal wastage. Renal anomalies are uncommon with a septate uterus and obstructive symptoms have been rarely reported. A complete septum with a noncommunicating hemicavity has been treated hysteroscopically (58) and by abdominal metroplasty (59).

Most studies report the highest incidence of SAB with this anomaly though it is difficult to compare results between studies. Many early studies failed to differentiate between a bicornuate uterus and a septate uterus when reporting pregnancy outcomes prior to or following surgery. Other studies did not specify if the losses were first- or second-trimester SAB or preterm labor. Many case series did not stratify for the type of surgical procedure used. The presurgery fetal wastage rate of a septate uterus may be an overestimate since most of the data are derived from surgical series in patients who were referred for poor reproductive outcome. Unlike the didelphic uterus, the septate uterus is rarely found on physical examination. Therefore, many patients with a septate uterus with uneventful pregnancies are not diagnosed.

The treatment of a uterine septum that is incidentally discovered during the investigation of infertility is controversial. While a septum is not a cause of infertility, it does increase the risk of pregnancy complications should conception occur. In a study of pre-clinical abortions after in vitro fertilization, Dicker et al. (60) reported that a uterine septa was the most common intracavitary lesion and recommended removal. Since in vitro fertilization is associated with significant cost and risk, and hysteroscopic division of the septum is a relatively minor outpatient procedure, we recommend performing it prior to initiating treatment with in vitro fertilization. A septum diagnosed during an investigation for recurrent pregnancy should be treated. Surgical management of a uterine septum can be accomplished by laparotomy or hysteroscopy.

Abdominal Technique

The Jones metroplasty (59) removes a wedge of tissue containing the septum (Fig. 3). It is initiated by outlining the wedge to be excised. A traction suture is placed in the fundus in the midline. Dilute vasopressin is injected into the incision site. The incisions begin at the fundus and continue anteriorly and posteriorly. The incision on the fundus should be at least 1 cm from the apparent insertion of the fallopian tubes. The triangular incision has the base at the fundus and the apex anteriorly and posteriorly. The position of the apex should be based on the calculated length of the septum. The endometrial cavity is identified as the incision is made. The uterus is closed side to side in three layers. The first layer includes the endometrium and part of the myometrium. The second includes the remainder of the myometrium and the third is to approximate the serosa. The main disadvantage of this procedure is the reduced size of the endometrial cavity. The insertion of the fallopian tubes will appear close to each other. The results of the procedure have been reported a live birth rate at term of 73%, comparable to other metroplasty procedures (61).

The Tompkins (62) procedure is performed by incising the septum from the fundus in the sagittal plane, then dividing the halves of the septum; thus no tissue is excised and the uterine volume is not reduced (Fig. 4). The myometrium is then reapproximated as with the Jones procedure. A fetal salvage rate of 77% has been reported (63). The Strassmann abdominal metroplasty, although applied to the septate uterus, is only indicated for the bicornuate uterus. The potential complications of the abdominal procedures are infection and hemorrhage. Uterine rupture has been reported after abdominal metroplasty and elective cesarean section is advised. Due to

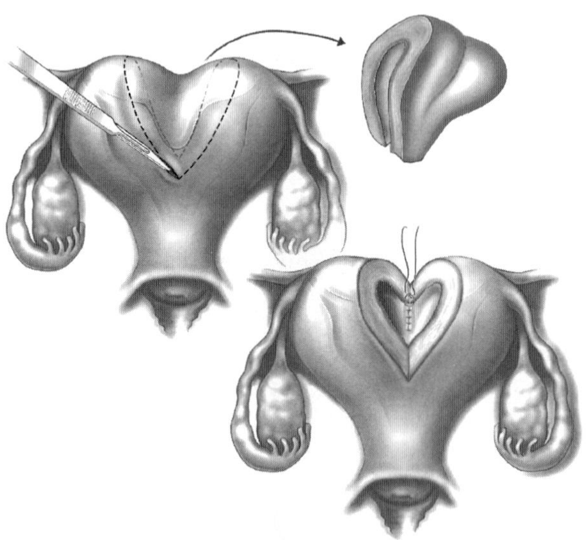

FIG. 3. Jones metroplasty.

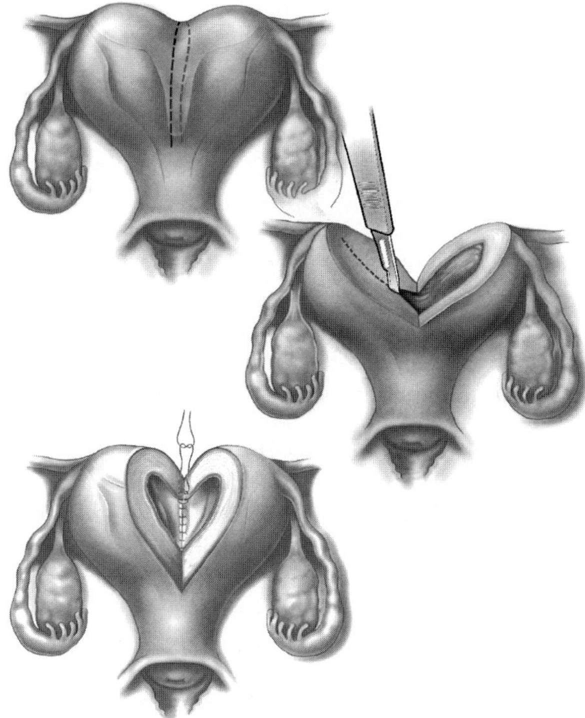

FIG. 4. Tompkins metroplasty.

the need for laparotomy, the risk of transfusion and postoperative adhesion formation, and the need for elective cesarean section, abdominal septoplasty is rarely performed. The hysteroscopic technique is the preferred method.

Hysteroscopic Technique

The advantages of this technique are outlined in Table 5. Hysteroscopic septoplasty requires no special preoperative preparation though some surgeons recom-

TABLE 5. *Advantages of
hysteroscopic septoplasy*

- No abdominal incision
- No myometrial incision
- Outpatient procedure
- No requirement for cesarean section
- No reduction in uterine cavity size
- Less postoperative morbidity
- Quicker recovery time
- No surgically induced pelvic adhesion

mend using a GnRH analog for 2 months to induce endometrial atrophy. The medication is expensive and associated with menopausal side effects and the early proliferative phase endometrium is adequately thin. We do not use it as a surgical adjunct for this procedure. We also have not felt it necessary to routinely perform LS concurrently to reduce the risk of uterine rupture. In cases where diagnostic LS is not indicated, such as recurrent pregnancy loss, we may rely on MRI to make the distinction between septate and bicornuate uteri without LS. However, if the anatomy is uncertain or the septum difficult to resect, LS is performed. Hysteroscopic septoplasty is performed as an outpatient procedure and may be accomplished under conscious sedation combined with a paracervical block.

The septum can be resected with hysteroscopic scissors, a resectoscope, or argon, KTP, or NdYAG lasers. Fedele et al. (64) compared the results of septoplasty with scissors, resectoscope, and argon laser. The reproductive outcome was not affected by the technique selected. The lasers are much more expensive and require special training and eye protection. The fiberoptic laser tips should never be air-cooled as deaths from air embolism have been reported. We prefer to use the resectoscope with a wire loop set to 50 to 70 W cutting (nonmodulated) current. A nonelectrolyte distending medium such as glycine is used. The loop is advanced and the electrical energy activated only under direct vision.

The septum is relatively avascular. However, contrary to classical teaching, the septum has been found to be mostly myometrial tissue rather than fibrous tissue (65,66). Nonetheless, the appearance of the septum is clearly different from the myometrium during the resection. It can be assumed that the organization of the myometrial tissue within the septum is different from the myometrial wall and is responsible for this apparent difference.

The division starts at the apex of the septum and is carried out horizontally (Fig. 5). During incision of the septum the anterior and posterior uterine walls move apart. There is a tendency to direct the dissection posteriorly. This must be avoided as it will result in bleeding from the myometrium. The septum incision is continued until both ostia are visualized in the panoramic view and no appreciable septum is left. An experienced hysteroscopist will recognize the myometrium at the fundus and stop the resection. The first sign of bleeding indicates that the myometrium has been reached. The advantage of the resectoscope over the hysteroscopic scissors is that this bleeding can be instantly coagulated to maintain a clear field of vision.

The most difficult cases are those with a broad-based septum. This has been defined differently, according to the experience of the hysteroscopists. Valle and Sciarra (67) defined it as a septum greater than 1 cm at its base. March and Israel (68) defined it as more than 3 cm at its base. With a wide septum the general principle is to resect the lateral margins of the septum first so as to diminish in small increments the width of the triangle. Incomplete resection of a uterine septum may sometimes occur. Fedele and colleagues (69) have shown that a residual septum of 1 cm or less will not influence the fertility, SAB, or live birth rates. Patients with a residual septum of more than 1 cm should undergo a repeat procedure to complete the resection.

The management of the cervical portion of a complete uterine septum is controversial. Some feel it prudent to spare the cervical portion of a complete septum to

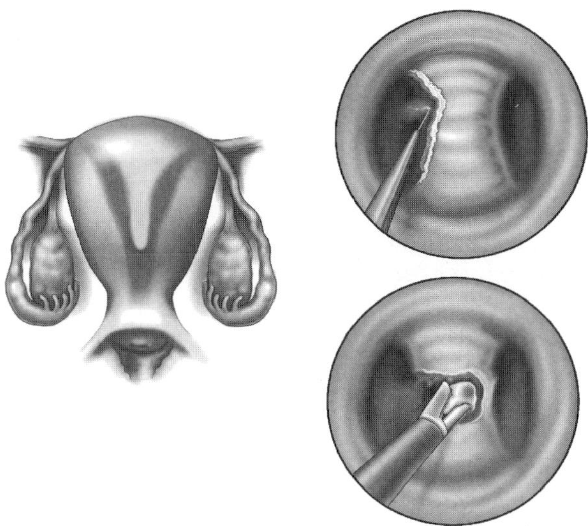

FIG. 5. Hysteroscopic resection of septum. The procedure can be performed with cautery or scissors.

avoid potential cervical incompetence or stenosis. Other authors advocate removing the cervical septum to facilitate the removal of the corporeal portion of the septum and reduce the risk of dystocia. Vercellini et al. (70) have reported excellent clinical outcome with removal of the cervical septum using simple Metzenbaum scissors followed by standard hysteroscopy with scissors to complete the remainder of the procedure. If the decision is made to retain the cervical portion of the septum, then the hysteroscopic dissection of the corporeal part of a complete septum should be performed with a balloon introduced into the second cervix to prevent the loss of distending media.

The main complications of hysteroscopic procedures are uterine perforation and fluid overload. Distending media other than normal saline may result in fatal hyponatremia. It is essential to carefully monitor fluid in and out volumes. Pregnancy should not be attempted for one or two menstrual cycles to allow complete coverage of the septal areas by the endometrium. As the incidence of intrauterine adhesion formation is very uncommon following hysteroscopic septoplasty, the prophylactic use of estrogens (71) and intrauterine Foley balloons or IUDs has not been shown to be of any value.

The pregnancy outcome after surgical treatment of a septum is excellent. Although there are many limitations in comparing the reproductive results after metroplasty in the published literature, an overview of several case series with a total of 359 cases (54,55,67,68,72–75) yielded the following summary statistics: SAB 14%, preterm delivery 12%, and term delivery rate of 74%. Some authors have reported the division of the uterine septum without hysteroscopic visualization with US guidance and endoscopic scissors inserted transcervically (76).

DIETHYLSTILBESTROL

History

Diethylstilbestrol (DES) is a synthetic nonsteroidal estrogen that was first synthesized in 1938. In 1948, Smith (77) reported that DES treatment initiated 6 to 7 weeks from the last menstrual period in 632 patients with threatened abortion or poor reproductive history reduced early pregnancy loss, intrauterine fetal demise, pregnancy-induced hypertension, and preterm delivery. It was believed that DES improved pregnancy outcome by increasing production of placental steroid hormones. In 1953, Dieckmann et al. (78) published the results of a prospective randomized double-blind placebo-controlled study with 1,646 patients that failed to confirm that DES was of any therapeutic value in reducing fetal wastage, PTD, or pregnancy-induced hypertension. Subsequent reanalysis of this study showed that DES actually increased the rates of SAB, PTD, and perinatal death (79). DES use was finally banned in 1971 following the finding of an association between vaginal clear cell adenocarcinoma and in utero DES exposure (80). The number of pregnant women treated with DES is unknown but estimates range from 2 million to 10 million (81,82).

Genital Malformations

Even with in utero DES exposure, vaginal clear cell adenocarcinoma is very rare. However, benign vaginal adenosis and structural cervical changes such as collars, hoods, septae, and cockscombs occur in a high percentage of DES daughters (81,83,84). DES also induces uterine malformations including hypoplastic cavity, T-shaped uteri, constriction bands, wide lower segment, and irregular borders. Kaufman et al. (83) reported that 69% of 267 DES daughters had uterine abnormalities on HSG. The most common abnormality was a hypoplastic T-shaped cavity in 31%. Cervical changes were present in 44% and of those, 86% had an abnormal HSG. Of the 67% with vaginal changes, 82% had a uterine abnormality. The presence of cervico-vaginal changes was associated with approximately a fivefold increase in abnormal HSGs.

Ectopic pregnancy, SAB, and PTD were increased, and the term delivery was reduced in DES patients with abnormal HSGs compared to DES patients with normal HSGs. Pregnancy outcome was worse in the DES group overall compared to normal controls (83). A larger follow-up study confirmed the increased incidence of poor pregnancy outcome if the HSG was abnormal, though no specific uterine abnormality was consistently associated with a particular adverse pregnancy outcome (85). It should be noted that the classic small T-shaped uterine cavity has also been found in women without in utero DES exposure (86). It is not known if the reproductive performance in these women is the same as in the DES daughters (48).

Kaufman et al. (85) reported that isolated areas of myometrial thickening produced indentations into the cavity. This was later confirmed with MRI (87). The embryologic mechanism for the anatomic alterations with DES is unknown (48). In a quantitative analysis of HSG images the uterine cavity area, upper uterine segment, and endocervical canal length were all significantly reduced in DES progeny (88). Again, an association between abnormal uterine cavities and cervicovaginal changes was observed. A subsequent study using transvaginal US confirmed a reduction in the uterine cavity area and cervical length and added that the uterine volume was also diminished with DES (89). HSG remains the gold standard for uterine cavity assessment for patients with infertility or fetal wastage (90). MRI was not as sensitive as HSG for detecting DES-associated uterine changes and US was completely incapable of diagnosing these defects (87,90).

DeCherney et al. (91) reported finding "withered" fallopian tubes, i.e., foreshortened, sacculated, and convoluted with a pinpoint os and constricted fimbria in 16 DES daughters. The tubes appeared normal on HSG and histologically there was thinning of the epithelium and increased connective tissue without inflammation. All of these patients had multiple peritubal cysts. Several of these patients did achieve an intrauterine pregnancy. The finding of withered tubes has not been confirmed by others, although Haney et al. (92) did note an increase in perifimbrial paratubal cysts. Unlike all of the other congenital uterine malformations, the DES uterus is not associated with an increase in renal anomalies (93,94).

Reproductive Function

There are conflicting studies regarding infertility and fetal wastage resulting from DES exposure. It is difficult to compare studies as they differ in patient selection, the degree to which other contributory conditions are ruled out and/or treated, and follow-up intervals. The studies also vary in how they established that the patients were in fact exposed to DES in utero. Tilley et al. (95) reported that 29% of DES-exposed mothers could not remember if they had taken DES and an additional 8% denied DES exposure when their charts indicated that they had taken it.

Three studies demonstrated reduced pregnancy rates in DES-exposed patients versus controls (Table 6). However, all three utilized the same database of patients from

TABLE 6. *Diethylstilbestrol (DES) and infertility*

Study	DES-exposed		Controls		Significant
	No. patients	% Pregs.[a]	No. patients	% Pregs.	
Bibbo (108)[b]	229	18	136	33	+
Herbst (107)	201	84	197	98	+
Senekijian (96)	138	82	203	95	+
Cousins (97)?	71	41	69	46	−
Barnes (108)	163	82	185	88	−
Berger (127)	69	67			
Schmidt (137)	106	71			
Kaufman (98)	367	82			
Combined	1,344	72	790	79	

Note: The first three studies are from Dieckmann's (78) data.

[a] "% Pregnant" = % ever pregnant during the study. Includes primary infertility patients who eventually conceived.

[b] Not stated how many patients were attempting to conceive.

the original Dieckmann study (78). Two additional controlled studies found no difference. The data in Table 1 are pregnancy rates, not infertility rates, i.e., the studies included patients with primary infertility who eventually conceived. Ultimately, an overall pregnancy rate of 72% was achieved by the DES progeny, which is similar to the 75% pregnancy rate in the control group.

Senekijian et al. (96) reported that cervicovaginal anomalies and abnormal HSGs were more common in DES patients with infertility compared with those who conceived. Cousins et al. (97) found no differences in pregnancy rates in DES patients with or without cervicovaginal changes and Kaufman et al. (98) noted that fertility was not decreased with an abnormal HSG unless there were constrictions in the upper segment. Berger and Alper (99) compared pregnancy rates in 50 DES patients (48 with abnormal HSGs) with 50 matched controls treated for primary infertility. Pregnancy was established in 44% of the controls but only in 4% of the DES patients, and none were viable. They concluded that primary infertility of 1 to 2 years in DES progeny with an abnormal HSG has a poor prognosis.

There are other factors that could potentially contribute to reduced fertility in DES daughters. Stillman (81) and Rosenfeld and Bronson (100) reported that poor cervical mucus may be more common with DES exposure. In the latter study only 13% of the DES patients with abnormal postcoital tests conceived, versus 80% of those with a normal test result. Other studies found no increase in poor cervical mucus or abnormal postcoital tests with DES (96,99,101).

Quantitative measures of DES uteri have shown that the endocervical canal was one third that of controls (88). This could potentially produce a relative outflow obstruction and retrograde menstruation leading to the increase in endometriosis noted by Berger and Alper (99) in primary infertility patients with DES exposure compared with matched controls. Other studies found similar rates of endometriosis in DES patients and controls (96,102) (Table 7). Haney and Hammond (101) reported that 9 of 11 patients with a history of cervical cryosurgery, electrocautery, or conization had cervical stenosis and 8 of those had endometriosis. Schmidt et al. (103) felt that abnormal healing of the DES cervix led to cervical stenosis in 35 of the 51 (75%) patients with a history of one of the minor cervical procedures noted above. They cautioned against attempting even minor gynecologic procedures on DES-exposed offspring.

Another factor that may postpone conception in DES progeny is altered menstrual function. Peress et al. (104) noted hirsutism in 72% and irregular menses in 50% of

TABLE 7. *Diethylstilbestrol (DES) and endometriosis (in infertility patients)*

Study	DES-exposed		Controls		Significance
	No. patients	% Endomet.	No. patients	% Endomet.	
Berger (99)	50	64	50	40	+
Stillman (102)	20	50	377	39	−
Senekijian (96)	24	21	9	44	−
Haney (101)	33	39			
Combined	127	47	436	39	

TABLE 8. *Diethylstilbestrol (DES) and menstrual dysfunction*

Study	DES-exposed		Controls		Significant
	No. patients	% Abnormal	No. patients	% Abnormal	
Bibbo (106)[a]	229	18	136	10	+
Herbst (107)[a]	338	32	298	15	+
Senekijian (96)[b]	61	38	27	56	−
Barnes (108)	218	16	158	10	−
Haney (88)	13	47			
Rosenfeld (100)	25	40			
Schmidt (137)	276	28			
Peress (104)	32	50			
Combined	1,192	32	619	15	

Note: The first three references used patients from the original Dieckmann's (78) study.
[a] Also significant decrease in duration of menstrual flow.
[b] Senekijian (96) limited patients to those with ovulatory factor primary infertility.

32 DES daughters and Assies et al. (105) found an increase in serum prolactin and testosterone levels in a small series of DES patients versus controls. There is disagreement as to whether menstrual irregularity is more common in DES-exposed women but overall there was a twofold increase associated with DES (Table 8). The most common menstrual abnormality was oligo-anovulation. Several studies also reported a reduction in the duration and qualitative assessment of volume in menstrual flow in DES daughters (97,106–109). The reduction in menstrual blood loss may be attributed to the smaller endometrial cavity area (88,89) as well as a reduction in endometrial thickness (89). Dysmenorrhea might also be increased (88,97).

Women with in utero DES exposure appear to carry a greater risk for adverse pregnancy outcome. Combining the ectopic pregnancy rates from the published studies yields a ninefold increased risk in the DES group (Table 9). SAB (Table 10) and PTD (Table 11) risks are each doubled in DES progeny. As a result of this propensity for poor pregnancy outcome in the DES group, the term delivery rate overall is about 1.5 times lower that of the controls; DES 54%, control 84% (Table 12). Similarly, the

TABLE 9. *Diethylstilbestrol (DES) and ectopic pregnancy rates*

Study	DES-exposed		Controls		Significant
	No. pregs.	% Ectopic	No. pregs.	% Ectopic	
Herbst (107)	212	6	254	0.3	+
Mangan (116)	179	5	337	0.3	+
Cousins (97)	43	5	56	0	−
Barnes (110)	220	4	224	1	−
Kaufman (83)	260	3	110	0	No analysis
Kaufman (85)	616	6			
Berger (127)	80	4			
Sandberg (138)	255	3			
Schmidt (137)	129	5			
Veridiano (120)	156	1			
Combined	2,150	5	981	0.5	

TABLE 10. *Diethylstilbestrol (DES) and spontaneous abortion rates*

	DES-exposed		Controls		
	No. pregs.	% SAB	No. pregs.	% SAB	Significance
Mangan (116)	164	18	308	8	+
Barnes (110)	220	26	224	16	+
Cousins (97)	27	19	39	21	−
Herbst (107)	212	27[a]	254	16[a]	−
Kaufman (83)	260	22	110	8	−
Kaufman (85)	616	18			
Berger (127)	62	31			
Schmidt (137)	93	24			
Veridiano (120)	96	24			
Combined	1,750	24	935	13	

Note: The number of pregnancies in all studies excludes elective abortions.
[a] Perinatal deaths were included with SABs.

TABLE 11. *Diethylstilbestrol (DES) and preterm delivery rates*

	DES-exposed		Controls		
	No. pregs.	% PTD	No. pregs.	% PTD	Significance
Linn (115)	200	18	12,240	7	+
Mangan (116)	164	7	308	2	+
Cousins (97)	27	30	39	0	+
Barnes (110)	220	8	224	5	−
Herbst (107)	212	15	254	3	−
Kaufman (83)	260	11	110	5	−
Kaufman (85)	616	15			
Berger (127)	62	13			
Schmidt (137)	93	13			
Sandberg (111)	164	17			
Veridiano (120)	96	15			
Combined	2,114	14	13,175	7	

Note: Pregnancies excluded elective abortions.

TABLE 12. *Diethylstilbestrol (DES) and term delivery rates*

	DES-exposed		Controls	
	No. pregs.	% Term	No. pregs.	% Term
Mangan (116)	164	60	308	89
Herbst (107)	212	2	254	81
Barnes (110)	220	62	224	78
Cousins (97)	27	44	39	80
Kaufman (83)	260	64	110	87
Kaufman (85)	616	60		
Berger (127)	62	34		
Schmidt (137)	93	50		
Veridiano (120)	96	59		
Sandberg (111)	164	57		
Combined	1,914	59	935	83

Note: Pregnancies excluded elective abortions.

overall live birth rate was 1.3 times lower for the DES group (Table 13). In the study by Barnes et al. (110), 81% of pregnant DES patients had at least one term live birth. No vaginal, cervical, or uterine abnormality, individually or in combination, has been shown to preclude term live births (111).

There are several potential explanations for the above findings. Salle et al. (89) demonstrated that the endometrial thickness was significantly less than that of the normal controls, particularly in the luteal phase. This may reflect insufficient endometrial support for the early conceptus leading to infertility or early SAB. This study also documented that the pulsatility index of the uterine arteries in the DES group was higher throughout the cycle and failed to undergo a decrease in the luteal phase. The higher pulsatility index indicates a greater impedance to blood flow suggesting that uterine perfusion is reduced, which may also lead to failed embryo implantation, SAB, and possibly intrauterine growth retardation and pregnancy induced hypertension (PIH). The authors advocated treating these patients with low-dose aspirin throughout the pregnancy. Many cases of recurrent SAB may be explained on an immune basis, i.e., the antiphospholipid antibody syndrome and possibly an alteration in natural killer cells. Noller et al. (112) reported that the lifetime history of autoimmune diseases was significantly higher in DES progeny though no single disease reached significance. Altered T-cell and natural killer cell functions have also been associated with in utero DES exposure (113,114).

Linn et al. (115) noted that other pregnancy complications such as PIH, premature rupture of the membranes, malpresentation, placenta previa, and low birth weight were significantly increased with DES exposure, whereas Mangan et al. (116) found no difference in malpresentation, placenta previa or abruption, cesarean section rates, or postpartum hemorrhage. In the study by Thorp et al. (117), there were no differences in PIH or premature rupture of the membranes. However, the cesarean section rate was higher and vaginal delivery was associated with greater blood loss and the need for manual placental extraction in the DES group. Labor curves were comparable between nulligravidas whereas parous DES progeny experienced significantly prolonged labors.

TABLE 13. *Diethylstilbestrol (DES) and live birth rates*

	DES-exposed		Controls	
	No. pregs.	% Live births	No. pregs.	% Live births
Mangan (116)	164	75	308	90
Herbst (107)	212	67	254	84
Cousins (97)	27	56	39	80
Kaufman (83)	260	74	110	92
Kaufman (85)	616	75		
Berger (127)	62	42		
Schmidt (137)	93	62		
Sandberg (111)	164	69		
Combined	1,632	76	711	92

Note: Pregnancies excluded elective abortions.

Treatment

Assisted reproductive techniques may be offered to infertile DES patients. Karande et al. (118) demonstrated that these patients had a similar number of oocytes retrieved and fertilized, and embryos replaced, to patients with tubal factor infertility. Pregnancy rates were also not significantly different though the DES patients had a poorer pregnancy outcome as expected. Consideration must be given to reducing the number of embryos transferred to avoid the complication of multiple pregnancy in the already compromised uterus. A successful gamete intrafallopian transfer (GIFT) pregnancy has also been reported in a DES patient (119). However, in vitro fertilization (IVF) should be the preferred procedure due to the higher risk of tubal pregnancy in DES women (84).

Treatment options for DES patients with fetal wastage are metroplasty or cervical cerclage. When assessing the success of any treatment it must be borne in mind that there is a trend toward a increase in duration of each successive pregnancy even without intervention. In patients who have achieved a term pregnancy, their future reproductive performance will not be compromised (120). Three very small studies reported performing metroplasty on the DES uterus. Khalifa et al. (121) stated that they performed a modification of the Jones abdominal metroplasty on three T-shaped uteri but provided no details of the procedure. It is difficult to envision this procedure or how removing a wedge of uterine fundus could be of benefit to patients with a uterus that is already hypoplastic to begin with. The two studies that performed operative hysteroscopy to achieve a more normal-appearing endometrial cavity included 13 women, 8 of whom had a history of in utero DES exposure (122,123). It cannot be determined if metroplasty of the DES uterus is of any clinical value based on these small numbers. Surgery to correct the anatomic abnormalities is not currently recommended (84).

The association of DES and cervical incompetence and the use of prophylactic cervical cerclage are still unresolved after long-standing debate. The definition of cervical incompetence is poorly established and the diagnosis commonly is uncertain and difficult to prove (111). The DES cervix may be predisposed to incompetency due to an increase in smooth muscle to collagen ratio (124), structural changes in collagen fibrils (125), and decreased elastin content (126). Unfortunately, these changes are not found uniformly and cannot be identified prospectively (48).

There are no randomized studies comparing prophylactic cerclage with expectant management. While a few small, uncontrolled series claimed that prophylactic cervical cerclage should be a universal practice, most authors advocate limiting cerclage to the standard clinical indications (81,85,107,110,127–129). In addition, two prospective randomized trials of prophylactic cerclage for patients at risk for preterm delivery found no benefit but significant risk associated with its use (130,131). DES patients with cervical changes may be particularly difficult to monitor for early signs of cervical incompetence (128) and cerclage may be technically challenging, requiring US guidance (132) or a transabdominal approach (133).

Ludmir et al. (125) performed a prospective, though not randomized, study in which 63 DES patients with a hypoplastic cervix or a history of second-trimester loss were treated by prophylactic cerclage or expectant management. Forty-three percent of the expectant management group required an emergency cerclage. Gestational age at delivery was comparable for the two cerclage groups and no perinatal deaths occurred. The 21 patients managed without cerclage delivered significantly earlier and 5 perinatal deaths occurred. Each of the 5 experienced premature rupture of membranes 3 to 7 days after a normal cervical examination. It is unknown if these could have been prevented by prophylactic cerclage.

In other prospective studies, Levine and Berkowitz (129) managed 120 pregnancies in 50 DES women with bimonthly cervical exams and bed rest if cervical change occurred. One patient with a history of cervical incompetence received a prophylactic cerclage in two pregnancies and another patient underwent an emergency cerclage. Overall, 92% of pregnancies resulted in a viable infant and 78% reached term. Michaels et al. (128) followed 21 pregnancies in 19 DES patients with weekly ultrasonograms. Five patients were treated with cerclage based on cervical changes. There were no second-trimester losses, deliveries before 36 weeks, or perinatal deaths. Thus, the decision to perform a prophylactic cerclage is a decision left up to the individual physician and patient.

REFERENCES

1. Simon C, Martinez L, Pardo P, Tortajada M, Pellicer A. Mullerian defects in women with normal reproductive outcome. *Fertil Steril* 1991;56:1192–3.
2. Ashton D, Amin HK, Richart RM, Neuwirth RS. The incidence of asymptomatic uterine anomalies in women undergoing transcervical tubal sterilization. *Obstet Gynecol* 1988;72:28–30.
3. Tho PT, Byrd JR, McDonough PG. Etiologies and subsequent reproductive performance of 100 couples with recurrent abortion. *Fertil Steril* 1979;32:389–395.
4. Harger JH, Archer DF, Marchese SG, et al. Etiology of recurrent pregnancy losses and outcome of subsequent pregnancies. *Obstet Gynecol* 1983;62:574–581.
5. Makino T, Hara T, Oka C, et al. Survey of 1120 Japanese women with a history of recurrent spontaneous abortions. *Eur J Obstet Gynecol Reprod Biol* 1992;44:123–130.
6. Raziel A, Arieli S, Bukovsky I. Investigation of the uterine cavity in recurrent aborters. *Fertil Steril* 1994;62:1080–1082.
7. Clifford K, Rai R, Watson H, Regan L. An informative protocol for the investigation of recurrent miscarriage: preliminary experience of 500 consecutive cases. *Hum Reprod* 1994;9:1328–1332.
8. Jurkovic D, Giepel A, Gruboeck K, et al. Three-dimensional ultrasound for the assessment of uterine anatomy and detection of congenital anomalies: a comparison with hysterosalpingography and two-dimensional sonography. *Ultrasound Obstet Gynecol* 1995;5:233.
9. Acien P. Uterine anomalies and recurrent miscarriage. *Clin N Am* 1996;49:944–955.
10. Meis PJ, Goldenberg RL, Mercer BM, et al. The preterm prediction study: risk factors for indicated preterm births. *Am J Obstet Gynecol* 1998;178:562–567.
11. Green LD, Harris RE. Uterine anomalies. Frequency of diagnosis and associated obstetric complications. *Obstet Gynecol* 1976;47:427–429.
12. Moutos DM, Damewood MD, Schlaff WD, Rock JA. A comparison of the reproductive outcome between women with a unicornuate uterus and women with a didelphic uterus. *Fertil Steril* 1992;58:88–93.
13. Tulandi T, Arronet GH, McInnes RA. Arcuate and bicornuate uterine anomalies and infertility. *Fertil Steril* 1980;34:362–364.
14. Maneschi F, Zupi E, Marconi D, Valli E, Romanini C, Mancuso S. Hysteroscopically detected asymptomatic Mullerian anomalies. Prevalence and reproductive implications. *J Reprod Med* 1995;40:684–688.

15. Acien P. Incidence of Mullerian defects in fertile and infertile women. *Hum Reprod* 1997;12:1372–1376.

16. Andrews MC, Jones HW. Impaired reproductive performance of the unicornuate uterus: intrauterine growth retardation, infertility, and recurrent abortion in five cases. *Am J Obstet Gynecol* 1982;144:173.

17. Golan A, Langer R, Bukovsky I, Caspi E. Congenital anomalies of the mullerian system. *Fertil Steril* 1989;51:747–755.

18. Abramovici H, Aktor JH, Ascal B. Congenital uterine malformations as indication for cervical suture (cerclage) in habitual abortion and premature delivery. *Int J Fertil* 1983;28:161.

19. Ludmir J, Samuels P, Brooks S, Mennuti MT. Pregnancy outcome of patients with uncorrected uterine anomalies managed in a high-risk obstetric setting. *Obstet Gynecol* 1990;75:906–910.

20. Fedele L, Zamberletti D, Vercellini P, Dorta M, Candiani GB. Reproductive performance of women with a unicornuate uterus. *Fertil Steril* 1987;47:416–419.

21. Rock JA, Schlaff WD. The obstetric consequences of uterovaginal anomalies. *Fertil Steril* 1985;43:681–692.

22. Raga F, Bauset C, Remohi J, Bonilla-Musoles F, Simon C, Pellicer A. Reproductive impact of congenital Mullerian anomalies. *Hum Reprod* 1997;12:2277–2281.

23. Rock JA. Surgery for anomalies of the mullerian ducts. In: Rock JA, Thompson JD, eds. *Te Linde's operative gynecology*, 8th ed. Philadelphia: Lippincott-Raven Publishers, 1997;687–730.

24. Stampe SS. Estimated prevalence of mullerian anomalies. *Acta Obstet Gynecol Scand* 1988;67:441–445.

25. Freedman MF. Uterine anomalies. *Semin Reprod Endocrinol* 1986;4:39–54.

26. Buttram VC, Gibbons WE. Mullerian anomalies: a proposed classification (an analysis of 144 cases). *Fertil Steril* 1979;32:40–46.

27. Musich JR, Behrman SJ. Obstetric outcome before and after metroplasty in women with uterine anomalies. *Obstet Gynecol* 1978;52:63–66.

28. Reuter KL, Daly DC, Cohen SM. Septate versus bicornuate uteri: errors in imaging diagnosis. *Radiology* 1989;172:749–752.

29. Wu MH, Hsu CC, Huang KE. Detection of congenital mullerian duct anomalies using three-dimensional ultrasound. *J Clin Ultrasound* 1997;25:487–492.

30. Carrington BM, Hricak H, Nuruddin RN, Secaf E, Laros RKJ, Hill EC. Mullerian duct anomalies: MR imaging evaluation. *Radiology* 1990;176:715–720.

31. Mintz MC, Thickman DI, Gussman D, Kressel HY. MR evaluation of uterine anomalies. *AJR* 1987;148:287–290.

32. Woodward PJ, Wagner BJ, Farley TE. MR imaging in the evaluation of female infertility. *Radiographics* 1993;13:293–310.

33. Fedele L, Dorta M, Brioschi D, et al. Magnetic resonance evaluation of double uteri. *Obstet Gynecol* 1989;74:844–847.

34. Letterie GS, Haggerty M, Lindee G. A comparison of pelvic ultrasound and magnetic resonance imaging as diagnostic studies for mullerian tract abnormalities. *Int J Fertil* 1995;40:34–38.

35. Thompson JP, Smith RA, Welch JS. Reproductive ability after metroplasy. *Obstet Gynecol* 1966;28:363.

36. Acien P. Reproductive performance of women with uterine malformations. *Hum Reprod* 1993;8:122–126.

37. Leible S, Munoz H, Walton R, Sabaj V, Cumsille F, Sepulveda W. Uterine artery blood flow velocity waveforms in pregnant women with mullerian duct anomaly: a biologic model for uteroplacental insufficiency. *Am J Obstet Gynecol* 1998;178:1048–1053.

38. Golan A, Langer R, Wexler S, Segev E, Niv D, David MP. Cervical cerclage—its role in the pregnant anomalous uterus. *Int J Fertil* 1990;35:164–170.

39. Stein AL, March CM. Pregnancy outcome in women with mullerian duct anomalies. *J Reprod Med* 1990;35:411–414.

40. Maneschi F, Marana R, Muzii L, Mancuso S. Reproductive performance in women with bicornuate uterus. *Acta Europaea Fertilitatis* 1993;24:117–120.

41. Oliva GC, Fratoni A, Genova M, Romanini C. Uterine motility in patients with bicornuate uterus. *Int J Gynaecol Obstet* 1992;37:7–12.

42. Winer CER. Uterine inversion associated with bicornuate uterus. *Br Med J* 1966;1:401–402.

43. Jain U, Agrawal SP. Torsion of a gravid horn of a bicornuate uterus. *J Ind Med Assoc* 1922;84:222.

44. Graham JMJ, Smith DW. Metopic craniostenosis as a consequence of fetal head constraint: two interesting experiments of nature. *Pediatrics* 1980;65:1000–1002.

45. Winter RM, Dearlove J, Jolly H, Pawson M, Wilson RG. Apparent microcephaly caused by a bicornuate uterus. *Br Med J Clin Res Ed* 1983;286:1640–1641.
46. Crabtree GS, Machin GA, Martin JM, Nicholson SF, Nimrod CA. Fetal deformation caused by uterine malformation. *Pediatr Pathol* 1984;2:305–312.
47. Zlotogora J, Arad I, Yarkoni S, Cohen T. Newborn with multiple joint contractures due to maternal bicornuate uterus. *Isr J Med Sci* 1985;21:454–455.
48. Patton PE. Anatomic uterine defects. *Clin Obstet Gynecol* 1994;37:705–721.
49. Buttram VC Jr. Mullerian anomalies and their management. *Fertil Steril* 1983;40:159–163.
50. Strassmann P. Die operative vereinigung eines doppelten uterus. *Zentralbl Gynakol* 1907;31:1322.
51. Pelosi MA. Laparoscopic-assisted transvaginal metroplasty for the treatment of bicornuate uterus: a case study. *Fertil Steril* 1996;65:886–890.
52. Strassmann EO. Plastic unification of double uterus. *Am J Obstet Gynecol* 1952;64:25–37.
53. Genell S, Sjovall A. The Strassmann operation results obtained in 58 cases. *Acta Obstet Gynecol Scand* 1959;38:477.
54. Candiani GB, Fedele L, Parazzini F, Zamberletti D. Reproductive prognosis after abdominal metroplasty in bicornuate or septate uterus: a life table analysis. *Br J Obstet Gynaecol* 1990;97:613–617.
55. Ayhan A, Yucel I, Tuncer ZS, et al. Reproductive performance after conventional metroplasty: an evaluation of 102 cases. *Fertil Steril* 1992;57:1194–1196.
56. Heinonen PK, Saarikoski S, Pystynen P. Reproductive performance of women with uterine anomalies. *Acta Obstet Gynecol Scand* 1982;61:157–162.
57. Blum M. Prevention of spontaneous abortion by cervical suture of the malformed uterus. *Int Surg* 1977;62:213–215.
58. Perino A, Chianchiano N, Simonaro C, Cittadini E. Endoscopic management of a case of complete septate uterus with a unilateral hematometra. *Hum Reprod* 1995;10:2171–2173.
59. Jones HW, Jones GE. Double uterus as an etiological factor in repeated abortion: indication for surgical repair. *Am J Obstet Gynecol* 1953;65:325–339.
60. Dicker D, Ashkenazi J, Dekel A, et al. The value of hysteroscopic evaluation in patients with preclinical in vitro fertilization abortions. *Hum Reprod* 1996;11:730–731.
61. Rock JA, Jones HW. The clinical management of the double uterus. *Fertil Steril* 1977;28:798.
62. Tompkins P. Comments on the bicornuate uterus and twinning. *Surg Clin N Am* 1962;42:1049–1055.
63. McShane PM, Reilly RJ, Schiff I. Pregnancy outcomes following Tompkins metroplsty. *Fertil Steril* 1983;40:190.
64. Fedele L, Arcaini LPF, Vercellini P, DiNola G. Reproductive prognosis after hysteroscopic metroplasty in 102 women: life table analysis. *Fertil Steril* 1993;59:768.
65. Dabirashrafi H, Bahadori M, Mohammad K, et al. Septate uterus: new idea on the histologic features of the septum in this abnormal uterus. *Am J Obstet Gynecol* 1995;172:105–107.
66. Zreik TG, Troiano RN, Ghoussoub RAD, Olive D, Arici A, McCarthy SM. Myometrial tissue in uterine septa. *J Am Assoc Gynecol Laparosc* 1998;5:155–160.
67. Valle RF, Sciarra JJ. Treatment of the septate uterus. *Obstet Gynecol* 1986;67:253–257.
68. March CM, Israel R. Hysteroscopic management of recurrent abortion caused by septate uterus. *Am J Obstet Gynecol* 1987;156:834–842.
69. Fedele L, Bianchi S, Marchini M, Mezzopane R, DiNola G, Tozzi L. Residual uterine septum of less than 1 cm after hysteroscopic metroplasty does not impair reproductive outcome. *Hum Reprod* 1996;11:727–729.
70. Vercellini P, DeGiorgi O, Cortesi I, Aimi G, Mazza P, Crosignani PG. Metroplasty for the complete septate uterus: does cervical sparing matter? *Am Assoc Gynecol Laparosc* 1996;3:509–514.
71. Dabirashrafi H, Mohammad K, Moghadami-Tabrizi N, Zandinejad K, Moghadami-Tabrizi M. Is estrogen necessary after hysteroscopic incision of the uterine septum. *J Am Assoc Gynecol Laparosc* 1996;3:623–625.
72. DeCherney AH, Russsell JB, Graebe RA, Polan ML. Resectoscope management of mullerian fusion defects. *Fertil Steril* 1986;45:726–728.
73. Perino A, Mencaglia L, Hamou J, Cittadini E. Hysteroscopy for metroplasty of uterine septa: report of 24 cases. *Fertil Steril* 1987;48:321–323.
74. Daly DC, Maier D, Soto-Albors C. Hysteroscopic metroplasty: six years experience. *Obstet Gynecol* 1989;73:201–205.
75. Colacurci N, DePlacido G, Mollo A, Carravetta C, DeFranciscis P. Reproductive outcome after hysteroscopic metroplasty. *Eur J Obstet Gynecol* 1996;66:147–150.

76. Ohl J, Bettahar-Lebugle K. Ultrasound guided transcervical resection of uterine septa: 7 years experience. *Ultrasound Obstet Gynecol* 1996;7:328–334.

77. Smith OW. Diethylstilbestrol in the prevention and treatment of complications of pregnancy. *Am J Obstet Gynecol* 1948;56:821–834.

78. Dieckmann WJ, Davis ME, Rynkiewicz LM, Pottinger RE. Does the administration of diethylstilbestrol during pregnancy have therapeutic value? *Am J Obstet Gynecol* 1953;66:1062–1081.

79. Brackbill Y, Berendes HW. Dangers of diethylstilbestrol: a review of a 1953 paper (letter). *Lancet* 1978;2:520.

80. Herbst AL, Ulfelder H, Poskanzer DC. Adenocarcinoma of the vagina: an association of maternal stilbestrol therapy with tumor appearing in young women. *N Engl J Med* 1971;284:878–881.

81. Stillman RJ. In utero exposure to diethylstilbestrol: adverse effects on the reproductive tract and reproductive performance and male and female offspring (review). *Am J Obstet Gynecol* 1982;142:905–921.

82. Giusti RM, Iwamoto K, Hatch EE. Diethylstilbestrol revisited: a review of the long-term health effects. *Ann Intern Med* 1995;122:778–788.

83. Kaufman RH, Adam E, Binder GL, Gerthoffer E. Upper genital tract changes and pregnancy outcome in offspring exposed in utero to diethylstilbestrol. *Am J Obstet Gynecol* 1980;137:299–308.

84. Mottla GL, Stillman RJ. Considering the role of assisted reproduction in infertile patients exposed in utero to diethylstilbestrol. *Assist Reprod Rev* 1992;2:173–183.

85. Kaufman RH, Noller K, Adam E, et al. Upper genital tract abnormalities and pregnancy outcome in diethylstilbestrol-exposed progeny. *Am J Obstet Gynecol* 1984;148:973–984.

86. Rennell CL. T-shaped uterus in diethylstilbestrol (DES) exposure. *AJR* 1979;132:979–980.

87. van Gils AP, Tham RT, Falke TH, Peters AA. Abnormalities of the uterus and cervix after diethylstilbestrol exposure: correlation of findings on MR and hysterosalpingography. *AJR* 1989;153:1235–1238.

88. Haney AF, Hammond CB, Soules MR, Creaseman WT. Diethylstilbestrol-induced upper genital tract abnormalities. *Fertil Steril* 1979;31:142–146.

89. Salle B, Sergeant P, Awada A, et al. Transvaginal ultrasound studies of vascular and morphological changes in uteri exposed to diethylstilbestrol in utero. *Hum Reprod* 1996;11:2531–2536.

90. Kipersztok S, Javitt M, Hill MC, Stillman RJ. Comparison of magnetic resonance imaging and transvaginal ultrasonography with hysterosalpingography in the evaluation of women exposed to diethylstilbestrol. *J Reprod Med* 1996;41:347–351.

91. DeCherney AH, Cholst I, Naftolin F. Structure and function of the fallopian tubes following exposure to diethylstilbestrol (DES) during gestation. *Fertil Steril* 1981;36:741–745.

92. Haney AF, Newbold RR, Fetter BF, McLachlan JA. Paraovarian cysts associated with prenatal diethylstilbestrol exposure. Comparison of the human with a mouse model. *Am J Pathol* 1986;124:405–411.

93. Kaufman RH, Adam E, Grey MP, Gerthoffer E. Urinary tract changes associated with exposure in utero to diethylstilbestrol. *Obstet Gynecol* 1980;56:330–332.

94. Gallup DG, Altaffer LF, Castle CA. Urinary tract evaluation of diethylstilbestrol-exposed female progeny followed in a colposcopy clinic. *J Reprod Med* 1984;29:717–721.

95. Tilley BC, Barnes AB, Bergstralh E, et al. A comparison of pregnancy history recall and medical records. Implications for retrospective studies. *Am J Epidemiol* 1985;121:269–281.

96. Senekijian EK, Potkul RK, Frey K, Herbst AL. Infertility among daughters either exposed or not exposed to diethylstilbestrol. *Am J Obstet Gynecol* 1988;158:493–498.

97. Cousins L, Karp W, Lacey C, Lucas WE. Reproductive outcome of women exposed to diethylstilbestrol in utero. *Obstet Gynecol* 1980;56:70–76.

98. Kaufman RH, Adam E, Noller K, Irwin JF, Gray M. Upper genital tract changes and infertility in diethylstilbestrol-exposed women. *Am J Obstet Gynecol* 1986;154:1312–1318.

99. Berger MJ, Alper MM. Intractable primary infertility in women exposed to diethylstilbestrol in utero. *J Reprod Med* 1986;31:231–235.

100. Rosenfeld DL, Bronson RA. Reproductive problems in the DES-exposed female. *Obstet Gynecol* 1980;55:453–456.

101. Haney AF, Hammond MG. Infertility in women exposed to diethylstilbestrol in utero. *J Reprod Med* 1983;28:851–856.

102. Stillman RJ, Miller LC. Diethylstilbestrol exposure in utero and endometriosis in infertile females. *Fertil Steril* 1984;41:369–372.

103. Schmidt G, Fowler WC Jr. Cervical stenosis following minor gynecologic procedures on DES-exposed women. *Obstet Gynecol* 1980;56:333–335.

104. Peress MR, Tsai CC, Mathur RS, Williamson HO. Hirsutism and menstrual patterns in women exposed to diethylstilbestrol in utero. *Am J Obstet Gynecol* 1982;144:135–140.

105. Assies J, Vonk J, Bleker O, Lumey L. Diethylstilbestrol (DES)–related endocrine disturbances in women. A story with no end, yet. *Ann NY Acad Sci* 1995;761:369–372.

106. Bibbo M, Haenszel WM, Wied GL, Hubby M, Herbst AL. A twenty-five-year follow-up study of women exposed to diethylstilbestrol during pregnancy. *N Engl J Med* 1978;298:763–767.

107. Herbst AL, Hubby MM, Azizi F, Makii MM. Reproductive and gynecologic surgical experience in diethylstilbestrol-exposed daughters. *Am J Obstet Gynecol* 1981;141:1019–1028.

108. Barnes AB. Menstrual history and fecundity of women exposed and unexposed in utero to diethylstilbestrol. *J Reprod Med* 1984;29:651–655.

109. Hornsby PP, Wilcox AJ, Weinberg CR, Herbst AL. Effects on the menstrual cycle of in utero exposure to diethylstilbestrol. *Am J Obstet Gynecol* 1994;170:709–715.

110. Barnes AB, Colton T, Gundersen J, et al. Fertility and outcome of pregnancy in women exposed in utero to diethylstilbestrol. *N Engl J Med* 1980;302:609–613.

111. Sandberg EC, Riffle NL, Higdon JV, Getman CE. Pregnancy outcome in women exposed to diethylstilbestrol in utero. *Am J Obstet Gynecol* 1981;140:194–205.

112. Noller KL, Blair PB, O'Brien PC, et al. Increased occurrence of autoimmune disease among women exposed in utero to diethylstilbestrol. *Fertil Steril* 1988;49:1080–1082.

113. Ford CD, Johnson GH, Smith WG. Natural killer cells in in utero diethylstilbestrol-exposed patients. *Gynecol Oncol* 1983;16:400–404.

114. Ways SC, Mortola JF, Zvaifler NJ, Weiss RJ, Yen SS. Alterations in immune responsiveness in women exposed to diethylstilbestrol in utero. *Fertil Steril* 1987;48:193–197.

115. Linn S, Lieberman E, Schoenbaum SC, et al. Adverse outcomes of pregnancy in women exposed to diethylstilbestrol in utero. *J Reprod Med* 1988;33:3–7.

116. Mangan CE, Borow L, Burtnett-Rubin MM, et al. Pregnancy outcome in 98 women exposed to diethylstilbestrol in utero, their mothers, and unexposed siblings. *Obstet Gynecol* 1982;59:315–319.

117. Thorp JMJ, Fowler WC, Donehoo R, Sawicki C, Bowes WA Jr. Antepartum and intrapartum events in women exposed in utero to diethylstilbestrol. *Obstet Gynecol* 1990;76:828–832.

118. Karande VC, Lester RG, Muasher SJ, Jones DL, Acosta AA, Jones HW Jr. Are implantation and pregnancy outcome impaired in diethylstilbestrol-exposed women after in vitro fertilization and embryo transfer? *Fertil Steril* 1990;54:287–291.

119. Alper MM, Oskowitz SP, Berger MJ, Thompson IE, Whitmyer J, Powers RD. Pregnancy after gamete intrafallopian transfer in a woman with primary infertility and in utero exposure to diethylstilbestrol. A case report. *J Reprod Med* 1988;33:489–491.

120. Veridiano NP, Delke I, Rogers J, Tancer ML. Reproductive performance of DES-exposed female progeny. *Obstet Gynecol* 1981;58:58–61.

121. Khalifa E, Toner JP, Jones HW Jr. The role of abdominal metroplasty in the era of operative hysteroscopy. *Surg Gynecol Obstet* 1993;176:208–212.

122. Nagel TC, Malo JW. Hysteroscopic metroplasty in the diethylstilbestrol-exposed uterus and similar nonfusion anomalies: effects on subsequent reproductive performance—a preliminary report. *Fertil Steril* 1993;59:502–506.

123. Garbin O, Dellenbach P. Metroplastie hysteroscopique d'agrandissement: un traitement des uterus DES et des hypolasies uterines? *J Gynecol Obstet Biol Reprod* 1996;25:41–46.

124. Buckingham JC, Buethe RA, Danforth DN. Collagen–muscle ratio in clinically normal and clinically incompetent cervices. *Am J Obstet Gynecol* 1965;91:231–237.

125. Ludmir J, Landon MB, Gabbe SG, Samuels P, Mennuti MT. Management of the diethylstilbestrol-exposed pregnant patient: a prospective study. *Am J Obstet Gynecol* 1987;157:665–669.

126. Leppert PC, Yu SY, Keller SK, Cerreta J, Mandl I. Decreased elastic fibers and desmosine content in incompetent cervix. *Am J Obstet Gynecol* 1987;157:1134–1139.

127. Berger MJ, Goldstein DP. Impaired reproductive performance in DES-exposed women. *Obstet Gynecol* 1980;55:25–27.

128. Michaels WH, Thompson HO, Schreiber FR, Berman JM, Ager J, Olson K. Ultrasound surveillance of the cervix during pregnancy in diethylstilbestrol-exposed offspring. *Obstet Gynecol* 1989;73:230–239.

129. Levine RU, Berkowitz KM. Conservative management and pregnancy outcome in diethylstilbestrol-exposed women with and without gross genital tract abnormalities. *Am J Obstet Gynecol* 1993;169:1125–1129.

130. Lazar P, Gueguen S, Dreyfus J, et al. Multicentered controlled trial of cervical cerclage in women at moderate risk of preterm delivery. *Br J Obstet Gynaecol* 1984;91:731–735.

131. Rush RW, Isaacs S, McPherson K, et al. A randomized controlled trial of cerclage in women at high risk of spontaneous preterm delivery. *Br J Obstet Gynaecol* 1984;91:724–730.
132. Ludmir J, Jackson GM, Samuels P. Transvaginal cerclage under ultrasound guidance in cases of severe cervical hypoplasia (see comments). *Obstet Gynecol* 1991;78:1067–1072.
133. Cammarano CL, Herron MA, Parer JT. Validity of indications for transabdominal cervicoisthmic cerclage for cervical incompetence. *Am J Obstet Gynecol* 1995;172:1871–1875.
134. Fedele L, Zamberletti D, D'Alberton A, Vercellini P, Candiani GB. Gestational aspects of uterus didelphys. *J Reprod Med* 1988;33:353–355.
135. Beernink FJ, Beernink HE, Chinn A. Uterus unicornis with a uterus solidaris. *Obstet Gynecol* 1976;47:651–653.
136. Capraro VJ, Chuang JT, Randall CL. Improved fetal salvage after metroplasty. *Obstet Gynecol* 1968;31:97.
137. Schmidt G, Fowler WCJ, Talbert LM, Edelman DA. Reproductive history of women exposed to diethylstilbestrol in utero. *Fertil Steril* 1980;33:21–24.
138. Sandberg EC, Christian JC. Diethylstilbestrol-exposed monozygotic twins discordant for cervicovaginal clear cell adenocarcinoma. *Am J Obstet Gynecol* 1980;137:220–228.

Congenital Malformations of the Female Genital Tract: Diagnosis and Management, edited by G. Gidwani and T. Falcone.
Lippincott Williams & Wilkins, Philadelphia © 1999.

12

Management of Associated Renal Anomalies

Jonathan H. Ross and Robert Kay

Department of Pediatric Urology, The Cleveland Clinic Foundation, Cleveland, Ohio 44195

The Mayer-Rokitansky-Küster-Hauser (MRKH) syndrome is typically described as vaginal agenesis associated with renal agenesis. However, a wide range of Müllerian and renal anomalies may occur in association with each other. In patients with Müllerian anomalies, an increased incidence of renal agenesis, renal ectopia, and renal fusion anomalies has been described. Ureteral ectopia may also be seen with some of these disorders. Careful evaluation of the urinary tract is an important component of the assessment of patients with Müllerian anomalies.

EMBRYOLOGIC CONSIDERATIONS

Development of the urinary tract and genital duct systems is intimately related in time and space. It is not surprising that anomalies of one are frequently associated with anomalies of the other. At the fourth week of gestation the ureteral bud arises from the mesonephric (Wolffian) duct (Fig. 1). The ureteral bud enters the adjacent metanephric blastema and induces it to develop into mature renal tissue. Branching of the ureteral bud forms the intrarenal collecting system. At approximately 6 weeks of gestation, while induction and differentiation of the kidney are occurring, the Müllerian duct migrates medially, crossing over the mesonephric duct. Careful studies of chick embryos have shown that induction and development of the Müllerian duct is dependent on a normal mesonephric duct (Fig. 2) (1). In human female embryos the mesonephric duct resorbs, leaving only the epoophoron and Gartner's duct as its cranial and caudal remnants. However, prior to its resorption, an abnormality affecting the mesonephric duct, and thereby renal development, could also interfere with normal Müllerian migration and fusion.

The cluster of anomalies seen in a given patient might depend on the timing and type of embryologic insult (2). A very early insult (prior to week 4) to the nephrogenic ridge could lead to unilateral agenesis of both the genital and urinary systems. A later insult (early week 4) could lead to maldevelopment of the ipsilateral urinary tract, and failure of migration of the ipsilateral Müllerian duct, resulting in a bifid genital duct system. Even later insults (weeks 4 to 6) would lead to failure of induc-

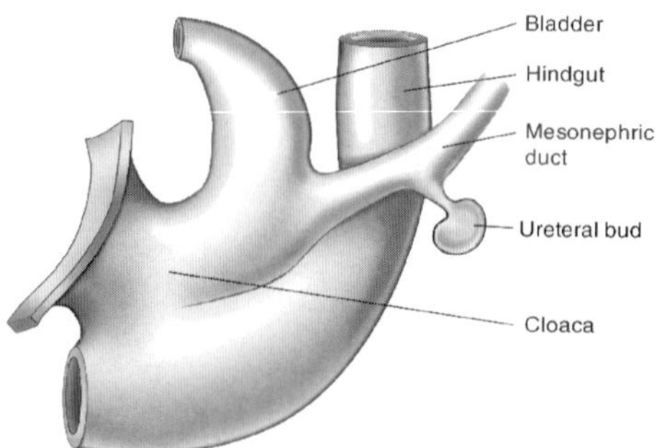

FIG. 1. The ureteral bud arises from the mesonephric duct and induces the nearby renal blastema.

tion of the metanephric blastema (resulting in renal agenesis) without any Müllerian abnormalities. Thus, disorders of medial fusion, such as bicornuate uterus, septated uterus, didelphic uterus, unicornuate uterus, and longitudinal vaginal septum, are frequently associated with renal anomalies (3,4). In contrast, disorders of vertical fusion such as transverse vaginal septum and imperforate hymen result from a primary failure of the Müllerian duct or vaginal plate. They are not typically associated with renal anomalies. Interestingly, when congenital absence of the vagina and uterus is associated with unilateral renal anomalies (classic MRKH), asymmetry of the uterine remnant or fallopian tube abnormalities are usually seen (5,6). When vaginal agenesis is associated with a symmetric uterine remnant and normal fallopian tubes, renal anomalies are usually absent. The latter, however, may be associated with hydronephrosis due to ureteral obstruction by the dilated Müllerian structures. Familial occurrences of the MRKH association have been described and a genetic basis for the association with an autosomal dominant inheritance has been proposed (7).

Some girls with Müllerian and renal anomalies also have abnormalities of the cervicothoracic somites (MURCS association). Some have occipital abnormalities as well. This has led to the hypothesis that in some cases a more global abnormality of

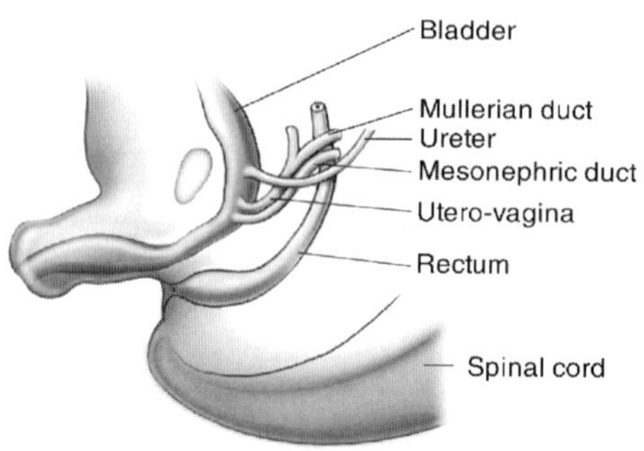

FIG. 2. In a 9-week embryo the Müllerian and mesonephric ducts are directly adjacent to each other.

the mesoderm affecting occipital, cervical, and thoracic somites and adjacent intermediate mesoderm may explain the associated anomalies (8).

RENAL AGENESIS

The classic association of renal and Müllerian anomalies is MRKH. Approximately one third of female patients with vaginal agenesis or other Müllerian anomalies of vertical fusion will have a renal anomaly (3,4,9–11). Conversely, as many as one third of female patients with unilateral renal agenesis will have a genital abnormality (Fig. 3) (12,13). Among 215 girls discovered to have renal agenesis during a mass screening with ultrasound, Sheih et al. reported 16 girls (7%) with unilateral occlusion of duplicated Müllerian ducts (14). Most of the Müllerian lesions were not apparent at presentation but were detected on follow-up ultrasounds around the time of menarche. They emphasize the importance of pelvic ultrasound in patients with unilateral renal agenesis. Patients detected prepubertally with initially normal pelvic ultrasounds should undergo a follow-up ultrasound at the age of menarche. In this way, the Müllerian anomalies can be treated early, thus reducing the risk of complications such as infertility.

Renal agenesis can occur because of a failure of the ureteral bud to properly induce the metanephric blastema to develop. Follow-up of prenatally detected renal anomalies has revealed that other cases of "renal agenesis" are due to in utero or neonatal regression of a hydronephrotic or multicystic dysplastic kidney (15,16). The association of Müllerian duct aplasia, renal aplasia, and cervicothoracic somite dysplasia (MURCS association) suggests that an unidentified regional teratogen may play a role in some patients. Indeed, the lower cervical–upper thoracic somites, arm buds, and pronephric ducts have an intimate spatial relationship at the end of the fourth

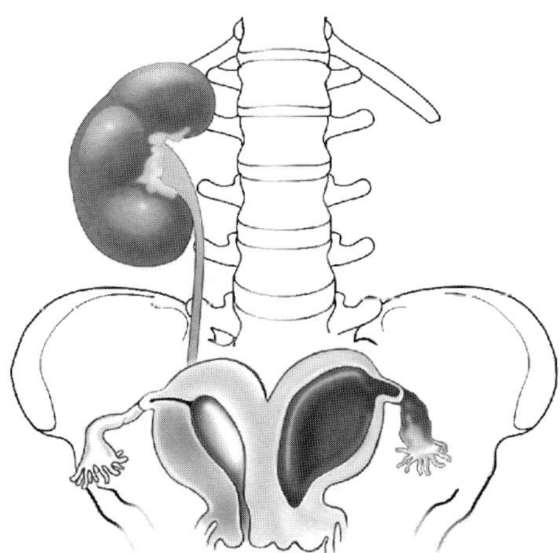

FIG. 3. Renal agenesis is commonly associated with Müllerian anomalies of vertical fusion and vaginal agenesis. The renal agenesis is ipsilateral to the obstructed or anomalous Müllerian moiety.

week of life (17). Finally, reports of Müllerian anomalies associated with renal agenesis occurring in first-degree relatives suggest that a genetic factor sometimes plays a role (18).

The adrenal gland arises from the coelomic mesothelium (adrenal cortex) and cells of the neural crest (adrenal medulla). It is not dependent on induction by mesonephric structures, and it is generally, though not always, present in patients with renal agenesis (19). In these cases the ipsilateral adrenal gland often has a "flattened" appearance on ultrasonography.

Bilateral renal agenesis is incompatible with life. From 16 weeks of gestation the urine is the major contributor to amniotic fluid. In the absence of renal parenchyma (and hence of urine) anhydramnios and Potter's syndrome results (20). Fetuses with Potter's syndrome have typical facies with a prematurely senile appearance, blunted nose, and flattened ears. Bowed legs and clubbed feet are typical. The skin appears excessively dry and loose. The anhydramnios, and perhaps absence of other renal substances, leads to fatal pulmonary hypoplasia (21).

Bilateral renal agenesis is less common in girls than boys, but when it occurs, associated genital anomalies are common (22). Other caudal anomalies such as imperforate anus are also common (22,23). However, since the bilateral renal agenesis is fatal, these associated anomalies are not of clinical significance.

Unilateral renal agenesis, which occurs in approximately one third of patients with Müllerian abnormalities, is more than an incidental finding. Its clinical significance relates to the increased incidence of urinary tract anomalies in a solitary kidney, the increased morbidity of renal trauma in a solitary kidney, and the possible long-term medical renal complications due to hyperfiltration in the solitary renal unit.

Although renal ectopia or malrotation may occur in a solitary kidney, significant renal anomalies are rare (24). The most common urinary tract abnormality is vesicoureteral reflux, which occurs in approximately one third of patients (25,26). Reflux is important because it allows the ascent of lower urinary tract infections, resulting in pyelonephritis and subsequent renal scarring. Diagnosis and treatment of reflux prior to any infections can reduce the risk of ultimate renal scarring. Therefore, it seems reasonable to screen children with a solitary kidney with a voiding cystourethrogram (VCUG) or nuclear cystogram. If reflux is detected, then the child may be placed on antibiotic prophylaxis until the reflux resolves or is corrected surgically. Other anomalies associated with a solitary kidney include ureteropelvic junction (UPJ) obstruction, obstructed megaureter, ectopic ureter, and renal hypodysplasia (25). However, selection undoubtedly plays a role in the rate of abnormalities reported in retrospective studies.

Loss of a solitary kidney is obviously of greater significance than renal loss in a patient with a normal contralateral kidney. Whether patients with unilateral renal agenesis should be advised to avoid high-risk activities, such as contact sports or skiing, is controversial. In a recent survey of the American Medical Society for Sports Medicine, 54.1% of respondents indicated that they would allow patients with a solitary kidney to participate fully in sports after a discussion of the possible risks (27). Epidemiologic data on sports-related injuries are not readily available and so an actual statistical risk cannot be assigned to sports participation. However, most renal injuries occur as a result of motor vehicle accidents or falls, and not from sports injuries (27–29). Admittedly, this may reflect the high level of exposure (nearly everyone rides in motor vehicles) rather than an intrinsically greater risk from motor vehicles compared to athletic participation. Still, actual loss of a kidney from a sports injury is rare (27,30,31).

Serious sports injuries to other solitary organs also occur but have not precluded sports participation. For example, catastrophic head injuries (always a solitary organ) occur at a rate of approximately 1 per 100,000 high school and college football players annually (32). The rate of head injuries from bicycle crashes requiring hospitalization is approximately 13 per 100,000 population (33). In professional hockey, head and back injuries are more common than abdominal injuries (34). In skiing, snowboarding, and tobogganing, central nervous system (CNS) injuries are five times more common than renal injuries (35,36).

In advising patients regarding participation in high-risk activities such as contact sports and skiing, the relative risk of serious injury to other organ systems should be considered. Since the risk of renal injury, and especially renal loss, is extremely low, and probably less than the risk to other major organ systems such as the CNS, recommending avoidance of these activities strictly because of a solitary kidney may not be reasonable. The psychological morbidity of limiting a child's activities and raising him or her with a sense of fragility must be taken into account. It seems that the most important advice for children with unilateral renal agenesis is to wear a seat-belt.

The long-term medical significance of a solitary kidney is unclear. Studies in animals and humans have demonstrated that a more than 50% loss of renal tissue leads to an increase in single-nephron glomerular filtration rate (37). This hyperfiltration at the single-nephron level can lead to proteinuria and loss of renal function. To what extent this phenomenon occurs when one kidney is absent but the other is normal is unclear.

Several studies have detected an increased incidence of hypertension, proteinuria, and renal insufficiency in adults with unilateral renal agenesis or a history of unilateral nephrectomy as a child (38). In 1986, Rugiu et al. reported a high rate of proteinuria, renal insufficiency, and hypertension in a small group of patients with renal agenesis and long-term follow-up (39). Subsequently, Argueso and colleagues reviewed the outcome of 138 children who underwent unilateral nephrectomy for a variety of diseases, with a normal contralateral kidney. The mean age at follow-up was 34 years. They detected a higher than expected incidence of proteinuria and renal insufficiency in these patients (40). In a similar study of patients with congenital absence of a kidney and a normal contralateral unit, comparable results were found, i.e., 47% of patients developed hypertension, 19% had proteinuria, and 13% had decreased renal function (41). Despite these findings, the overall survival rate was similar to that of controls. While the high incidence of complications in these studies may reflect a significant selection bias, there does seem to be an increased risk of hypertension, proteinuria, and medical renal disease in patients with a solitary kidney. Therefore, patients with unilateral renal agenesis should undergo annual blood pressure measurement and urinalysis (38). Serum creatinine should also be checked periodically. Some kindreds with renal agenesis have been reported, and ultrasound screening of first-degree relatives has been recommended (42).

RENAL FUSION ANOMALIES

Renal fusion anomalies occur more commonly in patients with Müllerian anomalies. However, the association is not as strong as with renal agenesis. The most common fusion anomaly is a horseshoe kidney (Fig. 4). Horseshoe kidneys are common in the general population with an incidence of approximately 1 in 500 (43). Because horseshoe kidney is so common, the incidence of Müllerian anomalies is very low in patients with a horseshoe kidney. Therefore, the presence of a fusion anomaly does not mandate a search for Müllerian abnormalities.

A horseshoe kidney results from fusion of the medial renal blastema of the two renal units between 4 and 8 weeks of embryogenesis. This fusion prevents migration of the renal units above the inferior mesenteric artery and prevents normal medial rotation of the kidneys. Thus the collecting systems of a horseshoe kidney assume an anterior, rather than posteromedial, position.

Why the fusion occurs is uncertain (44). One earlier theory attributes the renal fusion to an abnormally converging course of the ureters forcing the renal blastema toward the midline. Another theory ascribes the fusion to a tong-like effect of the umbilical arteries, forcing the areas of renal blastema to converge in the midline. Based on studies of embryos with horseshoe kidneys, Domenech-Mateu and Gonzalez-Compta proposed that cells from the posterior nephrogenic area fail to migrate normally, remaining in the midline and forming the parenchymal isthmus (44). They report that their embryologic findings are not consistent with the earlier hypotheses.

A horseshoe kidney may not be diagnosed by ultrasound because it is sometimes difficult to demonstrate the isthmus with this modality. Furthermore, the alteration in renal axes and the orientation of the collecting systems are not obvious. A horseshoe

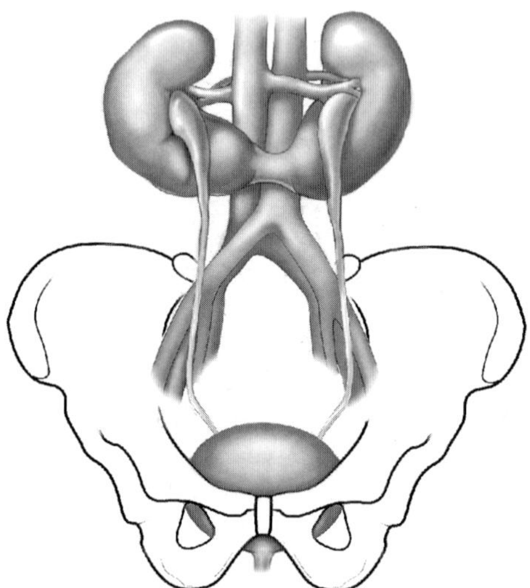

FIG. 4. Horseshoe kidney is the most common renal fusion anomaly associated with Müllerian anomalies.

kidney is readily apparent on intravenous urography (45). The renal axes deviate to or beyond the vertical, the collecting systems are unrotated, and the UPJs are more lateral than normal. The isthmus is often opacified with contrast. The horseshoe configuration is usually also evident on computed tomography (CT) and magnetic resonance imaging (MRI), which are commonly utilized in evaluation of the Müllerian anomaly.

Ureteropelvic junction obstruction is the most common congenital genitourinary abnormality found in association with a horseshoe kidney, occurring in approximately 15% of cases (46,47). While some of this increased incidence may be due to selection bias or an overdiagnosis of unobstructed hydronephrosis as UPJ obstruction in these patients, there does appear to be an intrinsic tendency for UPJ obstructions to occur in horseshoe kidneys.

Horseshoe kidneys frequently demonstrate pyelocaliectasis without obstruction. This could be due to a mild though inconsequential resistance to flow where the ureter crosses the isthmus, or may simply represent an associated dysmorphism analogous to megacalycosis. In any case, the tendency toward pyelectasis sometimes makes the diagnosis of a true UPJ obstruction problematic. Factors that argue against obstruction in a given patient are a mild, symmetric degree of hydronephrosis, a lack of symptoms, and normal parenchymal thickness and function. In equivocal cases a diuretic renal flow scan can be helpful (Fig. 5). Some studies have detected an increased incidence of vesicoureteral reflux in patients with a horseshoe kidney. Therefore, a VCUG should also be considered (48).

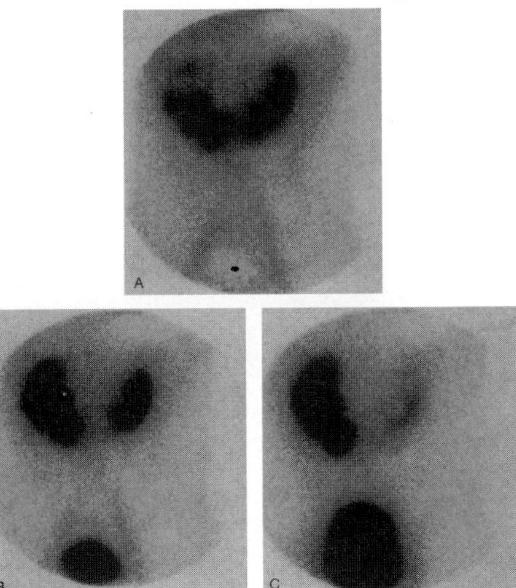

FIG. 5. A diuretic renal flow scan in a horseshoe kidney *(posterior view).* **A:** Early images demonstrate the horseshoe configuration. **B:** After initial uptake there is retention of radionuclide in both renal pelves. **C:** Following the administration of furosemide there is prolonged washout of radionuclide from the left renal moiety, confirming a true ureteropelvic junction obstruction on that side.

Once the diagnosis of a UPJ obstruction is made the options for correction are the same as in normal kidneys. The gold standard is a dismembered pyeloplasty. The operation may be performed essentially as it is in nonhorseshoe kidneys. However, because of the lower position of the kidney and the anteriorly located pelvis, modifications in the incision may be necessary. Due to concern that angulation and obstruction at the isthmus might occur, division of the isthmus and nephropexy to allow more dependent drainage of the UPJ have been proposed (46,49). However, the kidneys tend to revert to their previous orientation despite these maneuvers, and success can be achieved without dividing the isthmus (47).

For UPJ obstructions in a horseshoe kidney, ureterocalicostomy may be considered as an alternative to dismembered pyeloplasty (50). While ureterocalicostomy has been utilized predominantly for revisions of failed pyeloplasties, it has been successfully employed as a primary repair in markedly hydronephrotic horseshoe kidneys and is a reasonable approach for selected patients (51,52). Newer, minimally invasive techniques have also been successfully utilized for UPJ obstructions in horseshoe kidneys, albeit in small numbers. Antegrade endopyelotomy has been used successfully in seven of eight reported cases (53–56). Given the initial success of antegrade endopyelotomy, it is likely that retrograde endopyelotomy would also be effective for UPJ obstruction in a horseshoe kidney. An antegrade approach would be preferred for patients with associated renal calculi which were present in 22% of horseshoe kidneys in one series (47). Laparoscopic pyeloplasty is another alternative that we have successfully utilized in a horseshoe kidney.

Because of relative urinary stasis, urinary tract infections and renal calculi occur more commonly in horseshoe kidneys. When calculi occur, they may be managed by any of the standard techniques (57). An antegrade percutaneous approach may be utilized in those patients with a large stone burden or associated UPJ obstruction. Extracorporeal shock wave lithotripsy is successful in patients with a more moderate stone burden. Open surgery is reserved for select patients such as those with a large stone burden in a nonfunctioning moiety who might be best served by a nephrectomy.

In addition to an increased incidence of hydronephrosis and renal calculi, horseshoe kidneys are at a slightly increased risk for developing tumors. An increased incidence of Wilms' tumor, transitional cell carcinoma (TCC), and carcinoid tumor has been described (58). Reporting bias may play some role in these findings. Because the relative risk for Wilms' tumor and TCC is small and carcinoids are extremely rare, the risk for any given patient is not large enough to warrant routine screening. The risk of renal cell carcinoma—the most common renal tumor—does not appear to be increased in horseshoe kidneys.

Although a horseshoe kidney is the most common fusion anomaly to occur in patients with Müllerian abnormalities, crossed fused renal ectopia is also encountered. This anomaly is rare in the general population, occurring in 0.05% to 0.1%. Crossed fused ectopia occurs when one kidney crosses the midline during ascent and its renal parenchyma fuses with that of the contralateral kidney. The ureter inserts in the bladder on the original ipsilateral position. Whether fusion of the renal parenchyma from both sides occurs early and contributes to the crossed ectopia or, rather, results from it is unclear. Cook and Stephens theorize that crossed fused ectopia results from abnormal lateral flexion of the trunk and rotation of the hindgut during the time the ureteral buds are encountering the nephrogenic ridge and inducing development of the renal blastema. Due to this flexion and rotation, both ureteral buds could insert into nephrogenic blastema on the same side of the embryo. Furthermore, the flexion might result in an abnormal takeoff of the ureteral bud(s) from the mesonephric duct, resulting in the high incidence of reflux (due to a low takeoff) and ureteral ectopia (due to a high takeoff) seen in their series (59).

The most common anatomy in crossed fused ectopia has the upper pole of the crossed kidney fused with the lower pole of the orthotopic kidney (Fig. 6). However, the fused unit may assume other forms such as a sigmoid, disc, or L configuration. Because fusion impedes rotation, the renal pelves are usually anterior (59). Crossed ectopia may occur without fusion, though this is much less common (60). Solitary crossed ectopic kidneys have been described and are associated with Müllerian and other anomalies (61). Bilateral crossed ectopia can also occur.

Like other anomalous kidneys, crossed ectopic kidneys have an increased incidence of UPJ obstruction and vesicoureteral reflux (48). Patients with crossed fused ectopia should therefore undergo a VCUG and, if hydronephrosis is present, a diuretic renal flow scan. An ectopic ureter subtending the ectopic kidney occurs in approximately 2.5% of cases (60). The orthotopic moiety is usually normal. Anomalies outside the genitourinary tract are uncommon, although there is an increased incidence of imperforate anus, orthopedic and skeletal anomalies, and cardiac septal defects.

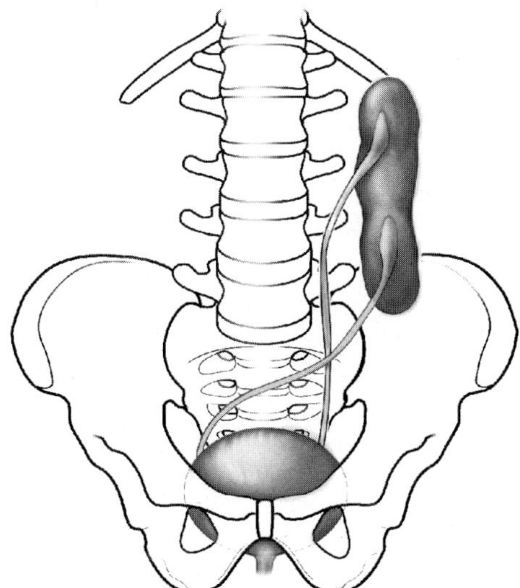

FIG. 6. The most common form of crossed fused ectopia with the crossed ectopic kidney inferior to the normal kidney.

RENAL ECTOPIA

An ectopic kidney is one that fails to ascend to its normal position in the renal fossa (Fig. 7). It is a rare disorder, occurring in 0.01% to 0.05% of patients (43). Fore et al. noted a 15% incidence of renal ectopia in 39 patients with Müllerian anomalies (62). Gleason et al. recently reviewed their experience with 82 ectopic kidneys (63). Of all patients (males and females), 26% had a genitourinary anomaly. Ectopic locations were pelvic (55%), crossed (32%), lumbar (12%), and thoracic (1%). When the ectopic kidney is also a solitary kidney the incidence of genital anomalies in girls is 66% (64).

The cause of renal ectopia remains unclear. Between weeks 4 and 8 of gestation the kidney ascends from its pelvic position and rotates medially as it ascends. Based on microdissection of chick embryos, Maizels and Stephens hypothesized that in some cases ectopia may result from a spinal defect that prevents renal ascent (65). The clinical association of spinal anomalies and renal ectopia might also reflect a regional insult to both systems during development. In any case, with failure of ascent, the kidney also fails to rotate normally, and the renal pelvis is generally in an anterior position, much like a horseshoe kidney. The adrenal is usually in its normal retroperitoneal position. In 10% of cases ectopia is bilateral. Thoracic kidneys are etiologically unrelated to the more common caudally ectopic kidneys and are not associated with genital anomalies.

The most common abnormality in an ectopic kidney is hydronephrosis. Half of the ectopic kidneys in Gleason's series were hydronephrotic (63). This probably overestimates the true incidence of hydronephrosis in ectopic kidneys since this was a retrospective review of mostly symptomatic patients. The cause of hydronephrosis was

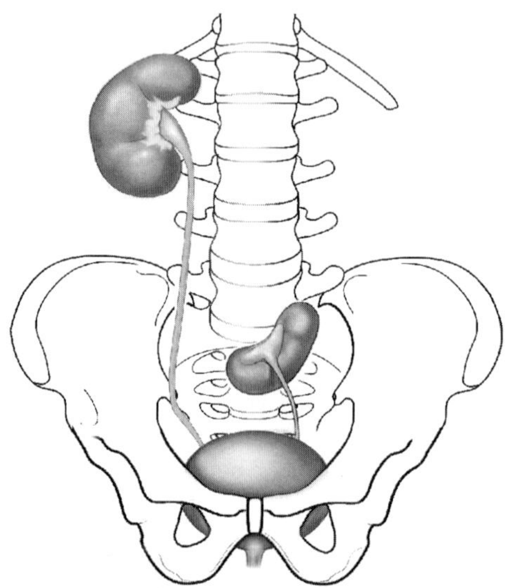

FIG. 7. The pelvis is the most common location for an ectopic kidney.

a UPJ obstruction in 37%. Other causes of hydronephrosis were vesicoureteral reflux (26%) and ureterovesical junction obstruction (15%). In 22% of cases, the hydronephrosis was unobstructed and felt to be due to abnormal position and malrotation alone. While ectopic kidneys are clearly at increased risk for UPJ obstruction, the high incidence of other causes of hydronephrosis demands a thorough evaluation including ultrasound and/or intravenous urography, VCUG, and diuretic renography. Cystoscopy with retrograde pyelography at the time of surgical correction might also be helpful. Thorough evaluation of the contralateral kidney is indicated because 25% of contralateral kidneys are hydronephrotic.

Surgical correction of UPJ obstructions occurring in ectopic kidneys requires special consideration (66–69). Most can be successfully repaired with a dismembered pyeloplasty. Because of the location of these kidneys, incisions must be tailored for direct access. A transabdominal approach is usually best for pelvic kidneys, whereas most crossed kidneys may be approached extraperitoneally. The associated malrotation requires special care in reconstructing a funneled dependent anastomosis. To avoid kinking or twisting of the anastomosis, extensive mobilization of the kidney is avoided. If an adequate positioning of the UPJ seems unlikely, ureterocalicostomy should be considered.

Alternatives to dismembered pyeloplasty or ureterocalicostomy include minimally invasive techniques, nephrectomy, and pyelovesicostomy. There is little experience with minimally invasive techniques for ectopic kidneys, although their location should make them amenable to a laparoscopic approach. While antegrade endopyelotomy might be difficult due to renal position, retrograde endopyelotomy seems a reasonable alternative (70). Reconstructive techniques are successful, so nephrectomy should be reserved for non-functioning kidneys. Pyelovesicostomy results in high-grade reflux and should be avoided as a primary repair. However, it may be useful in patients with failed prior reconstruction, those with extensive adhesions due to infection, and older patients with recurrent stone disease (71,72).

Other than hydronephrosis and vesicoureteral reflux, ectopic kidneys are not at increased risk for disease. Pelvic kidneys do not significantly increase the risk of obstetric complications, although dystocia from a pelvic kidney can rarely occur. When it does occur, cesarean section is indicated. Historically, an ectopic kidney was of interest to gynecologists because it could be misdiagnosed as a tumor or other pelvic mass (73). However, with modern imaging this should not occur.

ECTOPIC URETER AND URETEROCELE

In the general population ectopic ureters occur most commonly in duplicated collecting systems, subtending the upper pole. They are far less commonly associated with Müllerian anomalies than renal agenesis, fusion, and ectopia, but do occur in some cases (74–78).

An ectopic ureter results from an abnormally high takeoff of the ureteral bud from the mesonephric duct. As the mesonephric duct migrates into the bladder forming the trigone, the high bud will fail to make it to its normal position and will end up in-

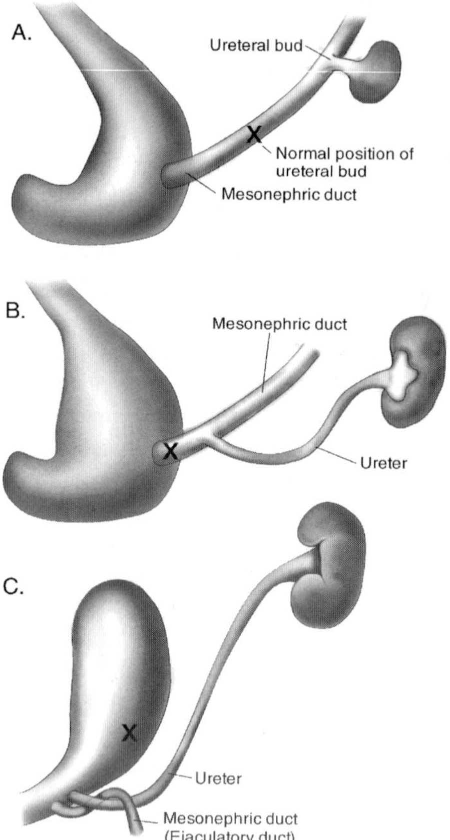

FIG. 8. A: Ectopic ureters occur as a result of a high takeoff of the ureteral bud from the mesonephric duct. **B, C:** As the mesonephric duct moves into the developing bladder to form the trigone, the ureter fails to migrate to its normal position and assumes an ectopic location inserting into the mesonephric duct structures or remnants.

serting at the bladder neck, proximal urethra, or along the mesonephric duct outside the urinary tract (Fig. 8) (79). In girls, the mesonephric duct remnant is the Gartner's duct. Ectopic ureters inserting into this remnant may ultimately drain in the anterolateral introitus or vagina. A persistent Gartner's duct cyst might be interposed between the ureter and its site of ultimate drainage, or the ectopic ureter subtending a dysplastic kidney might simply end at a Gartner's duct cyst without draining to the outside (76).

Li et al. reported 24 cases of duplicated uterus with unilateral uterine obstruction and unilateral renal anomalies (78). Twenty-two patients had renal agenesis, and two of these had ectopic ureters draining into Gartner's duct cysts. The other two patients had renal hypoplasia and dysplasia, both with ectopic ureters draining into Gartner's duct cysts. After initial evaluation with ultrasound, Li et al. found MRI most helpful in delineating the Müllerian and renal anomalies. Excision of the Gartner's duct cyst, ectopic ureter and kidney (if present) was undertaken in three of the four patients. This same group subsequently reported 10 cases of Gartner's duct cyst associated with renal dysgenesis and ipsilateral Müllerian duct obstruction (77). Again, they found MRI to best elucidate the anatomy. They recommended excision of the cyst and upper urinary tract only if it was symptomatic—usually with obstructive voiding symptoms. This was the case 50% of the time.

The management of an ectopic ureter depends on the age of the patient and the associated anomalies. In a child with a functioning renal moiety a ureteral reimplant or upper to lower pole ureteropyelostomy is appropriate (80,81). If the renal parenchyma draining through the ectopic ureter is dysplastic, then a heminephrectomy or nephrectomy (in a duplicated or single system, respectively) is appropriate. In some cases, reflux into the ectopic ureter or high-grade reflux into the ipsilateral lower pole might mandate reconstruction at the bladder level with ureteral reimplantation and/or complete excision of the ectopic ureter. Reimplantation is more easily accomplished in children over 1 year of age.

Ureteroceles are not associated with Müllerian anomalies but are in the differential diagnosis of an interlabial mass, which also includes an imperforate hymen. A ureterocele is a cystic dilatation of the intramural ureter associated with obstructive distention of the entire ureter (Fig. 9). A ureterocele may extend submucosally down the bladder neck and urethra, or it may prolapse through the urethra resulting in a bulging mass on the perineum. With careful inspection, a normal vagina can usually be identified, thereby excluding an imperforate hymen. When a ureterocele is suspected, it can be confirmed by ultrasonography of the kidneys and bladder. An ectopic ureter draining into a Gartner's duct cyst can bulge into the bladder and be mistaken for a ureterocele (82).

Ureteroceles are frequently treated with endoscopic incision, particularly in infants. This is often curative for intravesical ureteroceles. However, patients with ectopic ureteroceles often require heminephrectomy of the subtended upper pole, upper pole to lower pole ureteropyelostomy, or reconstruction at the bladder level (83).

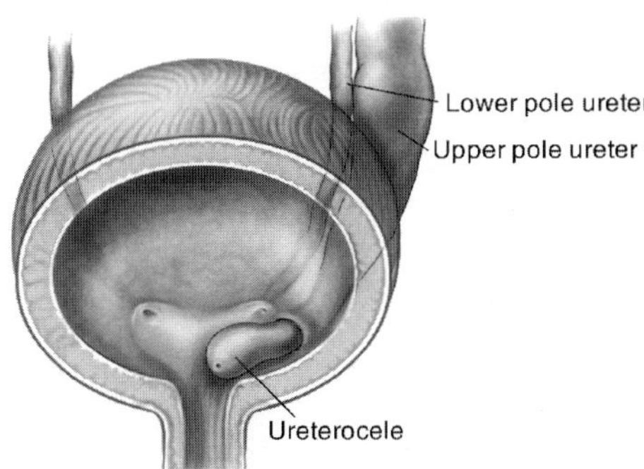

FIG. 9. A ureterocele is a cystic dilatation of the intramural ureter with obstructive hydronephrosis of the ureter it subtends.

MANAGEMENT OF HYDRONEPHROSIS IN PATIENTS WITH MÜLLERIAN ANOMALIES

Hydronephrosis in patients with Müllerian anomalies may be due to an associated primary uropathy or secondary to obstruction by a dilated Müllerian structure. Radiographic imaging of the Müllerian anomaly usually includes ultrasound and CT or MRI. These modalities will delineate the initial urologic anatomy. Management of the Müllerian anomaly invariably involves decompression of the obstructed Müllerian moiety, and intervention for urinary tract obstruction should be deferred until after Müllerian decompression. Follow-up ultrasound of the kidney(s) after Müllerian decompression may well demonstrate resolution of the hydronephrosis. If hydronephrosis persists, then further evaluation with intravenous urography and/or diuretic renography is indicated. The latter is particularly useful in distinguishing true UPJ obstructions from unobstructed dilatation in patients with renal ectopia or renal fusion anomalies. In selected cases, cystoscopy with retrograde pyelography may be needed. Treatment is then planned based on the results of these studies.

REFERENCES

1. Gruenwald P. The relation of the growing Müllerian duct to the Wolffian duct and its importance for the genesis of malformations. *Anat Rec* 1941;81:1–19.
2. Magee MC, Lucey DT, Fried FA. A new embryologic classification for uro-gynecologic malformations: the syndromes of mesonephric duct induced Müllerian deformities. *J Urol* 1979;121:265–267.
3. Woolf RB, Allen WM. Concomitant malformations: the frequent, simultaneous occurrence of congenital malformations of the reproductive and urinary tracts. *Obstet Gynecol* 1953;2:236–265.
4. Fedele L, Bianchi S, Agnoli B, Tozzi L, Vignali M. Urinary tract anomalies associated with unicornuate uterus. *J Urol* 1996;155:847–848.
5. Strubbe EH, Willemsen WNP, Lemmens JAM, Thijn CJP, Rolland R. Mayer-Rokitansky-Küster-Hauser syndrome: distinction between two forms based on excretory urographic, sonographic, and laparoscopic findings. *AJR* 1993;160:331–334.
6. Tarry WF, Duckett JW, Stephens FD. The Mayer-Rokitansky syndrome: pathogenesis, classification and management. *J Urol* 1986;136:648–652.
7. Battin J, Lacombe D, Leng JJ. Familial occurrence of hereditary renal adysplasia with Müllerian anomalies. *Clin Genet* 1993;43:23–24.
8. Lin HJ, Cornford ME, Hu B, Rutgers JKL, Beall MH, Lachman RS. Occipital encephalocele and MURCS association: case report and review of central nervous system anomalies in MURCS patients. *Am J Med Genet* 1996;61:59–62.
9. Griffin JE, Edwards C, Nadden JD, Harrod MJ, Wilson JD. Congenital absence of the vagina: the Mayer-Rokitansky-Küster-Hauser syndrome. *Ann Intern Med* 1976;85:224–236.
10. Pinsonneault O, Goldstein DP. Obstructing malformations of the uterus and vagina. *Fertil Steril* 1985;44:241–247.
11. Candiani GB, Fedele L, Candiani M. Double uterus, blind hemivagina, and ipsilateral renal agenesis: 36 cases and long-term follow-up. *Obstet Gynecol* 1997;90:26–32.
12. Thompson DP, Lynn HB. Genital anomalies associated with solitary kidney. *Mayo Clin Proc* 1966;41:539–548.
13. Bronshtein M, Bar-Hava I, Lightman A. The significance of early second-trimester sonographic detection of minor fetal renal anomalies. *Prenat Diagn* 1995;15:627–632.
14. Sheih CP, Li YW, Liao YJ, Chen WL, Lin JY, Chen SM. Early detection of unilateral occlusion of duplicated Müllerian ducts: the use of serial pelvic sonography for girls with renal agenesis. *J Urol* 1994;151:708–710.
15. Hitchcock R, Burge DM. Renal agenesis: an acquired condition? *J Pediatr Surg* 1994;29:454–455.
16. Mesrobian HGJ, Rushton HG, Bulas D. Unilateral renal agenesis may result from in utero regression of multicystic renal dysplasia. *J Urol* 1993;150:793–794.

17. Duncan PA, Shapiro LR, Stangel JJ, Klein RM, Addonizio JC. The MURCS association: Müllerian duct aplasia, renal aplasia, and cervicothoracic somite dysplasia. *J Pediatr* 1979;95:399–402.
18. Wiersma AF, Peterson LF, Justema EJ. Uterine anomalies associated with unilateral renal agenesis. *Obstet Gynecol* 1976;47:654–657.
19. Nakada T, Furuta H, Kazama T, Katayama T. Unilateral renal agenesis with or without ipsilateral adrenal agenesis. *J Urol* 1988;140:933–937.
20. Potter EL. Bilateral absence of ureters and kidneys: a report of 50 cases. *Obstet Gynecol* 1965;25:3-12.
21. Hislop A, Hey E, Reid L. The lungs in congenital bilateral renal agenesis and dysplasia. *Arch Dis Child* 1979;54:32–38.
22. Carpentier PJ, Potter EL. Nuclear sex and genital malformation in 48 cases of renal agenesis, with especial reference to nonspecific female pseudohermaphroditism. *Am J Obstet Gynecol* 1959;78:235–258.
23. Davidson WM, Ross GIM. Bilateral absence of the kidneys and related congenital anomalies. *J Pathol Bacteriol* 1954;68:459–474.
24. Longo VJ, Thompson GJ. Congenital solitary kidney. *J Urol* 1952;68:63–68.
25. Atiyeh B, Husmann D, Baum M. Contralateral renal abnormalities in patients with renal agenesis and noncystic renal dysplasia. *Pediatrics* 1993;91:812–815.
26. Song JT, Ritchey ML, Zerin JM, Bloom DA. Incidence of vesicoureteral reflux in children with unilateral renal agenesis. *J Urol* 1995;153:1249–1251.
27. Anderson CR. Solitary kidney and sports participation. *Arch Fam Med* 1995;4:885–888.
28. Kulmala R, Seppanen J, Heikkinen A, Auvinen O. Aetiology, diagnosis and treatment of patients with renal trauma. *Annales Chirurgiae Gynaecologiae* 1993;82:84–89.
29. Benchekroun A, Lachkar A, Soumana A, et al. Les traumatismes du rein: à propos de 30 cas. *Annales D'Urologie* 1997;31:237–242.
30. Borrero E. Left renal artery dissection caused by a football injury. *NY State J Med* 1991;91:550–552.
31. Skowvron O, Descotes JL, Frassinetti E, Coquilhat P, Michel A, Rambeaud JJ. Les traumatismes du rein à ski. *Progres en Urologie* 1995;5:361–369.
32. Clarke KS. Epidemiology of athletic head injury. *Clin Sports Med* 1998;17:1–12.
33. Zentner J, Franken H, Lobbecke G. Head injuries from bicycle accidents. *Clin Neurol Neurosurg* 1996;98:281–285.
34. Biasca N, Simmen HP, Bartolozzi AR, Trentz O. Review of typical ice hockey injuries: survey of the North American NHL and Hockey Canada versus European leagues. *Unfallchirurg* 1995;98:283–288.
35. Prall JA, Winston KR, Brennan R. Severe snowboarding injuries. *Injury* 1995;26:539–542.
36. Kim PCW, Haddock G, Bohn D, Wesson D. Tobogganing injuries in children. *J Pediatr Surg* 1995;30:1135–1137.
37. Brenner BM. Nephrology forum. Hemodynamically mediated glomerular injury and the progressive nature of kidney disease. *Kidney Int* 1983;23:647–655.
38. Robson WLM, Leung AKC, Rogers RC. Unilateral renal agenesis. *Adv Pediatr* 1995;42:575–592.
39. Rugiu C, Oldrizzi L, Lupo A, et al. Clinical features of patients with solitary kidneys. *Nephron* 1986;43:10–15.
40. Argueso LR, Ritchey ML, Boyle ET Jr, Milliner DS, Bergstralh EJ, Kramer SA. Prognosis of children with solitary kidney after unilateral nephrectomy. *J Urol* 1992;148:747–751.
41. Argueso LR, Ritchey ML, Boyle ET Jr, Milliner DS, Bergstralh EJ, Kramer SA. Prognosis of patients with unilateral renal agenesis. *Pediatr Nephrol* 1992;6:412–416.
42. Arfeen S, Rosborough D, Luger AM, Nolph KD. Familial unilateral renal agenesis and focal and segmental glomerulosclerosis. *Am J Kidney Dis* 1993;21:663–668.
43. Chelimsky GG, Gonzalez R. Abnormalities of the kidney. In: O'Donnell B, Koff SA, eds. *Pediatric urology*. London: Butterworths, 1997:339–354.
44. Domenech-Mateu JM, Gonzalez-Compta X. Horseshoe kidney: a new theory on its embryogenesis based on the study of a 16-mm human embryo. *Anat Rec* 1988;222:408–417.
45. Whitehouse GH. Some urographic aspects of the horseshoe kidney anomaly: a review of 59 cases. *Clin Radiol* 1975;25:107–114.
46. Das S, Amar D. Ureteropelvic junction obstruction with associated renal anomalies. *J Urol* 1984;131:872–874.
47. Pittis WR Jr, Muecke EC. Horseshoe kidneys: a 40-year experience. *J Urol* 1975;113:743–746.
48. Kelalis PP, Malek RS, Segura JW. Observations on renal ectopia and fusion in children. *J Urol* 1973;110:588–592.

49. Sharma SK, Bapna BC. Surgery of the horseshoe kidney: an experience of 24 patients. *Aust N Z J Surg* 1986;56:175–177.
50. Mesrobian HJ, Kelalis PP. Ureterocalicostomy: indications and results in 21 patients. *J Urol* 1989;142:1285–1287.
51. Levitt SB, Nabizadeh I, Javaid M, et al. Primary calycoureterostomy for pelviureteral junction obstruction: indications and results. *J Urol* 1981;126:382–386.
52. Mollard P, Braun P. Primary ureterocalycostomy for severe hydronephrosis in children. *J Pediatr Surg* 1980;15:87–92.
53. Bellman GC, Yamaguchi R. Special considerations in endopyelotomy in a horseshoe kidney. *Urology* 1996;47:582–586.
54. Koikawa Y, Naito S, Uozumi J, et al. Percutaneous endopyelotomy for ureteropelvic junction obstruction in a horseshoe kidney. *Scand J Urol Nephrol* 1996;30:145–147.
55. Nakamura K, Baba S, Tazaki H. Endopyelotomy in horseshoe kidneys. *J Endourol* 1994;8:203–206.
56. Salas M, Gelet A, Martin X, Sanseverino R, Viguier JL, Dubernard JM. Horseshoe kidney: the impact of percutaneous surgery. *Eur Urol* 1992;21:134–137.
57. Lampel A, Hohenfellner M, Schultz-Lampel D, Lazica M, Bohnen K, Thuroff JW. Urolithiasis in horseshoe kidneys: therapeutic management. *Urology* 1996;47:182–186.
58. Krishnan B, Truong LD, Saleh G, Sirbasku DM, Slawin KM. Horseshoe kidney associated with an increased relative risk of primary renal carcinoid tumor. *J Urol* 1997;157:2059–2066.
59. Cook WA, Stephens FD. Fused kidneys: morphologic study and theory of embryogenesis. *Birth Defects: Original Article Series* 1977;8:327–340.
60. Abeshouse BS, Bhisitkul I. Crossed renal ectopia with and without fusion. *Urol Int* 1959;9:63–91.
61. Kakei H, Kondo A, Ogisu BI, Mitsuya H. Crossed ectopia of solitary kidney: a report of two cases and a review of the literature. *Urol Int* 1976;31:470–475.
62. Fore SR, Hammond CB, Parker RT, Anderson EE. Urologic and genital anomalies in patients with congenital absence of the vagina. *Obstet Gynecol* 1975;46:410–416.
63. Gleason PE, Kelalis PP, Husmann DA, Kramer SA. Hydronephrosis in renal ectopia: incidence, etiology and significance. *J Urol* 1994;151:1660–1661.
64. Downs AR, Lane JW, Burns E. Solitary pelvic kidney: its clinical implications. *Urology* 1973;1:51–56.
65. Maizels M, Stephens FD. The induction of urologic malformations: understanding the relationship of renal ectopia and congenital scoliosis. *J Urol* 1979;17:209–217.
66. Czaplicki M, Krzeski T, Borkowski A, Niemierko M. Surgical treatment of stenosis of the pyeloureteral junction in pelvic kidney. *Eur Urol* 1984;10:377–379.
67. Donahoe PK, Hendren WH. Pelvic kidney in infants and children: experience with 16 cases. *J Pediatr Surg* 1980;15:486–495.
68. Felzenberg J, Nasrallah PF. Crossed renal ectopia without fusion associated with hydronephrosis in an infant. *Urology* 1991;38:450–452.
69. Kramer SA, Kelalis PP. Ureteropelvic junction obstruction in children with renal ectopia. *Journal d'Urologie* 1984;90:331–336.
70. Bales GT, Jarrard DF, Gerber GS. Ureteroscopic endopyelotomy in an ectopic kidney. *Urology* 1995;46:104–106.
71. Carini M, Selli C, Grechi G, Masini G. Pyelovesicostomy: an alternative to ureteropelvic junction-plasty in pelvic ectopic kidneys. *Urology* 1985;26:125–128.
72. Kumar A, Sharma SK, Vaidyanathan S, Goswami AK, Bapna BC. Vesicopyelostomy in the treatment of pelvic kidneys with pelviureteric junction obstruction: long-term follow-up. *Br J Urol* 1988;61:406–408.
73. Delson B. Ectopic kidney in obstetrics and gynecology. *NY State J Med* 1975;75:2522–2526.
74. Nasu K, Yoshimatsu J, Miyakawa I, Nakagawa M, Nomura Y. Absence of vagina and hypoplasia of the urethra and ectopia of the ureter. *J Obstet Gynecol* 1996;22:451–454.
75. Shibata T, Nonomura K, Kakizaki H, Murayama M, Seki T, Koyanagi T. A case of unique communication between blind-ending ectopic ureter and ipsilateral hemi-hematocopometrain uterus didelphys. *J Urol* 1995;153:1208–1210.
76. Sheih CP, Hung CS, Wei CF, Lin CY. Cystic dilatations within the pelvis in patients with ipsilateral renal agenesis or dysplasia. *J Urol* 1990;144:324–327.
77. Sheih, CP, Li YW, Liao YJ, Huang TS, Kao SP, Chen WJ. Diagnosing the combination of renal dysgenesis, Gartner's duct cyst and ipsilateral Mülerian duct obstruction. *J Urol* 1998;159:217–221.
78. Li YW, Sheih CP, Chen WJ. Unilateral occlusion of duplicated uterus with ipsilateral renal anomaly in young girls: a study with MRI. *Pediatr Radiol* 1995;25S1:S54–59.

79. Tanagho EA. Embryologic basis for lower ureteral anomalies: a hypothesis. *Urology* 1976; 7:451–464.
80. Ghoneimi AE, Miranda J, Truong T, Monfort G. Ectopic ureter with complete ureteric duplication: conservative surgical management. *J Pediatr Surg* 1996;31:467–472.
81. Plaire JC, Pope JC IV, Kropp BP, et al. Management of ectopic ureters: experience with the upper tract approach. *J Urol* 1997;158:1245–1247.
82. Sumfest JM, Burns MW, Mitchell ME. Pseudoureterocele: potential for misdiagnosis of an ectopic ureter as a ureterocele. *Br J Urol* 1995;75:401–405.
83. Coplen DE, Duckett JW. The modern approach to ureteroceles. *J Urol* 1995;153:166–171.

13

Psychosocial Aspects of Congenital Female Tract Anomalies

*Vanessa K. Jensen and **Stephanie L. Reiter

*Section of Pediatric Psychology, The Cleveland Clinic Children's Hospital, Cleveland, Ohio 44195, and **Department of Pediatrics, Rainbow Babies and Children's Hospital, Cleveland, Ohio 44106-1736*

It is well established that both nature and nurture play a part in the psychological and social functioning of an individual. Similarly, sexuality, sexual identity, sex role, and sexual behavior are multidetermined, with clear impact of genetics, hormones, anatomy, and environment. While this multidetermined causality is generally accepted in many areas (e.g., intelligence, personality), society places an additional symbolic meaning on the etiology of a person's anatomy and sexual behavior. Sex role, sexual identity, and sexual functioning are different concepts, and each must be considered in addressing the psychosocial functioning of children, adolescents, and adults with vaginal anomalies. Development in these areas varies across the age span, with different issues and needs at different stages, for both the patient and her family.

Congenital vaginal anomalies fall into two primary groups: those with associated chromosomal and hormonal abnormalities, primarily congenital adrenal hyperplasia (CAH), and those with normal chromosomal and hormonal functioning but without a functional vaginal tract, such as Mayer-Rokitansky-Küster-Hauser syndrome (MRKH). Although there are distinct differences between these two groups, some issues transcend the specific diagnosis. For both groups, parents and patients are affected by the diagnosis. Particularly when diagnosed in infancy or childhood, parents may be faced with a number of decisions that will impact the child and family for the long term. Parents must cope with having a child with differences of varying degrees, which may require a range of surgeries and treatments. For those patients requiring surgery, especially those pursuing vaginal reconstruction, a long-term commitment to the use of dilators and/or regular sexual intercourse is necessary. For those with CAH, a commitment to hormone therapy is also necessary. As such, issues of compliance with treatment and general coping must be openly addressed. Moreover, all must be viewed in the context of child and adolescent developmental needs and stages.

Despite the above similarities, patients with CAH and MRKH differ significantly in their psychosocial and developmental issues and their needs vary considerably.

For this reason, CAH and MRKH will be addressed separately, reviewing the psychosocial issues of each at various developmental levels and recommending strategies for the physician in assisting patients with these conditions.

CONGENITAL ADRENAL HYPERPLASIA

Congenital adrenal hyperplasia is a family of disorders associated with errors in cortisol biosynthesis that is transmitted by autosomal recessive genes (1–4) and affects 1 in 20,000 newborn girls (5). There are several clinical variants, i.e., simple virilizing CAH (SV), salt-wasting CAH (SW), late onset CAH (virilizing not before puberty), and cryptic form (with biochemical but no clinical alterations). The most common type of CAH is 21-hydroxylase deficiency, occurring in 90% to 95% of the cases (6). Children born with CAH have a deficiency in one of the enzymes (e.g., 21-hydroxylase) necessary for the synthesis of cortisol (6), causing increased adrenocorticotropic hormone (ACTH) secretion and subsequent accumulation of androgenic metabolites, including androstenedione and testosterone (7). The increased levels of androgens have virilizing effects on the developing female fetus and may result in the ambiguous appearance of the external genitalia. The degree of virilization ranges from clitoromegaly to partial labial fusion to complete development of a scrotum and incorporation of the urethra into a penis (8). Thus, although normal in chromosome complement, CAH patients of both sexes are exposed to adrenal-derived androgens until proper treatment is instituted.

Psychosocial Management and Diagnosis in Infancy and Early Childhood

Children born with CAH are most often identified at birth. In the newborn infant, a precise diagnosis is achieved by combining the results of the physical examination with laboratory tests. When all information from the physical examination, laboratory, imaging studies, and, rarely, exploratory laparotomy is available, the sex of the child can be assigned with greater confidence (9). Although most experts agree that a patient's first reconstructive surgery should be performed within the first 3 months of life, there are different opinions about when plastic surgery of the introitus and vagina should be performed (10,11). The male role is elected for all genotypical males born with hypospadias and undescended testicles. For a small subgroup of genotypic males who are born with hypoplasia of the penis, the current standard of care is to raise them as girls (9). All of the genotypically female patients with CAH, as well as females with clitoromegaly from other causes, are typically reared as girls (i.e., 90% of the entire cohort with intersexual malformation). In current practice, regardless of the genotype, most children with ambiguous genitalia are assigned to female upbringing, with the crucial determinant being the size of the phallus. Fewer than 10% of patients born with intersex anomalies will be directed to a male sex assignment.

Assigning a gender, however, may not be as simple as it appears. Gender identity represents a person's recognition of himself or herself as male or female and is influenced by both environmental and hormonal factors; gender role is illustrated by different behaviors within a given culture that make a person recognizable as male or female (e.g., dress, speech, play, work); and gender orientation refers to the choice of sexual partner (i.e., heterosexual, homosexual, or bisexual) (12). Human psychosexual differentiation is more than just a reflection of nurturance and social cues (8). Rather, the greater frequency of bisexuality and homosexuality in children and adolescents with CAH supports the theory that elevated levels of androgens in the female pseudohermaphrodite create a male psychosexuality just as they create a male anatomy (13). Others found that although girls with CAH exhibited a higher incidence of atypical female gender role activities, none were uncertain about their female identity (12,14). Clearly, CAH has physical and physiologic effects. What is also apparent, however, are potential psychological, emotional, social, and sexual consequences.

Regardless of what decision is made concerning gender assignment, experts agree that physicians must take every precaution not to expose the parents to internal disagreements among members of the health care team about the child's initial sex (15). Rather, medical professionals should explain that the child's sex is incompletely developed and has not yet been fully determined (12). In addition to diagnosis, parents must be given information regarding genetic transmission. Genetic counseling with these parents must weigh statistical considerations, morbidity risks specific to the syndrome, as well as therapeutic prognosis. Because CAH is an autosomal recessive disorder, 25% are homozygous, 50% heterozygous, and 25% homozygous unaffected. Moreover, all of these issues must be examined in light of the family's personal, emotional, religious, and ethical beliefs.

At this initial diagnostic stage, parents will also likely have numerous questions regarding treatment. Treatment usually consists of medical therapy with glucocorticoids and mineral corticoids in cases of salt loss, as well as surgical correction of the virilized external genitals (16). In addition to providing a clear explanation of their child's condition with the necessary clinical vocabulary, parents of children who undergo sex reassignment will also need guidance as to how to deal with the reannouncement of their baby's sex and the explanation of their child's condition to others. Money (15) recommends using the book *Sex Errors of the Body* (17) and giving the parents a beginning course in the embryology of sexual differentiation. This book can also be used as a reference for parents and can be used to explain the infant's condition to older siblings and again in later years to help explain the disorder to the child.

Psychosocial Management in Early to Middle Childhood

Explaining her status at birth to the patient and what treatments and surgeries she has had and may need is an issue that parents usually must address during early to middle childhood. As the patient may begin asking difficult questions related to her medical status, it is important for medical specialists to assist parents with these questions. Likewise, consultation with a pediatric psychologist to address psychological and emotional issues might be necessary. The patient may feel different from other children, both emotionally and behaviorally. Females (who are exposed to male hormones) and males reassigned as females may be more interested in traditionally male-oriented activities and feel isolated or different from their peers. A child who is frequently teased or not allowed to pursue certain sex-stereotyped leisure activities will develop an identity and behavioral responses very different from those of a child who does not have these experiences. Associations have been suggested between gender transposition and stigmatization as a child (18). Physicians and parents should also be alerted to a potential rise in compliance problems as the patient attempts to diminish her differentness.

As the patient begins to learn more about her disorder, typically her peers may also begin to ask questions. Preparing the patient for these questions can facilitate her adjustment to the diagnosis. In addition to the basic dissemination of information and its impact on the child's personal and interpersonal growth, the patient is also faced with normal sexual development issues. Children at this age have an increasing awareness of their own bodies and curiosity of others' bodies. However, because of the influence of male hormones and possible physical differences in external genitalia, patients with CAH might experience these developmental changes differently. Like a typically developing child, a patient with CAH should be supported in keeping her body private, and any questions should be answered at a developmentally appropriate level.

Psychosocial Management in Adolescence

The emergence of adolescence can raise additional issues and challenges for patients with CAH. At this age, many patients may begin to explore sexual relationships with others. Normal sexual exploration, however, may be complicated by the physical appearance of the patient's genitalia, as well as the need for additional reconstructive surgeries. As discussed, there is still debate regarding the best time to pursue a second reconstructive surgery. However, studies have shown better success rates for patients over the age of 16 (61% versus 12%) who were either interested in sexual activity and/or willing to follow postoperative dilator exercises (5). Furthermore, although many studies have shown positive anatomic and functional results following reconstructive surgery (16,19), very few researchers have looked at the psychological and emotional adjustment of patients with CAH. Although reconstructive surgery may have produced functionally and anatomically adequate genitalia, this does not assume adequate psychosexual functioning. It is clear that patients with CAH are often confronted with questions regarding their sexuality, including both their gender identity and sexual orientation. Genotypically male patients raised as girls, as well as genotypical females exposed to virilizing hormones, may have several different reactions. They may identify more with their genotype, regardless of their phenotype, or they may be attracted to either a genotypically or phenotypically similar partner. CAH may begin to influence their relationships in a more fundamental way than previous platonic friendships as they explore sexual relationships. Feelings of differentness (physically and psychologically) may be amplified, relative to their level of cognitive development. Physicians may be called on to assist the patient with when, what, and how to tell their partners about their condition. Lastly, although most adolescents are not actively planning to start a family, they may be starting to think about their future as parents, and physicians might need to address different questions related to fertility (discussed in more detail in the following section).

In addition to social issues, adolescents with CAH are required to follow a strict regimen of hormone treatments and may be required to undergo subsequent reconstructive surgeries. Their desire to assert their independence and autonomy, as well as possible ambiguity regarding their sex role, gender identity, and sexual orientation, may contribute to noncompliance with hormonal treatment and follow-up care from surgery. Poor compliance may also reflect both past hormonal influences on the brain and the ongoing effects of hormones (8). Because of compliance problems, some health care teams recommend waiting until the adolescent is at least 16 years old to perform repeat operations (5). The greater success of repeat surgeries at this age (likely due to greater interest in sexual functioning) reduces the likelihood of additional surgeries, which predicts better psychological outcome.

Psychosocial Management in Adulthood

As patients with CAH enter adulthood, it appears that there are difficulties with entering and/or maintaining long-term relationships. Compared to 90% of healthy adults, only 50% of simple-type adrenal hyperplastics and 12.5% of salt-losing type were married (8). In addition, while only 5% of healthy adults had no sexual experience, 30% of simple and 60% of salt-losing adults had no sexual experiences. These results indicate that adults with CAH may have significantly delayed and/or limited sexual and/or intimate experiences (5,20), which many speculate is attributable to their atypical gender roles and gender identity (16). Their reasons for not entering into long-term intimate relationship may be quite variable as well. While some women may be hesitant to commit because of physical malformations, others may be uncertain of their gender identity and/or gender orientation, or be involved in relationships other than the traditional heterosexual relationship.

Even if a patient with CAH is able to achieve satisfactory sexual functioning, issues regarding fertility remain. Although 60% of one sample of women with CAH involved in heterosexual relationships were able to conceive (6), many women with CAH are not able to conceive without intervention and must consider other options. For those who are genotypically female and involved in either heterosexual or homosexual relationships, options may include artificial insemination, adoption, surrogacy, and stepchildren. For those who are genotypically male yet phenotypically female, adoption and stepchildren are two alternatives.

Finally, a small percentage of patients with CAH experience gender dysmorphic feelings and opt for gender transposition surgery. Patients undergoing this process must be involved in a comprehensive program involving extensive medical and psychological evaluation and intervention.

CONGENITAL ABSENCE OF THE VAGINA

The congenital absence of the vagina, most commonly due to MRKH, is relatively rare (1:4,000 to 1:20,000 live female births), yet MRKH is the second most common cause of primary amenorrhea (21). In this syndrome, usually both the vagina and the uterus are absent. Some patients may have uterine remnants and there may or may not be a rudimentary vaginal opening. Patients with MRKH are chromosomally normal and usually have at least one functional ovary. Thus they develop as typical females with expected secondary sexual characteristics. Although there is a greater than expected incidence of urinary tract anomalies (22), in general, patients with MRKH have essentially a hidden disability. There is nothing unusual about their external appearance, and often patients are not diagnosed until adolescence or later.

Patients with MRKH occasionally present in infancy or early childhood, primarily if there are obvious external genital differences or associated urinary anomalies. A small number are also diagnosed in early adolescence with clinical symptoms of abdominal pain and/or mass. Most commonly, patients are diagnosed in late adolescence when they present with primary amenorrhea. In each case, there are numerous issues to be addressed by the patient and her family, including coping with the initial diagnosis and its implications, weighing treatment options, managing intervention, and coping with long-term issues after treatment, particularly infertility. It is important for physicians and other health care professionals to realize that to date there are no data suggesting that women with MRKH have any greater or lesser degree of psychological distress than other females. However, from a developmental perspective, there are times and events that should be proactively addressed in order to optimize future functioning.

Psychosocial Management and Diagnosis in Infancy and Early Childhood

When a child is diagnosed with MRKH in infancy, parents will be faced with the global issue of having a child with a congenital abnormality, along with specific questions about the disorder. Short-term questions include whether the infant is completely female and if the child will experience future complications or discomfort. Longer term, perhaps more worrisome, questions include issues of adolescent development, menstruation, future sexual functioning, and fertility. Parents are also faced with the prospect of future intervention(s) and how and when to discuss this with the child.

Parents of infants or young children diagnosed with MRKH should be provided with information about congenital absence of the vagina, including treatment options, preferably both in discussion and in writing. Parents must be reassured that the child is a chromosomally normal female who will develop typical female secondary sexual characteristics, but will not experience menses due to absence of a vagina. Females with MRKH most commonly do not have a functional uterus and thus pregnancy is not possible. If at least one functional ovary is present, as is usually the case, there is the option of surrogacy, although this is controversial (23). For the patient diagnosed in infancy or early childhood, treatment options may change greatly by the time intervention is recommended, possibly 10 to 20 years later.

After the diagnosis is made clear to the family, little may be necessary from a psychological point of view for a child with MRKH until middle to late childhood when the normal exploration of her body might raise questions. However, there are currently no clear guidelines regarding when and how to tell a child about her physical differences. Anecdotal information suggests that it may be most prudent for parents not to hide this information from the child, but rather to deal with her medical condition routinely as questions arise and as situations naturally occur, such as during routine medical checkups or science classes in elementary school. As she becomes increasingly concerned about her body and about sexuality (typically late childhood or early adolescence), more information should be provided. The child should be gradually introduced to the idea that she will not menstruate like other girls. If surgical treatment is anticipated, it should be discussed that later she will need to have an operation to allow her body to work better (including review of the role of the vagina in intercourse as she becomes familiar with those terms). Depending on the child's emotional, social, and physical development, information about future sexuality and fertility should be introduced during late childhood or early adolescence. While these topics may not yet be salient for the child, the more comfortable the patient and parents are, and the more routinely such issues are discussed, the more the child is likely to feel safe expressing her feelings and raising concerns.

As the patient is learning about the reproductive organs and the process of conception and childbirth, many questions will arise that she may or may not feel comfortable discussing with parents. Depending on the child's relationship with her parents and health care provider(s), specific consultation with others may be helpful in explaining these concepts to the child at her level. Parental comfort with the topic and parental coping with the child's diagnosis and future treatment will impact on the child's coping (24). The child should be supported in keeping information about her body private and helped to feel comfortable bringing any questions or concerns to parents or health care providers.

Psychosocial Management and Diagnosis in Early to Mid-Adolescence

In patients with a partially functional uterus, congenital absence of the vagina may first become apparent in early adolescence when the patient presents with abdominal pain and/or a mass due to reabsorbed menstrual fluids. Developmentally, this is a time when increasing interest is developing regarding sexuality but reasoning is still at a less than adult level. At this age, many girls have engaged in some exploration of their bodies (possibly including same-sex body exploration), and this should be openly and supportively discussed, particularly if the child experienced distress or concerns about what was noticed. A girl at this age may not have a clear sense of what she is supposed to have and may require an explanation to understand why she requires medical evaluations and/or treatments. In the girl with clinical symptoms, intervention may be necessary earlier than is usual with expected issues of body integrity, privacy, and coping with dilatation and/or surgery.

For girls diagnosed in infancy, early adolescence may be the first time that they must face being different. At the same time, some girls may express relief that they do not have to address the issue of menstruation. As other girls start their periods, the patient may feel that there is something wrong with her. Parents should respond calmly and reassure the young teen that she is completely female and no different from any other girl other than a part of her body on the inside. It may be helpful to remind her that no one else can see her differences and that she alone can decide with whom she wishes to share this information. Peer pressure and the desire to be like everyone else are powerful at this age. Self-esteem may be problematic in the early adolescent years, as it is for many girls, particularly if the child overfocuses on her physical differences or if early or extensive surgical intervention is required.

For patients requiring early surgical intervention because of clinical symptoms, intensive patient and parent education and counseling should be mandatory. Compliance with postsurgical care and patient motivation are considered key in the functional outcome of surgery, and these are issues that may be more difficult for a young adolescent. Physician support and reassurance can be helpful in creating a sense of confidence in the patient and family.

Psychosocial Management and Diagnosis in Late Adolescence or Adulthood

Most commonly, patients are first diagnosed with absence of the vagina in later adolescence or early adulthood when they contact a physician due to primary amenorrhea or difficulty with intercourse. Until diagnosis, there is often no indication of any abnormality, and the patient has developed typically with the exception of primary amenorrhea.

For parents, this later diagnosis may raise feelings that they missed something about their child. Like parents of younger children, parents of adolescents might respond first with shock and disbelief, then with anger and confusion. Eventual acceptance will likely be blended with decisions regarding treatment and coping with short- and long-term issues. Parents may also express frustration or anger at the medical professionals involved with the patient, some of whom may have offered reassurance in the past that the patient's amenorrhea was not abnormal.

Adolescent females often face struggles regarding their identity, relationships, and the future, all of which may be affected by the diagnosis of MRKH and its treatment. Little has been written in the professional literature regarding the general coping of patients with MRKH. These adolescents and young women may have concerns about whether they are abnormal, and may experience doubts about their identity as a female or their sexuality in general. Patients are likely to express a range of emotions, including shock, denial, anger, fear, sadness, and anxiety.

By early adulthood, many patients will have experienced some degree of intimacy in relationships, possibly experiencing frustration or embarrassment at attempts at intercourse. As part of the diagnostic process, and certainly prior to treatment, these experiences should be discussed, supporting the patient's feelings and frustrations. The role of the vagina and other female sex organs (including the clitoris) in sexual activities should be discussed, with reassurance to the patient that her diagnosis does not preclude her from experiencing sexual pleasure or orgasm. Her ability to have satisfactory sexual intercourse will depend, however, on her individual anatomy and the outcome of intervention. Information about the relative success of treatment for most patients should be offered to assist in keeping her hopeful about the future. Nevertheless, some degree of sadness and loss is normal and should be supported (24).

Due to the intense commitment of time and emotional energy required for successful treatment, the timing of intervention is important. It has been suggested that the individual's psychological and physical maturity are key in the decision regarding when to intervene, for both dilatation and surgery (21). The patient must be compliant with dilatation and postsurgical care, capable of coping with the scrutiny and lack of privacy regarding her body, and accepting of her physical differentness. In retrospect, one study of women after intervention for MRKH indicated that 18 to 20 years of age was the ideal time for surgery (25). However, individual factors make this a very case-specific decision.

Studies to date suggest that regardless of specific surgical procedure, most women are quite satisfied with the outcome of treatment and enjoy satisfactory sexual relationships (21,24,26,27). Compliance with dilatation and/or the early establishment of regular sexual intercourse are related to long-term outcomes (21). Additional factors in successful treatment appear to be patient and parent adjustment to the congenital abnormality, involvement in an ongoing sexual relationship, overall physical and psychological maturity of the patient, and a strong desire to be sexually active (21,23,24,26). The supportive services typically provided, however, may not be adequate for optimal outcome in some patients (21,27).

The issue of infertility remains a major issue for many women, even if satisfactory sexual activity is achieved (21,27). Even for those diagnosed earlier in childhood or adolescence, the reality of infertility is likely to first become salient in later adolescence or early adulthood as decisions regarding family life are considered. The reassurance that "you can always adopt" is inappropriate as it only serves to minimize and trivialize the patient's very real distress. When the patient is ready, however, counseling regarding fertility options may be helpful for some patients, including the possibility of adoption and, for some women, surrogacy.

RESOURCES FOR PATIENTS AND FAMILIES

Patients and families should be referred to both local and national resources for patients with congenital vaginal anomalies. Specific examples are listed in Table 1. A recent survey of women with MRKH involved in an internet on-line support group suggests that the help and understanding of others with similar issues may provide emotional support and may decrease the sense of isolation that some women feel in dealing with such a personal and private condition (27). The women also expressed the desire for more written information on MRKH and for detailed information on the

TABLE 1. *Resources for patients and families*[a]

Friends Health Connection (http://www.48friend.com). Nonprofit organization that connects people who are experiencing or who have overcome a similar disease, allowing communication and mutual support.
MAGIC Foundation for Children's Growth (http://www.magicfoundation.org). Nonprofit organization providing support and education regarding growth disorders in children and including CAH (708-383-0808).
MRKH Listserv (http://www.surrogacy.com/online_support/mrkh/index.html). A confidential listserv for women with MRKH.
MRKH Resource List (http://www.execpc.com~pdefrain). Resource list compiled for and about women with MRKH.
National Adrenal Diseases Foundation (NADF; http://medhlp.org/nadf). A nonprofit organization dedicated to providing support, information, and education to those with adrenal diseases (including CAH). Also provides a pen-pal program for children with CAH (516-487-4992).
National Organization for Rare Disorders (NORD; http://www.rarediseases.org). A federation of voluntary health organizations with the goal of helping persons with rare, "orphan" diseases (800-999-6673).

CAH, congenital adrenal hyperplasia; MRKH, Mayer-Rokitansky-Küster-Hauser syndrome.
[a] These are examples of currently available resources. Such programs and addresses change from time to time and a general library or Internet search may yield more information in the future.

various treatment and fertility options available to them. Physicians and other health care specialists working with patients and families should be familiar with these resources in order to assist those who choose to utilize them.

SUMMARY

It has been suggested that all patients with genital tract anomalies have a psychological component to their condition (28), referring to the profound impact that such a difference may have on an individual's psychological functioning. The issues and needs of girls (and their families) with vaginal anomalies vary dramatically depending on the diagnosis, age at diagnosis, required treatment, and subsequent outcome. Overall, data suggest that most women with MRKH go on to experience relatively normal sexual and interpersonal relationships and are generally satisfied with the outcome of intervention. Women with CAH, on the other hand, experience a more complex set of issues related to hormonal, chromosomal, and structural differences and have a substantially more varied outcome. In both cases, when a child or adolescent is diagnosed with a vaginal tract anomaly, referral for evaluation and treatment by a pediatric or adolescent psychologist experienced in dealing with congenital differences is essential for both the patient and her family. Similarly, when MRKH is diagnosed in adulthood, referral to a psychologist familiar with the disorder may be key in a successful adjustment and outcome. All health professionals can be most helpful to women and their families by providing early and accurate information regarding the anomaly and options for treatment, non-judgmental support and encouragement for a woman's choices, and caring and compassionate medical services.

REFERENCES

1. Migeon CJ. Diagnosis and treatment of adrenogenital disorders. In: DeGroot LJ, Besser GM, Cahill GF Jr, et al., eds. *Endocrinology,* Vol 2, 2nd ed. Philadelphia: WB Saunders, 1989:1676–1704.
2. New MI, ed. Congenital adrenal hyperplasia. *Ann NY Acad Sci* 1985;485.
3. New MI, Levine LS. Adrenal hyperplasia in intersex states. In: Josso N, ed. *The intersex child.* Basel: Karger, 1981:51–64.
4. Sinforiani E, Livieri C, Mauri M, Biso P, Sibilla L, Chiesa L, Martelli A. Cognitive and neuroradiological findings in congenital adrenal hyperplasia. *Psychoneuroendocrinology* 1994;19:55–64.
5. Azziz R, Mulaikal RM, Migeon CJ, Jones HW Jr, Rock JA. Congenital adrenal hyperplasia: long term results following vaginal reconstruction. *Fertil Steril* 1986;46:1011–1014.
6. Mulaikal RM, Migeon CJ, Rock JA. Fertility rates in female patients with congenital adrenal hyperplasia due to 21-hydroxylase deficiency. *N Engl J Med* 1987;316:178–182.
7. Gordon AH, Lee PA, Dulcan MK, Finegold DH. Behavioral problems, social competency, and self perception among girls with congenital adrenal hyperplasia. *Child Psychiatry Hum Dev* 1986;17:129–138.
8. Federman DD. Psychosexual adjustment in congenital adrenal hyperplasia. *N Engl J Med* 1987;316:209–211.
9. Newman K, Randolph J, Anderson K. The surgical management of infants and children with ambiguous genitalia. *Ann Surg* 1991;215:644–653.
10. Gonzalez R, Fernandes ET. Single-stage feminization genitoplasty. *J Urol* 1990;143:776–778.
11. Ulrich T, Hinderer MD. Reconstruction of the external genitalia in the adrenogenital syndrome by means of a personal one-stage procedure. *Plast Reconstr Surg* 1989;17:21–31.
12. Izquierdo G, Glassberg KI. Gender assignment and gender identity in patients with ambiguous genitalia. *Urology* 1993;42:232–242.
13. Money J, Schwartz M, Lewis VG. Adult erotosexual status and fetal hormonal masculinization and demasculinization: 46,XX congenital virilizing adrenal hyperlasia and 46,XY androgen-insensitivity syndrome compared. *Psychoneuroendocrinology* 1984;9:405–414.
14. Money J, Ehrhardt AA. *Man and woman, boy and girl: differentiation and dimorphism of the gender identity from conception to maturity.* Baltimore: Johns Hopkins University Press, 1972.
15. Money J. Psychologic considerations in patients with ambisexual development. *Semin Reprod Endocrinol* 1987;5:307–313.
16. Slijper FME, van der Kamp HJ, Brandenburg H, de Muinck Keizer-Schrama, SMPF, Drop SLS, Molenaar JC. Evaluation of psychosexual development of young women with congenital adrenal hyperplasia: a pilot study. *J Sex Educ Ther* 1992;18:200–207.
17. Money J: *Sex errors of the body: dilemmas, education, counseling.* Baltimore: Johns Hopkins University Press, 1968.
18. Money J, Norman BF. Gender identity and gender transposition: longitudinal outcome study of 24 hermaphrodites assigned as boys. *J Sex Marital Ther* 1987;13:75–92.
19. Newman K, Randolph J, Parson S. Functional results in young women having clitoral reconstruction as infants. *J Pediatr Surg* 1992;27:180–184.
20. Kinsey AC, Pomeroy WB, Martin CE, Gebhard PH. *Sexual behavior in the human female.* Philadelphia: WB Saunders, 1953.
21. Mobus VJ, Kortenhorn K, Kreienberg R, and Friedberg V. Long-term results after operative correction of vaginal aplasia. *Am J Obstet Gynecol* 1996;175:617–624.
22. Meyers RL. Congenital anomalies of the vagina and their reconstruction. *Clin Obstet Gynecol* 1997;40:168–180.
23. American Academy of Pediatrics. Ethical issues in surrogate motherhood. *AAP News* 1992;9(7).
24. Hecker BR, McGuire LS. Psychosocial function in women treated for vaginal agenesis. *Am J Obstet Gynecol* 1977;129:543–547.
25. Lamont E. Congenital absence of the vagina: diagnosis and plastic surgical reconstruction. *Ann Plast Surg* 1978;1:380–391.
26. Alessandrescu D, Peltecu GC, Buhimschi CS, Buhimschi IA. Neocolpopoiesis with split-thickness skin graft as a surgical treatment of vaginal agenesis: retrospective review of 201 cases. *Am J Obstet Gynecol* 1996;175:131–138.
27. Jensen VK. The experiences of women with MRKH. Unpublished data, 1998.
28. Spence JE. Vaginal and uterine anomalies in the pediatric and adolescent patient. *Pediatr Adol Gynecol* 1998;11:3–11.

Subject Index